KU-441-591

DClinPsy
2014

CANCELLED 21 DEC 2023

Maria Henderson Library
Gartnavel Royal Hospital
Glasgow G12 0XH Scotland

GARTNAVEL ROYAL HOSPITAL

GRH009734

CANCELLED 21 DEC 2023

COGNITIVE BEHAVIOR THERAPY

DO NOT

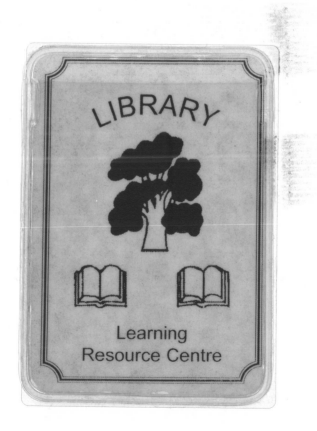

LIBRARY

Learning
Resource Centre

DO NO

COGNITIVE BEHAVIOR THERAPY

Basics and Beyond

SECOND EDITION

Judith S. Beck

Foreword by Aaron T. Beck

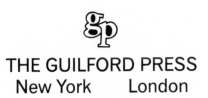

THE GUILFORD PRESS
New York   London

© 2011 Judith S. Beck
Published by The Guilford Press
A Division of Guilford Publications, Inc.
72 Spring Street, New York, NY 10012
www.guilford.com

All rights reserved

Except as indicated, no part of this book may be reproduced, translated, stored
in a retrieval system, or transmitted, in any form or by any means, electronic,
mechanical, photocopying, microfilming, recording, or otherwise, without written
permission from the publisher.

Printed in the United States of America

This book is printed on acid-free paper.

Last digit is print number: 9 8 7 6 5 4 3 2

LIMITED PHOTOCOPY LICENSE

These materials are intended for use only by qualified mental health professionals.

The Publisher grants to individual purchasers of this book nonassignable permission to reproduce all materials for which photocopying permission is specifically
granted in a footnote. This license is limited to you, the individual purchaser, for
personal use or use with individual clients. This license does not grant the right to
reproduce these materials for resale, redistribution, electronic display, or any other
purposes (including but not limited to books, pamphlets, articles, video- or audio-
tapes, blogs, file-sharing sites, Internet or intranet sites, and handouts or slides for
lectures, workshops, webinars, or therapy groups, whether or not a fee is charged).
Permission to reproduce these materials for these and any other purposes must
be obtained in writing from the Permissions Department of Guilford Publications.

The author has checked with sources believed to be reliable in her effort to
provide information that is complete and generally in accord with the standards
of practice that are accepted at the time of publication. However, in view of the
possibility of human error or changes in behavioral, mental health, or medical
sciences, neither the author, nor the editor and publisher, nor any other party who
has been involved in the preparation or publication of this work warrants that
the information contained herein is in every respect accurate or complete, and
they are not responsible for any errors or omissions or the results obtained from
the use of such information. Readers are encouraged to confirm the information
contained in this book with other sources.

Library of Congress Cataloging-in-Publication Data
Beck, Judith S.
  Cognitive behavior therapy : basics and beyond / Judith S. Beck.–2nd ed.
    p. cm.
  Rev. ed. of: Cognitive therapy. c1995.
  Includes bibliographical references and index.
  ISBN 978-1-60918-504-6 (hardcover)
  1. Cognitive therapy. I. Beck, Judith S. Cognitive therapy. II. Title.
  RC489.C63B43 2011
  616.89′1425—dc22

                                                              2011002830

To my father,
Aaron T. Beck, MD

ABOUT THE AUTHOR

Judith S. Beck, PhD, is President of the Beck Institute for Cognitive Behavior Therapy (*www.beckinstitute.org*) and Clinical Associate Professor of Psychology in Psychiatry at the University of Pennsylvania School of Medicine. She has written nearly 100 articles and chapters as well as several books for professionals and consumers; has made hundreds of presentations, nationally and internationally, on topics related to cognitive behavior therapy; and is the codeveloper of the Beck Youth Inventories and the Personality Belief Questionnaire. Dr. Beck is a founding fellow and past president of the Academy of Cognitive Therapy.

FOREWORD

I am delighted that the success of the first edition of *Cognitive Therapy: Basics and Beyond* has prompted this revision. It offers readers fresh insights into this approach to psychotherapy, and, I trust, will be welcomed by those who are versed in cognitive behavior therapy as well as students new to the field. Given the tremendous amount of new research and expansion of ideas that continue to move the field in exciting new directions, I applaud the efforts to expand this volume to incorporate some of the different ways of conceptualizing and treating our patients.

I would like to take the reader back to the early days of cognitive therapy and its development since then. When I first started treating patients with a set of therapeutic procedures that I subsequently labeled "cognitive therapy" (and now refer to as "cognitive behavior therapy"), I had no idea where this approach—which departed so strongly from my psychoanalytic training—would lead me. Based on my clinical observations and some systematic clinical studies and experiments, I theorized that there was a thinking disorder at the core of the psychiatric syndromes such as depression and anxiety. This disorder was reflected in a systematic bias in the way the patients interpreted particular experiences. By pointing out these biased interpretations and proposing alternatives—that is, more probable explanations—I found that I could produce an almost immediate lessening of the symptoms. Training the patients in these cognitive skills helped to sustain the improvement. This concentration on here-and-now problems appeared to produce almost total alleviation of symptoms in 10 to 14 weeks. Later clinical trials by my own group and clinicians/investigators elsewhere supported the efficacy of this approach for anxiety disorders, depressive disorders, and panic disorder.

By the mid-1980s, I could claim that cognitive therapy had attained the status of a "system of psychotherapy." It consisted of (1) a theory of personality and psychopathology with solid empirical findings to support its basic postulates; (2) a model of psychotherapy, with sets of principles and strategies that blended with the theory of psychopathology; and (3) solid empirical findings based on clinical outcome studies to support the efficacy of this approach.

Since my earlier work, a new generation of therapists/researchers/teachers has conducted basic investigations of the conceptual model of psychopathology and applied cognitive behavior therapy to a broad spectrum of psychiatric disorders. The systematic investigations explore the basic cognitive dimensions of personality and the psychiatric disorders, the idiosyncratic processing and recall of information in these disorders, and the relationship between vulnerability and stress.

The applications of cognitive behavior therapy to a host of psychological and medical disorders extend far beyond anything I could have imagined when I treated my first few cases of depression and anxiety with cognitive therapy. On the basis of outcome trials, investigators throughout the world, but particularly the United States, have established that cognitive behavior therapy is effective in conditions as diverse as posttraumatic stress disorder, obsessive–compulsive disorder, phobias of all kinds, and eating disorders. Often in combination with medication, it has been helpful in the treatment of bipolar disorder and schizophrenia. Cognitive therapy has also been found to be beneficial in a wide variety of chronic medical disorders such as low back pain, colitis, hypertension, and chronic fatigue syndrome.

With a smorgasbord of applications of cognitive behavior therapy, how can an aspiring therapist begin to learn the nuts and bolts of this therapy? Extracting from *Alice in Wonderland*, "Start at the beginning." This now brings us back to the question at the beginning of this foreword. The purpose of this book by Dr. Judith Beck, one of the foremost second-generation cognitive behavior therapists (and who, as a teenager, was one of the first to listen to me expound on my new theory), is to provide a solid basic foundation for the practice of cognitive behavior therapy. Despite the formidable array of different applications of cognitive behavior therapy, they all are based on fundamental principles outlined in this volume. Even experienced cognitive behavior therapists should find this book quite helpful in sharpening their conceptualization skills, expanding their repertoire of therapeutic techniques, planning more effective treatment, and troubleshooting difficulties in therapy.

Of course, no book can substitute for supervision in cognitive behavior therapy. But this book is an important volume and can be supplemented by supervision, which is readily available from a network of trained cognitive therapists (see Appendix B).

Dr. Judith Beck is eminently qualified to offer this guide to cognitive behavior therapy. For the past 25 years, she has conducted numerous workshops and trainings in cognitive behavior therapy, supervised both beginners and experienced therapists, helped develop treatment protocols for various disorders, and participated actively in research on cognitive behavior therapy. With such a background to draw on, she has written a book with a rich lode of information to apply this therapy, the first edition of which has been the leading cognitive behavior therapy text in most graduate psychology, psychiatry, social work, and counseling programs.

The practice of cognitive behavior therapy is not simple. I have observed a number of participants in clinical trials, for example, who can go through the motions of working with "automatic thoughts," without any real understanding of the patients' perceptions of their personal world or any sense of the principle of "collaborative empiricism." The purpose of Dr. Judith Beck's book is to educate, to teach, and to train both the novice and the experienced therapist in cognitive behavior therapy, and she has succeeded admirably in this mission.

AARON T. BECK, MD
Beck Institute for Cognitive Behavior Therapy
Department of Psychiatry, University of Pennsylvania

PREFACE

The past two decades have been an exciting time in the field of cognitive therapy. With the explosion of new research, cognitive behavior therapy has become the treatment of choice for many disorders,
not only because it reduces people's suffering quickly and moves them
toward remission, but also because it helps them stay well. A central
mission of our nonprofit organization, the Beck Institute for Cognitive
Behavior Therapy, is to provide state-of-the-art training to health and
mental health professionals in Philadelphia and throughout the world.
But exposure to this type of psychotherapy through workshops and various training programs is not enough. Having trained many thousands
of people in the past 25 years, I still find that people need a basic manual to read and to which they can repeatedly refer if they are to master
the theory, principles, and practice of cognitive behavior therapy.

This book is designed for a broad audience of health and mental
health professionals, from those who have never been exposed to cognitive behavior therapy before to those who are quite experienced but
wish to improve their skills, including how to conceptualize patients
cognitively, plan treatment, employ a variety of techniques, assess the
effectiveness of their treatment, and specify problems that arise in a
therapy session. To present the material as simply as possible, I have
chosen one patient (whose name and identifying characteristics I have
changed) to use as an example throughout the book. Sally is an ideal
patient in many ways, and her treatment clearly exemplifies "standard"
cognitive behavior therapy for uncomplicated, single-episode depression. Although the treatment described is for a straightforward case of

depression with anxious features, the techniques presented also apply to patients with a wide variety of problems. References for other disorders are provided so that the reader can learn to tailor treatment appropriately.

The first edition of this book was published in more than 20 languages, and I received feedback from all over the world, much of which I have incorporated into this new edition. I have included new material on evaluation and behavioral activation, the Cognitive Therapy Rating Scale (used in many research studies and training programs to measure therapist competency), and a Cognitive Case Write-Up (based on the template provided by the Academy of Cognitive Therapy as a prerequisite to receiving certification). I have also integrated a greater emphasis on the therapeutic relationship, guided discovery and Socratic questioning, eliciting and using patients' strengths and resources, and homework. I have been guided by my clinical practice, teaching, and supervision; by research and publications in the field; and by discussions with students and colleagues, from novice to expert, from many different countries, who specialize in various aspects of cognitive behavior therapy and in many different disorders.

This book could not have been written without the groundbreaking work of the father of cognitive therapy, Aaron T. Beck, who is also my father and an extraordinary scientist, theorist, practitioner, and person. I have also learned a great deal from every supervisor, supervisee, and patient with whom I have worked. I am grateful to them all.

JUDITH S. BECK, PhD

CONTENTS

Chapter 1. Introduction to Cognitive Behavior Therapy   1

What Is Cognitive Behavior Therapy?   2
What Is the Theory Underlying
    Cognitive Behavior Therapy?   3
What Does the Research Say?   4
How Was Beck's Cognitive Behavior
    Therapy Developed?   5
What Are the Basic Principles of Treatment?   6
What Is a Therapy Session Like?   11
Developing as a Cognitive Behavior Therapist   12
How to Use This Book   14

Chapter 2. Overview of Treatment   17

Developing the Therapeutic Relationship   17
Planning Treatment and Structuring Sessions   21
Identifying and Responding
    to Dysfunctional Cognitions   22
Emphasizing the Positive   26
Facilitating Cognitive and Behavioral Change
    between Sessions (Homework)   27

Chapter 3. Cognitive Conceptualization   29

The Cognitive Model   30
Beliefs   32
Relationship of Behavior to Automatic Thoughts   36

xv

Chapter 4. The Evaluation Session   46

Goals of the Assessment Session   47
Structure of the Assessment Session   48
Starting the Evaluation Session   48
The Assessment Phase   49
Final Part of the Assessment   53
Involving a Family Member   53
Relating Your Impressions   53
Setting Initial Goals for Treatment and Relating Your
     Treatment Plan   54
Expectations for Treatment   56
Devising an Initial Cognitive Conceptualization
     and Treatment Plan   57

Chapter 5. Structure of the First Therapy Session   59

Goals and Structure of the Initial Session   59
Setting the Agenda   60
Doing a Mood Check   62
Obtaining an Update   63
Discussing the Diagnosis   65
Problem Identification and Goal Setting   68
Educating the Patient about the Cognitive Model   70
Discussion of Problem or Behavioral Activation   74
End-of-Session Summary and Setting of Homework   74
Feedback   76

Chapter 6. Behavioral Activation   80

Conceptualization of Inactivity   80
Conceptualization of Lack of Mastery or Pleasure   81
Using the Activity Chart to Assess the Accuracy
     of Predictions   97

Chapter 7. Session 2 and Beyond: Structure and Format   100

The First Part of the Session   101
The Middle Part of the Session   112
Final Summary and Feedback   118
Session 3 and Beyond   120

Chapter 8. Problems with Structuring the Therapy Session   123

Therapist Cognitions   123
Interrupting the Patient   124
Socializing the Patient   125
Engaging the Patient   125
Strengthening the Therapeutic Alliance   126
Mood Check   127
Brief Update   129

Bridge between Sessions   130
Review of Homework   133
Discussion of Agenda Items   133
Setting New Homework   134
Final Summary   135
Feedback   135

Chapter 9. Identifying Automatic Thoughts   137

Characteristics of Automatic Thoughts   137
Explaining Automatic Thoughts to Patients   140
Eliciting Automatic Thoughts   142
Teaching Patients to Identify Automatic Thoughts   155

Chapter 10. Identifying Emotions   158

Distinguishing Automatic Thoughts from Emotions   159
Difficulty in Labeling Emotions   162
Rating Degrees of Emotion   164
Using Emotional Intensity to Guide Therapy   165

Chapter 11. Evaluating Automatic Thoughts   167

Selecting Key Automatic Thoughts   167
Questioning to Evaluate an Automatic Thought   170
Assessing the Outcome of the Evaluation Process   176
Conceptualizing Why the Evaluation of an Automatic
    Thought Was Ineffective   176
Using Alternate Methods to Help Patients Examine
    Their Thinking   178
When Automatic Thoughts Are True   182
Teaching Patients to Evaluate Their Thinking   184
Taking a Shortcut: Not Using the Questions at All   185

Chapter 12. Responding to Automatic Thoughts   187

Reviewing Therapy Notes   188
Evaluating and Responding to Novel Automatic Thoughts
    between Sessions   192
Responding to Automatic Thoughts in Other Ways   197

Chapter 13. Identifying and Modifying Intermediate Beliefs   198

Cognitive Conceptualization   199
Modifying Beliefs   214

Chapter 14. Identifying and Modifying Core Beliefs   228

Categorizing Core Beliefs   231
Identifying Core Beliefs   233
Presenting Core Beliefs   235

Educating Patients about Core Beliefs and Monitoring
    Their Operation   235
Developing a New Core Belief   239
Strengthening New Core Beliefs   240
Modifying Negative Core Beliefs   241
The Core Belief Worksheet   242

Chapter 15. Additional Cognitive and Behavioral Techniques   256

Problem Solving and Skills Training   256
Making Decisions   258
Refocusing   260
Measuring Moods and Behavior Using
    the Activity Chart   263
Relaxation and Mindfulness   263
Graded Task Assignments   264
Exposure   265
Role-Playing   267
Using the "Pie" Technique   268
Self-Comparisons and Credit Lists   272

Chapter 16. Imagery   277

Identifying Images   277
Educating Patients about Imagery   279
Responding to Spontaneous Images   280
Inducing Imagery as a Therapeutic Tool   289

Chapter 17. Homework   294

Setting Homework Assignments   295
Increasing Homework Adherence   299
Conceptualizing Difficulties   308
Reviewing Homework   315

Chapter 18. Termination and Relapse Prevention   316

Early Activities   316
Activities Throughout Therapy   318
Near Termination Activities   322
Booster Sessions   327

Chapter 19. Treatment Planning   332

Accomplishing Broad Therapeutic Goals   333
Planning Treatment across Sessions   333
Creating a Treatment Plan   334
Planning Individual Sessions   336
Deciding Whether to Focus on a Problem   340
Modifying Standard Treatment for Specific Disorders   344

Chapter 20. Problems in Therapy 346

Uncovering the Existence of a Problem 346
Conceptualizing Problems 348
Stuck Points 355
Remediating Problems in Therapy 356

Chapter 21. Progressing as a Cognitive Behavior Therapist 358

Appendix A. Cognitive Case Write-Up 361

Appendix B. Cognitive Behavior Therapy Resources 366

Training Programs 366
Therapist and Patient Materials and Referrals 366
Assessment Materials 366
Cognitive Behavior Therapy
   Professional Organizations 367

Appendix C. Cognitive Therapy Rating Scale 368

References 375

Index 381

Chapter 1

INTRODUCTION TO
COGNITIVE BEHAVIOR THERAPY

A revolution in the field of mental health was initiated in the early 1960s by Aaron T. Beck, MD, then an assistant professor in psychiatry at the University of Pennsylvania. Dr. Beck was a fully trained and practicing psychoanalyst. A scientist at heart, he believed that in order for psychoanalysis to be accepted by the medical community, its theories needed to be demonstrated as empirically valid. In the late 1950s and early 1960s, he embarked on a series of experiments that he fully expected would produce such validation. Instead, the opposite occurred. The results of Dr. Beck's experiments led him to search for other explanations for depression. He identified distorted, negative cognition (primarily thoughts and beliefs) as a primary feature of depression and developed a short-term treatment, one of whose primary targets was the reality testing of patients' depressed thinking.

In this chapter, you will find the answers to the following questions:

- What is cognitive behavior therapy?
- How was it developed?
- What does research tell us about its effectiveness?
- What are its basic principles?
- How can you become an effective cognitive behavior therapist?

WHAT IS COGNITIVE BEHAVIOR THERAPY?

Aaron Beck developed a form of psychotherapy in the early 1960s that he originally termed "cognitive therapy." "Cognitive therapy" is now used synonymously with "cognitive behavior therapy" by much of our field and it is this latter term that will be used throughout this volume. Beck devised a structured, short-term, present-oriented psychotherapy for depression, directed toward solving current problems and modifying dysfunctional (inaccurate and/or unhelpful) thinking and behavior (Beck, 1964). Since that time, he and others have successfully adapted this therapy to a surprisingly diverse set of populations with a wide range of disorders and problems. These adaptations have changed the focus, techniques, and length of treatment, but the theoretical assumptions themselves have remained constant. In all forms of cognitive behavior therapy that are derived from Beck's model, treatment is based on a cognitive formulation, the beliefs and behavioral strategies that characterize a specific disorder (Alford & Beck, 1997).

Treatment is also based on a conceptualization, or understanding, of individual patients (their specific beliefs and patterns of behavior). The therapist seeks in a variety of ways to produce cognitive change—modification in the patient's thinking and belief system—to bring about enduring emotional and behavioral change.

Beck drew on a number of different sources when he developed this form of psychotherapy, including early philosophers, such as Epictetus, and theorists, such as Karen Horney, Alfred Adler, George Kelly, Albert Ellis, Richard Lazarus, and Albert Bandura. Beck's work, in turn, has been expanded by current researchers and theorists, too numerous to recount here, in the United States and abroad.

There are a number of forms of cognitive behavior therapy that share characteristics of Beck's therapy, but whose conceptualizations and emphases in treatment vary to some degree. These include rational emotional behavior therapy (Ellis, 1962), dialectical behavior therapy (Linehan, 1993), problem-solving therapy (D'Zurilla & Nezu, 2006), acceptance and commitment therapy (Hayes, Follette, & Linehan, 2004), exposure therapy (Foa & Rothbaum, 1998), cognitive processing therapy (Resick & Schnicke, 1993), cognitive behavioral analysis system of psychotherapy (McCullough, 1999), behavioral activation (Lewinsohn, Sullivan, & Grosscup, 1980; Martell, Addis, & Jacobson, 2001), cognitive behavior modification (Meichenbaum, 1977), and others. Beck's cognitive behavior therapy often incorporates techniques from all these therapies, and other psychotherapies, within a cognitive framework. Historical overviews of the field provide a rich description of how the different streams of cognitive behavior therapy originated and grew (Arnkoff & Glass, 1992; A. Beck, 2005; Clark, Beck, & Alford, 1999; Dobson & Dozois, 2009; Hollon & Beck, 1993).

Cognitive behavior therapy has been adapted for patients with diverse levels of education and income as well as a variety of cultures and ages, from young children to older adults. It is now used in primary care and other medical offices, schools, vocational programs, and prisons, among other settings. It is used in group, couple, and family formats. While the treatment described in this book focuses on individual 45-minute sessions, treatment can be briefer. Some patients, such as those who suffer from schizophrenia, often cannot tolerate a full session, and some practitioners can use cognitive therapy techniques, without conducting a full therapy session, within a medical or rehabilitation appointment or medication check.

WHAT IS THE THEORY UNDERLYING COGNITIVE BEHAVIOR THERAPY?

In a nutshell, the *cognitive model* proposes that dysfunctional thinking (which influences the patient's mood and behavior) is common to all psychological disturbances. When people learn to evaluate their thinking in a more realistic and adaptive way, they experience improvement in their emotional state and in their behavior. For example, if you were quite depressed and bounced some checks, you might have an *automatic thought*, an idea that just seemed to pop up in your mind: "I can't do anything right." This thought might then lead to a particular reaction: you might feel sad (emotion) and retreat to bed (behavior). If you then examined the validity of this idea, you might conclude that you had overgeneralized and that, in fact, you actually do many things well. Looking at your experience from this new perspective would probably make you feel better and lead to more functional behavior.

For lasting improvement in patients' mood and behavior, cognitive therapists work at a deeper level of cognition: patients' basic beliefs about themselves, their world, and other people. Modification of their underlying dysfunctional beliefs produces more enduring change. For example, if you continually underestimate your abilities, you might have an underlying belief of incompetence. Modifying this general belief (i.e., seeing yourself in a more realistic light as having both strengths and weaknesses) can alter your perception of specific situations that you encounter daily. You will no longer have as many thoughts with the theme, "I can't do anything right." Instead, in specific situations where you make mistakes, you will probably think, "I'm not good at this [specific task]."

WHAT DOES THE RESEARCH SAY?

Cognitive behavior therapy has been extensively tested since the first outcome study was published in 1977 (Rush, Beck, Kovacs, & Hollon, 1977). At this point, more than 500 outcome studies have demonstrated the efficacy of cognitive behavior therapy for a wide range of psychiatric disorders, psychological problems, and medical problems with psychological components (see, e.g., Butler, Chapman, Forman, & Beck, 2006; Chambless & Ollendick, 2001). Table 1.1 lists many of the disorders and problems that have been successfully treated with cognitive behavior therapy. A more complete list may be found at *www.beckinstitute.org.*

Studies have been conducted that demonstrate the effectiveness of cognitive behavior therapy in community settings (see, e.g., Shadish, Matt, Navarro & Philips, 2000; Simons et al., 2010; Stirman, Buchhofer, McLaulin, Evans, & Beck, 2009). Other studies have found computer-assisted cognitive behavior therapy to be effective (see, e.g., Khanna & Kendall, 2010; Wright et al., 2002). And several researchers have demonstrated that there are neurobiological changes associated with cognitive behavior therapy treatment for various disorders (see, e.g.,

TABLE 1.1. Partial List of Disorders Successfully Treated by Cognitive Behavior Therapy

Psychiatric disorders	Psychological problems	Medical problems with psychological components
Major depressive disorder	Couple problems	Chronic back pain
Geriatric depression	Family problems	Sickle cell disease pain
Generalized anxiety disorder	Pathological gambling	Migraine headaches
Geriatric anxiety	Complicated grief	Tinnitus
Panic disorder	Caregiver distress	Cancer pain
Agoraphobia	Anger and hostility	Somatoform disorders
Social phobia		Irritable bowel syndrome
Obsessive–compulsive disorder		Chronic fatigue syndrome
Conduct disorder		Rheumatic disease pain
Substance abuse		Erectile dysfunction
Attention-deficit/hyperactivity disorder		Insomnia
Health anxiety		Obesity
Body dysmorphic disorder		Vulvodynia
Eating disorders		Hypertension
Personality disorders		Gulf War syndrome
Sex offenders		
Habit disorders		
Bipolar disorder (with medication)		
Schizophrenia (with medication)		

Goldapple et al., 2004). Hundreds of research studies have also validated the cognitive model of depression and of anxiety. A comprehensive review of these studies can be found in Clark and colleagues (1999) and in Clark and Beck (2010).

HOW WAS BECK'S COGNITIVE BEHAVIOR THERAPY DEVELOPED?

In the late 1950s and early 1960s, Dr. Beck decided to test the psychoanalytic concept that depression is the result of hostility turned inward toward the self. He investigated the dreams of depressed patients, which, he predicted, would manifest greater themes of hostility than the dreams of normal controls. To his surprise, he ultimately found that the dreams of depressed patients contained *fewer* themes of hostility and far greater themes of defectiveness, deprivation, and loss. He recognized that these themes paralleled his patients' thinking when they were awake. The results of other studies Beck conducted led him to believe that a related psychoanalytic idea—that depressed patients have a need to suffer—might be inaccurate (Beck, 1967). At that point, it was almost as if a stacked row of dominoes began to fall. If these psychoanalytic concepts were not valid, how else could depression be understood?

As Dr. Beck listened to his patients on the couch, he realized that they occasionally reported two streams of thinking: a free-association stream and quick, evaluative thoughts about themselves. One woman, for example, detailed her sexual exploits. She then reported feeling anxious. Dr. Beck made an interpretation: "You thought I was criticizing you." The patient disagreed: "No, I was afraid I was boring you." Upon questioning his other depressed patients, Dr. Beck recognized that all of them experienced "automatic" negative thoughts such as these, and that this second stream of thoughts was closely tied to their emotions. He began to help his patients identify, evaluate, and respond to their unrealistic and maladaptive thinking. When he did so, they rapidly improved.

Dr. Beck then began to teach his psychiatric residents at the University of Pennsylvania to use this form of treatment. They, too, found that their patients responded well. The chief resident, A. John Rush, MD, now a leading authority in the field of depression, discussed conducting an outcome trial with Dr. Beck. They agreed that such a study was necessary to demonstrate the efficacy of cognitive therapy to others. Their randomized controlled study of depressed patients, published in 1977, established that cognitive therapy was as effective as imipramine, a common antidepressant. This was an astounding study. It was one of the first times that a talk therapy had been compared to a medication. Beck, Rush, Shaw, and Emery (1979) published the first cognitive therapy treatment manual 2 years later.

Important components of cognitive behavior therapy for depression include a focus on helping patients solve problems; become behaviorally activated; and identify, evaluate, and respond to their depressed thinking, especially to negative thoughts about themselves, their worlds, and their future. In the late 1970s Dr. Beck and his postdoctoral fellows at the University of Pennsylvania began to study anxiety, and found that a somewhat different focus was necessary. Patients with anxiety needed to better assess the risk of situations they feared, to consider their internal and external resources, and improve upon their resources. They also needed to decrease their avoidance and confront situations they feared so they could test their negative predictions behaviorally. Since that time, the cognitive model of anxiety has been refined for each of the various anxiety disorders, cognitive psychology has verified these models, and outcome studies have demonstrated the efficacy of cognitive behavior therapy for anxiety disorders (Clark & Beck, 2010).

Fast-forward several decades. Dr. Beck, his fellows, and other researchers worldwide continue to study, theorize, adapt, and test treatments for patients who suffer from an ever-growing list of problems. Cognitive therapy or cognitive behavior therapy is now taught in most graduate schools in the United States and in many other countries.

WHAT ARE THE BASIC PRINCIPLES OF TREATMENT?

Although therapy must be tailored to the individual, there are, nevertheless, certain principles that underlie cognitive behavior therapy for all patients. Throughout the book, I use a depressed patient, Sally, to illustrate these central tenets and to demonstrate how to use cognitive theory to understand patients' difficulties and how to use this understanding to plan treatment and conduct therapy sessions. Sally is a nearly ideal patient and allows me to present cognitive behavior therapy in a straightforward manner. I make some note of how to vary treatment for patients who do not respond as well as she, but the reader must look elsewhere (e.g., J. S. Beck, 2005; Kuyken, Padesky & Dudley, 2009; Needleman, 1999) to learn how to conceptualize, strategize, and implement techniques for patients with diagnoses other than depression or for patients whose problems pose a challenge in treatment.

"Sally" was an 18-year-old single female when she sought treatment with me during her second semester of college. She had been feeling quite depressed and anxious for the previous 4 months and was having difficulty with her daily activities. She met criteria for a major depressive episode of moderate severity according to DSM-IV-TR (the *Diagnostic and Statistical Manual of Mental Disorders, Fourth Edition, Text Revision*; American Psychiatric Association, 2000). A fuller portrait of Sally is provided in Appendix A.

The basic principles of cognitive behavior therapy are as follows:

Principle No. 1. Cognitive behavior therapy is based on an ever-evolving formulation of patients' problems and an individual conceptualization of each patient in cognitive terms. I consider Sally's difficulties in three time frames. From the beginning, I identify her *current thinking* that contributes to her feelings of sadness ("I'm a failure, I can't do anything right, I'll never be happy"), and her *problematic behaviors* (isolating herself, spending a great deal of unproductive time in her room, avoiding asking for help). These problematic behaviors both flow from and in turn reinforce Sally's dysfunctional thinking. Second, I identify *precipitating factors* that influenced Sally's perceptions at the onset of her depression (e.g., being away from home for the first time and struggling in her studies contributed to her belief that she was incompetent). Third, I hypothesize about key *developmental events* and her *enduring patterns of interpreting* these events that may have predisposed her to depression (e.g., Sally has had a lifelong tendency to attribute personal strengths and achievement to luck, but views her weaknesses as a reflection of her "true" self).

I base my conceptualization of Sally on the cognitive formulation of depression and on the data Sally provides at the evaluation session. I continue to refine this conceptualization at each session as I obtain more data. At strategic points, I share the conceptualization with Sally to ensure that it "rings true" to her. Moreover, throughout therapy I help Sally view her experience through the cognitive model. She learns, for example, to identify the thoughts associated with her distressing affect and to evaluate and formulate more adaptive responses to her thinking. Doing so improves how she feels and often leads to her behaving in a more functional way.

Principle No. 2. Cognitive behavior therapy requires a sound therapeutic alliance. Sally, like many patients with uncomplicated depression and anxiety disorders, has little difficulty trusting and working with me. I strive to demonstrate all the basic ingredients necessary in a counseling situation: warmth, empathy, caring, genuine regard, and competence. I show my regard for Sally by making empathic statements, listening closely and carefully, and accurately summarizing her thoughts and feelings. I point out her small and larger successes and maintain a realistically optimistic and upbeat outlook. I also ask Sally for feedback at the end of each session to ensure that she feels understood and positive about the session. See Chapter 2 for a lengthier description of the therapeutic relationship in cognitive behavior therapy.

Principle No. 3. Cognitive behavior therapy emphasizes collaboration and active participation. I encourage Sally to view therapy as teamwork; together we decide what to work on each session, how often we should meet, and what Sally can do between sessions for therapy homework. At first, I am more active in suggesting a direction for therapy sessions and in summarizing what we've discussed during a session. As Sally becomes less depressed and more socialized into treatment, I encourage her to become increasingly active in the therapy session: deciding which problems to talk about, identifying the distortions in her thinking, summarizing important points, and devising homework assignments.

Principle No. 4. Cognitive behavior therapy is goal oriented and problem focused. I ask Sally in our first session to enumerate her problems and set specific goals so both she and I have a shared understanding of what she is working toward. For example, Sally mentions in the evaluation session that she feels isolated. With my guidance, Sally states a goal in behavioral terms: to initiate new friendships and spend more time with current friends. Later, when discussing how to improve her day-to-day routine, I help her evaluate and respond to thoughts that interfere with her goal, such as: *My friends won't want to hang out with me. I'm too tired to go out with them.* First, I help Sally evaluate the validity of her thoughts through an examination of the evidence. Then Sally is willing to test the thoughts more directly through behavioral experiments (pages 217–218) in which she initiates plans with friends. Once she recognizes and corrects the distortion in her thinking, Sally is able to benefit from straightforward problem solving to decrease her isolation.

Principle No. 5. Cognitive behavior therapy initially emphasizes the present. The treatment of most patients involves a strong focus on current problems and on specific situations that are distressing to them. Sally begins to feel better once she is able to respond to her negative thinking and take steps to improve her life. Therapy starts with an examination of here-and-now problems, regardless of diagnosis. Attention shifts to the past in two circumstances. One, when patients express a strong preference to do so, and a failure to do so could endanger the therapeutic alliance. Two, when patients get "stuck" in their dysfunctional thinking, and an understanding of the childhood roots of their beliefs can potentially help them modify their rigid ideas. ("Well, no wonder you still believe you're incompetent. Can you see how almost any child—who had the same experiences as you—would grow up believing she was incompetent, and yet it might not be true, or certainly not completely true?")

For example, I briefly turn to the past midway through treatment to help Sally identify a set of beliefs she learned as a child: "If I achieve highly, it means I'm worthwhile," and "If I don't achieve highly, it means I'm a failure." I help her evaluate the validity of these beliefs both in the past and present. Doing so leads Sally, in part, to develop more functional and more reasonable beliefs. If Sally had had a personality disorder, I would have spent proportionally more time discussing her developmental history and childhood origin of beliefs and coping behaviors.

Principle No. 6. Cognitive behavior therapy is educative, aims to teach the patient to be her own therapist, and emphasizes relapse prevention. In our first session I educate Sally about the nature and course of her disorder, about the process of cognitive behavior therapy, and about the cognitive model (i.e., how her thoughts influence her emotions and behavior). I not only help Sally set goals, identify and evaluate thoughts and beliefs, and plan behavioral change, but I also teach her how to do so. At each session I ensure that Sally takes home therapy notes—important ideas she has learned—so she can benefit from her new understanding in the ensuing weeks and after treatment ends.

Principle No. 7. Cognitive behavior therapy aims to be time limited. Many straightforward patients with depression and anxiety disorders are treated for six to 14 sessions. Therapists' goals are to provide symptom relief, facilitate a remission of the disorder, help patients resolve their most pressing problems, and teach them skills to avoid relapse. Sally initially has weekly therapy sessions. (Had her depression been more severe or had she been suicidal, I may have arranged more frequent sessions.) After 2 months, we collaboratively decide to experiment with biweekly sessions, then with monthly sessions. Even after termination, we plan periodic "booster" sessions every 3 months for a year.

Not all patients make enough progress in just a few months, however. Some patients require 1 or 2 years of therapy (or possibly longer) to modify very rigid dysfunctional beliefs and patterns of behavior that contribute to their chronic distress. Other patients with severe mental illness may need periodic treatment for a very long time to maintain stabilization.

Principle No. 8. Cognitive behavior therapy sessions are structured. No matter what the diagnosis or stage of treatment, following a certain structure in each session maximizes efficiency and effectiveness. This structure includes an introductory part (doing a mood check, briefly reviewing the week, collaboratively setting an agenda for the session), a middle part (reviewing homework, discussing problems on the agenda, setting new homework, summarizing), and a final part (eliciting feedback). Following this format makes the process of therapy more understandable to patients and increases the likelihood that they will be able to do self-therapy after termination.

Principle No. 9. Cognitive behavior therapy teaches patients to identify, evaluate, and respond to their dysfunctional thoughts and beliefs. Patients can have many dozens or even hundreds of automatic thoughts a day that affect their mood, behavior, and/or physiology (the last is especially pertinent to anxiety). Therapists help patients identify key cognitions and adopt more realistic, adaptive perspectives, which leads patients to feel better emotionally, behave more functionally, and/or decrease their physiological arousal. They do so through the process of *guided discovery*, using questioning (often labeled or mislabeled as "Socratic questioning") to evaluate their thinking (rather than persuasion, debate, or lecturing). Therapists also create experiences, called *behavioral experiments*, for patients to directly test their thinking (e.g., "If I even look at a picture of a spider, I'll get so anxious I won't be able to think"). In these ways, therapists engage in *collaborative empiricism.* Therapists do not generally know in advance to what degree a patient's automatic thought is valid or invalid, but together they test the patient's thinking to develop more helpful and accurate responses.

When Sally was quite depressed, she had many automatic thoughts throughout the day, some of which she spontaneously reported and others that I elicited (by asking her what was going through her mind when she felt upset or acted in a dysfunctional manner). We often uncovered important automatic thoughts as we were discussing one of Sally's specific problems, and together we investigated their validity and utility. I asked her to summarize her new viewpoints, and we recorded them in writing so that she could read these adaptive responses throughout the week to prepare her for these or similar automatic thoughts. I did not encourage her to uncritically adopt a more positive viewpoint, challenge the validity of her automatic thoughts, or try to convince her that her thinking was unrealistically pessimistic. Instead we engaged in a collaborative exploration of the evidence.

Principle No. 10. Cognitive behavior therapy uses a variety of techniques to change thinking, mood, and behavior. Although cognitive strategies such as Socratic questioning and guided discovery are central to cognitive behavior therapy, behavioral and problem-solving techniques are essential, as are techniques from other orientations that are implemented within a cognitive framework. For example, I used Gestalt-inspired techniques to help Sally understand how experiences with her family contributed to the development of her belief that she was incompetent. I use psychodynamically inspired techniques with some Axis II patients who apply their distorted ideas about people to the therapeutic relationship. The types of techniques you select will be influenced by your conceptualization of the patient, the problem you are discussing, and your objectives for the session.

These basic principles apply to all patients. Therapy does, however, vary considerably according to individual patients, the nature of their difficulties, and their stage of life, as well as their developmental and intellectual level, gender, and cultural background. Treatment also varies depending on patients' goals, their ability to form a strong therapeutic bond, their motivation to change, their previous experience with therapy, and their preferences for treatment, among other factors.

The *emphasis* in treatment also depends on the patient's particular disorder(s). Cognitive behavior therapy for panic disorder involves testing the patient's catastrophic misinterpretations (usually life- or sanity-threatening erroneous predictions) of bodily or mental sensations (Clark, 1989). Anorexia requires a modification of beliefs about personal worth and control (Garner & Bemis, 1985). Substance abuse treatment focuses on negative beliefs about the self and facilitating or permission-granting beliefs about substance use (Beck, Wright, Newman, & Liese, 1993).

WHAT IS A THERAPY SESSION LIKE?

The structure of therapy sessions is quite similar for the various disorders, but interventions can vary considerably from patient to patient. (The website of the Academy of Cognitive Therapy [*www.academyofct. org*] posts a list of books that describe the cognitive formulation, major emphases, strategies, and techniques for a wide range of diagnoses, patient variables, and treatment formats and settings.) Below is a general description of treatment sessions and the course of treatment, especially for patients who are depressed.

At the beginning of sessions, you will reestablish the therapeutic alliance, check on patients' mood, symptoms, and experiences in the past week, and ask them to name the problems they most want help in solving. These difficulties may have arisen during the week and/or they may be problems patients expect to encounter in the coming week(s). You will also review the self-help activities ("homework" or "action plan") patients engaged in since the previous session. Then, in the context of discussing a specific problem patients have put on the agenda, you will collect data about the problem, cognitively conceptualize patients' difficulties (asking for their specific thoughts, emotions, and behaviors associated with the problem), and collaboratively plan a strategy. The strategy most often includes straightforward problem solving, evaluating patients' negative thinking associated with the problem, and/or behavior change.

For example, Sally, the college student, is having difficulty studying. She needs help evaluating and responding to her thoughts ("What's the use? I'll probably flunk out anyway") before she is able to fully engage in solving her problem with studying. I make sure Sally has adopted a more accurate and adaptive view of the situation and has decided which solutions to implement in the coming week (e.g., starting with relatively easier tasks, mentally summarizing what she has read after every page or two of reading, planning shorter study sessions, going for walks when she takes breaks, and asking the teaching assistant for help). Our session sets the stage for Sally to make changes in her thinking and behavior during the coming week that, in turn, lead to an improvement in her mood and functioning.

Having discussed a problem and collaboratively set therapy homework, Sally and I turn to a second problem she has put on the agenda and repeat the process. At the end of the session we review important points from the session. I make sure that Sally is highly likely to do the homework assignments, and I elicit her feedback about the session.

DEVELOPING AS A COGNITIVE BEHAVIOR THERAPIST

To the untrained observer, cognitive behavior therapy sometimes appears deceptively simple. The *cognitive model*, the proposition that one's thoughts influence one's emotions and behavior, is quite straightforward. Experienced cognitive behavior therapists, however, accomplish many tasks at once: conceptualizing the case, building rapport, socializing and educating the patient, identifying problems, collecting data, testing hypotheses, and summarizing. The novice cognitive behavior therapist, in contrast, usually needs to be more deliberate and structured, concentrating on fewer elements at one time. Although the ultimate goal is to interweave these elements and conduct therapy as effectively and efficiently as possible, beginners must first learn the skill of developing the therapeutic relationship, the skill of conceptualization, and the techniques of cognitive behavior therapy, all of which is best done in a step-by-step manner.

Developing expertise as a cognitive behavior therapist can be viewed in three stages. (These descriptions assume that the therapist is already proficient in basic counseling skills: listening, empathy, concern, positive regard, and genuineness, as well as accurate understanding, reflection, and summarizing. Therapists who do not already possess these skills often elicit a negative reaction from patients.) In Stage 1 you learn basic skills of conceptualizing a case in cognitive terms based on an intake evaluation and data collected in session. You also learn to structure the session, use your conceptualization of a patient and good common sense to plan treatment, and help patients solve problems and view their dysfunctional thoughts in a different way. You also learn to use basic cognitive and behavioral techniques.

In Stage 2 you become more proficient at integrating your conceptualization with your knowledge of techniques. You strengthen your ability to understand the flow of therapy. You become more easily able to identify critical goals of treatment and more skillful at conceptualizing patients, refining your conceptualization during the therapy session itself, and using the conceptualization to make decisions about interventions. You expand your repertoire of techniques and become more proficient in selecting, timing, and implementing appropriate techniques.

In Stage 3 you more automatically integrate new data into the conceptualization. You refine your ability to make hypotheses to confirm or revise your view of the patient. You vary the structure and techniques of basic cognitive behavior therapy as appropriate, particularly for patients with personality disorders and other difficult disorders and problems.

If you already practice in another psychotherapeutic modality, it will be important for you to make a collaborative decision with patients to introduce the cognitive behavior therapy approach, describing what you would like to do differently and providing a rationale. Most patients agree to such changes when they are phrased positively, to the patient's benefit. When patients are hesitant, you can suggest the institution of a change (such as setting an agenda) as an "experiment," rather than a commitment, to motivate them to try it.

THERAPIST: Mike, I was reading an important book on making therapy more effective and I thought of you.

PATIENT: Oh?

THERAPIST: Yes, and I have some ideas about how we can help you get better faster. [being collaborative] Is it okay if I tell you about it?

PATIENT: Okay.

THERAPIST: One thing I read was called "setting the agenda." That means at the beginning of sessions, I'm going to ask you tell me the names of problems you want my help in solving during the session. For example, you might say that you're having a problem with your boss, or with getting out of bed on weekends, or that you've been feeling really anxious about your finances. (*pause*) By asking you the names of problems up front, we can figure out how to spend our time in session better. (*pause*) [eliciting feedback] How does that sound?

HOW TO USE THIS BOOK

This book is intended for individuals at any stage of experience and skill development who lack mastery in the fundamental building blocks of cognitive conceptualization and treatment. It is critical to have mastered the basic elements of cognitive behavior therapy in order to understand how and when to vary standard treatment for individual patients.

Your growth as a cognitive behavior therapist will be enhanced if you start applying the tools described in this book to yourself. First, as you read, begin to conceptualize your own thoughts and beliefs. Start paying attention to your own shifts in affect. When you notice that your mood has changed or intensified in a negative direction (or when you notice that you are engaging in dysfunctional behavior or are experiencing bodily sensations associated with negative affect), ask yourself what emotion you are feeling, as well as the cardinal question of cognitive behavior therapy:

> **"What was just going through my mind?"**

In this way, you will teach yourself to identify your own automatic thoughts. Teaching yourself the basic skills of cognitive behavior therapy using yourself as the subject will enhance your ability to teach your patients these same skills.

It will be particularly useful to identify your automatic thoughts as you are reading this book and trying techniques with your patients. If, for instance, you find yourself feeling slightly distressed, ask yourself, "What was just going through my mind?" You may uncover automatic thoughts such as:

> "This is too hard."
> "I may not be able to master this."
> "This doesn't feel comfortable to me."
> "What if I try it and it doesn't work?"

Experienced therapists whose primary orientation has not been cognitive may be aware of a different set of automatic thoughts:

"This won't work."

"The patient won't like it."

"It's too superficial/structured/unempathic/simple."

Having uncovered your thoughts, you can note them and refocus on your reading, or turn to Chapters 11 and 12, which describe how to evaluate and respond to automatic thoughts. By turning the spotlight on your own thinking, not only can you boost your cognitive behavior therapy skills, but you can also take the opportunity to modify dysfunctional thoughts and positively influence your mood (and behavior), making you more receptive to learning.

A common analogy used for patients also applies to the beginning cognitive behavior therapist. Learning the skills of cognitive behavior therapy is similar to learning any other skill. Do you remember learning how to drive or how to use a computer? At first, did you feel a little awkward? Did you have to pay a great deal of attention to small details and motions that now come smoothly and automatically to you? Did you ever feel discouraged? As you progressed, did the process make more and more sense, and feel more and more comfortable? Did you finally master it to the point where you were able to perform the task with relative ease and confidence? Most people have had just such an experience learning a skill in which they are now proficient.

The learning process is the same for the beginning cognitive behavior therapist. As you will learn to do for your patients, keep your goals small, well-defined, and realistic. Give yourself credit for small gains. Compare your progress to your ability level before you started reading this book, or to the time you first started learning about cognitive behavior therapy. Be cognizant of opportunities to respond to negative thoughts in which you unfairly compare yourself to experienced cognitive behavior therapists, or in which you undermine your confidence by contrasting your current level of skill with your ultimate objectives.

If you feel anxious about starting to use cognitive behavior therapy with patients, make yourself a "coping card," an index card on which you have written statements that are important to remember. My psychiatric residents often have unhelpful thoughts before they see their first outpatient. I ask them to create a card that addresses these thoughts. The card is individualized but generally says something such as:

My goal is not to cure this patient today. No one expects me to.

My goal is to establish a good working alliance, to do some problem

solving if I can, and to sharpen my cognitive behavior therapy skills.

Reading this card helps reduce their anxiety so that they can focus on their patients and be more effective.

Finally, the chapters of this book are designed to be read in the order presented. You might be eager to skip over introductory chapters in order to jump to the sections on techniques. The sum of cognitive behavior therapy, however, is not merely the employment of cognitive and behavioral techniques. Among other attributes, it entails the artful selection and effective utilization of a wide variety of techniques based on one's conceptualization of the patient. The next chapter provides an overview of treatment, followed by an initial chapter on conceptualization. Chapter 4 describes the evaluation process, and Chapters 5–8 focus on how to structure and what to do in therapy sessions. Chapters 9–14 describe the basic building blocks of cognitive behavior therapy: identifying cognitions and emotions and adaptively responding to automatic thoughts and beliefs. Additional cognitive and behavioral techniques are provided in Chapter 15, and imagery is discussed in Chapter 16. Chapter 17 describes homework. Chapter 18 outlines issues of termination and relapse prevention. These preceding chapters lay the groundwork for Chapters 19 and 20: planning treatment and diagnosing problems in therapy. Finally, Chapter 21 offers guidelines in progressing as a cognitive behavior therapist.

Chapter 2

OVERVIEW OF TREATMENT

This chapter briefly describes cognitive behavior therapy treatment and introduces several essential streams that run through each therapy session. They are:

- Developing the therapeutic relationship.
- Planning treatment and structuring sessions.
- Identifying and responding to dysfunctional cognitions.
- Emphasizing the positive.
- Facilitating cognitive and behavioral change between sessions (homework).

You will also learn more about each of these elements in future chapters.

DEVELOPING THE THERAPEUTIC RELATIONSHIP

It is essential to start building trust and rapport with patients from your first contact with them. Research demonstrates that positive alliances are correlated with positive treatment outcomes (Raue & Goldfried, 1994). This ongoing process is easily accomplished with most patients (although it can be more difficult with patients with severe mental illness or those with strong Axis II pathology). To accomplish this goal, you will:

- Demonstrate good counseling skills and accurate understanding.
- Share your conceptualization and treatment plan.
- Collaboratively make decisions.
- Seek feedback.
- Vary your style.
- Help patients solve their problems and alleviate their distress.

Demonstrating Good Counseling Skills

You will continuously demonstrate your commitment to and understanding of patients through your empathic statements, choice of words, tone of voice, facial expressions, and body language. As I tell my trainees, you strive to be a nice human being in the room with patients. You treat them the way *you* would like to be treated. You demonstrate empathy and accurate comprehension of their problems and ideas through your thoughtful questions, reflections, and statements, which leads to their feeling valued and understood. You will try to impart the following implicit (and sometimes explicit) messages, but only when you genuinely endorse them:

"I care about you and value you."
"I want to understand what you are experiencing and help you."
"I'm confident we can work well together and that cognitive behavior therapy will help."
"I'm not overwhelmed by your problems, even though you might be."
"I've helped other patients much like you."

If you cannot honestly endorse these messages, you may need help from a supervisor to respond to your automatic thoughts about the patient, about cognitive behavior therapy, or about yourself.

Through the relationship, you can indirectly help depressed patients:

- Feel likeable, when you are warm, friendly, and interested.
- Feel less alone, when you describe the process of working together as a team to solve their problems and work toward their goals.
- Feel more optimistic, as you present yourself as realistically hopeful that treatment will help.
- Feel a greater sense of self-efficacy, when you help them see how much credit they deserve for solving problems, doing homework, and engaging in other productive activities.

A common myth about cognitive behavior therapy, held by people who have not read the seminal books or watched videotapes of master clinicians, is that it is conducted in a cold, mechanical fashion. This is simply inaccurate. In fact, the earliest cognitive behavior therapy manual (Beck et al., 1979) stressed the importance of developing a good therapeutic relationship.

Sharing Your Conceptualization and Treatment Plan

You will continuously share your conceptualization with patients and ask them whether it "rings true." For example, a patient may have just described a problem with her mother. You have questioned her to fill in the cognitive model. Then you conceptualize aloud, in summary form. "Okay, I want to make sure I understand. The situation was that your mother yelled at you on the phone for not calling your brother, and your automatic thought was, 'She doesn't realize how busy I am. She doesn't blame *him* for not calling *me*.' These thoughts led you to feel hurt and angry, but you didn't say anything back to her [behavior].... Did I get that right?" If your conceptualization is accurate, the patient invariably says, "Yes, I think that's right." If you are wrong, the patient usually says, "No, it's not exactly like that. It's more like ..." Eliciting patients' feedback strengthens the alliance and allows you to more accurately conceptualize them and conduct effective treatment.

Making Collaborative Decisions

While you guide patients during sessions, you will also actively enlist their participation. You will help them prioritize the problems they want help in solving during a session. You will provide rationales for interventions and elicit their approval ("I think it may reduce your stress if you take a rest a couple of times a day—is it okay if we talk about that?").

You may suggest, and elicit their reaction to, some self-help activities they can try at home. You continuously act as a team.

Seeking Feedback

You will be continuously alert for your patients' emotional reactions throughout the session, observing their facial expressions, body language, choice of words, and tone of voice. When you recognize that patients are experiencing increased distress, you will often address the issue at the time: "You look upset. What was just going through your mind?" You may find that patients express negative thoughts about themselves, the process of therapy, or you. As described in Chapter 8, it is important to positively reinforce patients for providing feedback, then conceptualize the problem and plan a strategy to solve it. Failure to identify and address patients' negative feedback reduces their ability to focus on solving their real-life difficulties and feel better. They may even decide not to return to therapy the following week. (See J. S. Beck, 2005, for an extensive discussion of solving problems in the therapeutic relationship.)

Even when you discern that your alliance with patients is strong, you will still elicit feedback from them at the end of sessions: "What did you think about the session? Was there anything that bothered you, or you thought I misunderstood? Is there anything you want to do differently next time?" Asking these questions can strengthen the alliance significantly. You may be the first health or mental health professional who has ever asked the patient for feedback. Patients usually feel honored and respected by your genuine concern for their reactions.

Varying Your Style

Most patients will respond positively to you when you are warm, empathic, and caring. However, an occasional patient might have a negative reaction. For example, a patient may perceive you as being overly caring or too "touchy-feely." Watching for patients' emotional reactions in the session can alert you to ask questions to elicit a problem such as this, so you can change how you present yourself and help the patient feel more comfortable working with you.

Helping Patients Alleviate Their Distress

One of the best ways to strengthen the therapeutic relationship is by being an effective and competent cognitive behavior therapist. Research has demonstrated that the therapeutic alliance becomes strengthened when patients' symptomatology is reduced (DeRubeis & Feeley, 1990; Feeley, DeRubeis, & Gelfand, 1999).

In general, you will spend enough time developing the therapeutic relationship to engage patients in working effectively with you as a team, and you will use the therapeutic alliance to provide evidence to patients that their core beliefs are incorrect. If the alliance is sound, you will avoid spending additional unnecessary time in order to maximize the time you spend helping patients solve problems they will face in the coming week. Some patients, particularly those with personality disorders, do require a far greater emphasis on the therapeutic relationship and advanced strategies to forge a good working alliance (Beck, Freeman, Davis, & Associates, 2004; J. S. Beck, 2005; Young, 1999).

PLANNING TREATMENT AND STRUCTURING SESSIONS

A major goal of treatment is to make the process of therapy understandable to you and the patient. You will try to conduct therapy as efficiently as possible, so you can alleviate the patient's suffering as quickly as possible. Adhering to a standard format (as well as teaching the tools of therapy to the patient) facilitates these objectives. But, as noted above, you will not deliver treatment in a rote or impersonal way—if you did, you would not be very effective.

Most patients feel more comfortable when they know what to expect from therapy, when they clearly understand what you want them to do, when they feel that you and they are a team, and when they have a concrete idea of how therapy will proceed, both within a session and over the course of treatment. You will maximize the patient's understanding by explaining the general structure of sessions and then adhering (flexibly at times) to that structure.

You will begin to plan treatment for a session before patients enter your office. You will quickly review their chart, especially their goals for treatment and the therapy notes and homework assignments from the previous session(s). As noted above, you will have a general idea of how you intend to structure the session. The overarching therapeutic goal is to improve the patient's mood during the session and to create a plan so the patient can feel better and behave more functionally during the week. What you will do specifically in the session will be influenced by patients' symptoms, your conceptualization, the strength of the therapeutic alliance, their stage of treatment, and, especially, the problems they put on the agenda.

Your goal in the first part of a therapy session is to reestablish the therapeutic alliance and collect data so you and the patient can collaboratively set and prioritize the agenda. In the second part of a session, you and the patient will discuss the problems on the agenda. In the context of solving these problems, you will teach the patient relevant cognitive, behavioral, problem-solving, and other skills. You will continually reinforce the cognitive model, help patients evaluate and respond to their automatic thoughts, do problem solving, and ask them to summarize their new understandings.

These kinds of discussions and interventions naturally lead to homework assignments, which usually involve having patients remind themselves of their new, more realistic way of thinking about the problem and implementing solutions during the week. One important ongoing assignment is to have patients identify and respond to their dysfunctional thinking throughout the week, when they notice their mood is getting worse, they are behaving in a dysfunctional way, and/or they are experiencing significant physiological arousal.

In the final part of the session, you will elicit from patients what they thought were the most important points of the session, ensure that these ideas are written down, review (and modify if necessary) the homework assignments, and elicit and respond to patients' feedback about the session. While experienced cognitive behavior therapists may deviate from this format at times, novice therapists are usually more effective when they follow the specified structure. Further descriptions of the structure of therapy sessions appear in Chapters 5, 7, and 8.

To structure sessions effectively, you will need to *gently* interrupt patients: "Oh, can I interrupt you for a moment? Are you saying...?" Strategically and skillfully interrupting patients is illustrated in later chapters. If you initially feel awkward with a more tightly structured session, you will most likely find that the process gradually becomes second nature, especially when you note the positive results.

IDENTIFYING AND RESPONDING TO DYSFUNCTIONAL COGNITIONS

An important part of nearly every therapy session is to help patients respond to their inaccurate or unhelpful ideas: their automatic thoughts, images (mental pictures), and/or underlying beliefs. You can identify important automatic thoughts in several ways (see Chapter 9), but you will usually ask a basic question when a patient is reporting a distressing situation or emotion, or dysfunctional behavior:

> *"What is going through your mind right now?"*

Next, you will help patients evaluate their thinking in two major ways:

- You will engage in a process of *guided discovery* to help patients develop a more adaptive and reality-based perspective.
- You will jointly design *behavioral experiments* to test patients' predictions whenever feasible.

Guided Discovery

Usually in the context of discussing a problem, you elicit patients' cognitions (automatic thoughts, images, and/or beliefs). You will often ascertain which cognition or cognitions are most upsetting to patients, then ask them a series of questions to help them gain distance (i.e., see their cognitions as ideas, not necessarily as truths), evaluate the validity and utility of their cognitions, and/or decastastrophize their fears. Questions such as the following are often helpful:

> "What is the evidence that your thought is true? What is the evidence on the other side?"
>
> "What is an alternative way of viewing this situation?"
>
> "What is the worst that could happen, and how could you cope if it did? What's the best that could happen? What's the most realistic outcome of this situation?"
>
> "What is the effect of believing your automatic thought, and what could be the effect of changing your thinking?"
>
> "If your [friend or family member] were in this situation and had the same automatic thought, what advice would you give him or her?"
>
> "What should you do?"

As described in Chapter 11, not all these questions apply to all automatic thoughts, and you might often use a different line of questioning altogether. But these questions are a useful guide, and are illustrated in the following transcript, excerpted from Sally's fourth therapy session. I help Sally specify a problem that is important to her, identify and evaluate an associated dysfunctional idea, devise a reasonable plan, and assess the effectiveness of the intervention.

THERAPIST: Okay, Sally, you said you wanted to talk about a problem with finding a part-time job?

PATIENT: Yeah. I need the money ... but I don't know.

THERAPIST: (*noticing that Sally looks more dysphoric*) What's going through your mind right now?

PATIENT: [automatic thought] I won't be able to handle a job.

THERAPIST: [labeling her idea as a thought and linking it to her mood] And how does that thought make you feel?

PATIENT: [emotion] Sad. Really low.

THERAPIST: [beginning to evaluate the thought] What's the evidence that you won't be able to work?

PATIENT: Well, I'm having trouble just getting through my classes.

THERAPIST: Okay. What else?

PATIENT: I don't know ... I'm still so tired. It's hard to make myself even go and *look* for a job, much less go to work every day.

THERAPIST: In a minute we'll look at that. [suggesting an alternative view] Maybe it's actually harder for you at this point to go out and *investigate* jobs than it would be for you to go to a job that you already had. In any case, is there any other evidence that you couldn't handle a job, assuming that you can get one?

PATIENT: ... No, not that I can think of.

THERAPIST: Any evidence on the other side? That you *might* be able to handle a job?

PATIENT: I did work last year. And that was on top of school and other activities. But this year ... I just don't know.

THERAPIST: Any other evidence that you could handle a job?

PATIENT: I don't know.... It's possible I could do something that doesn't take much time. And that isn't too hard.

THERAPIST: What might that be?

PATIENT: A sales job, maybe. I did that last year.

THERAPIST: Any ideas of where you could work?

PATIENT: Actually, maybe the [university] bookstore. I saw a notice that they're looking for new clerks.

THERAPIST: Okay. And what would be the *worst* that could happen if you did get a job at the bookstore?

PATIENT: I guess if I couldn't do it.

THERAPIST: And if that happened, how would you cope?

PATIENT: I guess I'd just quit.

THERAPIST: And what would be the *best* that could happen?

PATIENT: Uh ... that I'd be able to do it easily.

THERAPIST: And what's the most *realistic* outcome?

PATIENT: It probably won't be easy, especially at first. But I might be able to do it.

THERAPIST: Sally, what's the effect of believing your thought, "I won't be able to handle a job"?

PATIENT: Makes me feel sad.... Makes me not even try.

THERAPIST: And what's the effect of changing your thinking, of realizing that possibly you could work in the bookstore?

PATIENT: I'd feel better. I'd be more likely to apply for the job.

THERAPIST: So what do you want to do about this?

PATIENT: Go to the bookstore. I could go this afternoon.

THERAPIST: How likely are you to go?

PATIENT: Oh, I guess I will. I will go.

THERAPIST: And how do you feel now?

PATIENT: A little better. A little more nervous, maybe. But a little more hopeful, I guess.

Here Sally is easily able to identify and evaluate her dysfunctional thought, "I won't be able to handle a job," with standard questions. Many patients, though, may require far more therapeutic effort before they are willing to follow through behaviorally. Had Sally been hesitant, I might have asked her to summarize what we had discussed and then we may have jointly composed a coping card based on her summary, that might have said something such as:

If I avoid going to the bookstore, remind myself that I probably could handle a job there and I could always quit if it didn't work out. It's not a big deal.

Behavioral Experiments

Whenever possible, you will collaboratively design experiments that patients can conduct right in the therapy session itself (as well as between sessions). Discussing the validity of patients' ideas, as described above, can help them change their thinking, but the change may be significantly more profound if the cognition is amenable to a behavioral test, that is, if the patient can have an experience that disconfirms its validity (Bennett-Levy et al., 2004). Suitable cognitions are usually linked to patients' negative predictions. A depressed patient, for example, might have the automatic thought, "If I try to read anything, I won't be able to concentrate well enough to understand it." You might ask the patient to read a short passage from a book in your office to see to what degree this thought is valid. An anxious patient may express the thought, "If I tell you about the abuse, I'll be so upset, I'll fall apart," or "If I get anxious and my heart starts to pound, I'll have a heart attack." You will collaboratively design experiments to test these kinds of ideas.

At the beginning of treatment, you will generally focus on situation-specific thoughts, which are usually amenable to change. Toward the middle of therapy, you will continue to work at the automatic thought level, but you will also focus on modifying patients' more generalized cognitions: their underlying assumptions and core beliefs. (These various levels of cognition are described at length in the next chapter.) Treatment continues, ideally, until patients' disorders are in remission and they have learned the necessary skills to prevent relapse.

EMPHASIZING THE POSITIVE

Most patients, especially those with depression, tend to focus unduly on the negative. When they are in a depressive mode, they automatically (i.e., without conscious awareness) and selectively attend to and put great emphasis on negative experience, and they either discount or fail to recognize more positive experience. Their difficulty in processing positive data in a straightforward manner leads them to develop a distorted sense of reality. To counteract this feature of depression, you will continually help patients attend to the positive.

At the evaluation, you will elicit patients' strengths ("What are some of your strengths and positive qualities?"). From the first session on, you will elicit positive data from the preceding week ("What positive things happened since I saw you last? What positive things did you do?"). You will orient sessions toward the positive, helping patients have a better week. You will use the therapeutic alliance to demonstrate that you view patients as valuable human beings ("I think it's great that you talked to the teacher [of the child you were tutoring] to see whether he could get more help"). You will ask patients for data that is contrary to their negative automatic thoughts and beliefs ("What's the [positive] evidence on the other side, that perhaps your automatic thought isn't true?").

You will point out the positive data you hear as patients discuss problems and ask what this data means about them ("What does this say about you, that you got the job in the bookstore?"). You will be on alert for, and note aloud, instances of positive coping that patients may allude to throughout the session ("What a good idea, to solve the problem by asking Allison to study with you"). You will collaboratively set homework assignments with patients to facilitate their experiencing a sense of pleasure and achievement. Methods of conceptualizing and incorporating patients' strengths as well as building resilience are described in Kuyken et al. (2009).

FACILITATING COGNITIVE AND BEHAVIORAL CHANGE BETWEEN SESSIONS (HOMEWORK)

An important aim of treatment is to help patients feel better by the end of the session and to set them up to have a better week. To achieve this objective, you will:

> - Help patients evaluate and respond to automatic thoughts that they are likely to experience between sessions.
> - Help patients devise solutions to their problems to implement during the week.
> - Teach patients new skills to practice during the week.

Because patients tend to forget much of what occurs in therapy sessions, it is important that anything you want them to remember be recorded so they can review it at home. Either you or they should write down their self-help assignments in a therapy notebook (which you can photocopy and attach to your treatment notes) or on carbonless paper (available from office supply stores or printers). Homework usually consists of:

> - Behavioral changes as a result of problem solving and/or skills training in session (e.g., problem of isolation might lead to behavioral solution of calling friends; problem of being overloaded

at work might lead to patient's assertively discussing the difficulty with a supervisor).

• Identifying automatic thoughts and beliefs when patients notice a dysfunctional change in affect, behavior, or physiology, and then evaluating and responding to their cognitions through Socratic questioning, behavioral experiments, and/or reading therapy notes that address their cognitions. For example:

> If I start to think that I can't clean up the kitchen, remind myself that I'm only going to do it for 10 minutes, that it may be difficult but probably won't be impossible, and that the first minute or two will probably be the hardest, and then it's likely to get easier.

Homework naturally flows from the discussion of each problem, because the patient will have things to remember (changes in cognition) and/or things to do. It is of utmost importance to plan homework assignments carefully, crafting them for your patient based on your conceptualization of what will help most, along with the patient's agreement. It is also essential to review homework the following week. An important early assignment for patients with depression is scheduling activities. See Chapter 6 for a detailed description of activity scheduling and Chapter 17 for detailed guidelines in setting and reviewing homework.

Chapter 3

COGNITIVE CONCEPTUALIZATION

A cognitive conceptualization provides the framework for understanding a patient. To initiate the process of formulating a case, you will ask yourself the following questions:

"What is the patient's diagnosis(es)?"

"What are his current problems? How did these problems develop and how are they maintained?"

"What dysfunctional thoughts and beliefs are associated with the problems? What reactions (emotional, physiological, and behavioral) are associated with his thinking?"

Then you will hypothesize how the patient developed this particular psychological disorder:

"How does the patient view himself, others, his personal world, his future?"

"What are the patient's underlying beliefs (including attitudes, expectations, and rules) and thoughts?"

"How is the patient coping with his dysfunctional cognitions?"

"What stressors (precipitants) contributed to the development of his current psychological problems, or interfere with solving these problems?"

"If relevant, what early experiences may have contributed to the patient's current problems? What meaning did the patient glean from these experiences, and which beliefs originated from, or became strengthened by, these experiences?"

"If relevant, what cognitive, affective, and behavioral mechanisms (adaptive and maladaptive) did the patient develop to cope with these dysfunctional beliefs?"

You begin to construct a cognitive conceptualization during your first contact with a patient and continue to refine your conceptualization throughout treatment. This organic, evolving formulation helps you plan for efficient and effective therapy (Kuyken et al., 2009; Needleman, 1999; Persons, 2008; Tarrier, 2006). In this chapter I describe the cognitive model, the theoretical basis of cognitive behavior therapy. I then discuss the relationship of thoughts and beliefs and present the case example of Sally, used throughout this book.

THE COGNITIVE MODEL

Cognitive behavior therapy is based on the *cognitive model*, which hypothesizes that people's emotions, behaviors, and physiology are influenced by their perception of events.

Situation/event
↓
Automatic thoughts
↓
Reaction (emotional, behavioral, physiological)

It is not a situation in and of itself that determines what people feel, but rather how they *construe* a situation (Beck, 1964; Ellis, 1962). Imagine, for example, a situation in which several people are reading a basic text on cognitive behavior therapy. They have quite different emotional and behavioral responses to the same situation, based on what is going through their minds as they read.

Reader A thinks, "This really makes sense. Finally, a book that will really teach me to be a good therapist!" Reader A feels mildly excited and keeps reading.

Reader B, on the other hand, thinks, "This approach is too simplistic. It will never work." Reader B feels disappointed and closes the book.

Reader C has the following thoughts: "This book isn't what I expected. What a waste of money." Reader C is disgusted and discards the book altogether.

Reader D thinks, "I really need to learn all this. What if I don't understand it? What if I never get good at it?" Reader D feels anxious and keeps reading the same few pages over and over.

Reader E has different thoughts: "This is just too hard. I'm so dumb. I'll never master this. I'll never make it as a therapist." Reader E feels sad and turns on the television.

The way people feel emotionally and the way they behave are associated with how they interpret and think about a situation. *The situation itself does not directly determine how they feel or what they do*; their emotional response is mediated by their perception of the situation. Cognitive behavior therapists are particularly interested in the level of thinking that may operate simultaneously with a more obvious, surface level of thinking.

For example, while you are reading this text, you may notice two levels in your thinking. Part of your mind is focusing on the information in the text; that is, you are trying to understand and integrate the information. At another level, however, you may be having some quick, evaluative thoughts. These thoughts are called *automatic thoughts* and are not the result of deliberation or reasoning. Rather, these thoughts seem to spring up spontaneously; they are often quite rapid and brief. You may barely be aware of these thoughts; you are far more likely to be aware of the emotion or behavior that follows. Even if you are aware of your thoughts, you most likely accept them uncritically, believing that they are true. You don't even think of questioning them. You can learn, however, to identify your automatic thoughts by attending to your shifts in affect, your behavior, and/or your physiology. Ask yourself, "What was just going through my mind?" when:

- You begin to feel dysphoric.
- You feel inclined to behave in a dysfunctional way (or to avoid behaving in an adaptive way).
- You notice distressing changes in your body or mind.

Having identified your automatic thoughts, you can, and probably already do to some extent, evaluate the validity of your thinking. For example, if you have a lot to do, you may have the automatic thought, "I'll never get it all finished." But you may do an automatic reality check, recalling past experiences and reminding yourself, "It's okay. You know you always get done what you need to." When you find your interpretation of a situation is erroneous and you correct it, you probably discover that your mood improves, you behave in a more functional way, and/or your physiological arousal decreases. In cognitive terms, when dysfunctional thoughts are subjected to objective reflection, one's emotions, behavior, and physiological reaction generally change. Chapter 11 offers specific guidelines on how to evaluate automatic thoughts.

But where do automatic thoughts spring from? What makes one person construe a situation differently from another person? Why may the same person interpret an identical event differently at one time than at another? The answer has to do with more enduring cognitive phenomena: beliefs.

BELIEFS

Beginning in childhood, people develop certain ideas about themselves, other people, and their world. Their most central or *core beliefs* are enduring understandings so fundamental and deep that they often do not articulate them, even to themselves. The person regards these ideas as absolute truths—just the way things "are" (Beck, 1987). For example, Reader E, who thought he was too unintelligent to master this text, frequently has a similar concern when he has to engage in a new task (e.g., learning a new skill on the computer, figuring out how to put together a bookcase, or applying for a bank loan). He seems to have the core belief, "I'm incompetent." This belief may operate only when he is in a depressed state, or it may be activated much of the time. When this core belief is activated, Reader E interprets situations through the lens of this belief, even though the interpretation may, on a rational basis, be patently invalid.

Reader E tends to focus selectively on information that confirms his core belief, disregarding or discounting information to the contrary. For example, Reader E did not consider that other intelligent, competent people might not fully understand the material in their first reading. Nor did he entertain the possibility that the author had not presented the material well. He did not recognize that his difficulty in comprehension could be due to a lack of concentration, rather than a lack of brainpower. He forgot that he often had difficulty initially when presented with a body of new information, but later had a good track record of mastery. Because his incompetence belief was activated, he automatically interpreted the situation in a highly negative, self-critical way. In this way, his belief is maintained, even though it is inaccurate and dysfunctional. It is important to note that he is not purposely trying to process information in this way; it occurs automatically.

Figure 3.1 illustrates this distorted way of processing information. The circle with a rectangular opening represents Reader E's schema. In Piagetian terms, the schema is a hypothesized mental structure that organizes information. Within this schema is Reader E's core belief: "I'm incompetent." When Reader E is presented with negative data this schema becomes activated, and the data, contained in negative rectangles, are immediately processed as confirming his core belief, which makes the belief stronger.

But a different process occurs when Reader E is presented with positive data (such as analyzing which health care plan would be best for his family). Positive data are encoded in the equivalent of positive triangles, which cannot fit into the schema. His mind automatically discounts the data ("I chose a health care plan, *but* it took me a long time.") When his boss praised him, he immediately thought, "My boss is wrong. I didn't do that project well. I didn't deserve it [his praise]." These interpretations, in essence, change the shape of the data from positive triangles to negative rectangles. Now the data fit into the schema and, as a result, strengthen the negative core belief.

There are also positive data that Reader E just does not notice. He does not negate some evidence of competence, such as paying his bills on time or fixing a plumbing problem. Rather, he does not seem to process these positive data at all; they bounce off the schema. Over time, Reader E's core belief of incompetence becomes stronger and stronger.

Sally, too, has a core belief of incompetence. Fortunately, when she is not depressed a different schema (which contains the core belief, "I'm reasonably competent") is activated much, but not all, of the time. But when she is depressed, the incompetence schema predominates. One important part of therapy is to help Sally view negative data in a more realistic and adaptive way. Another important part of therapy is to help her identify and process positive data in a straightforward way.

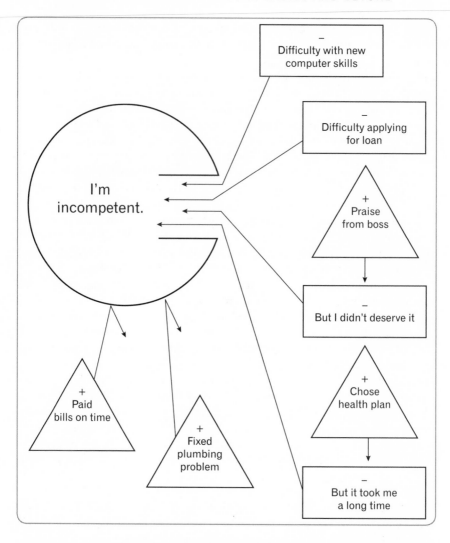

FIGURE 3.1. Information-processing model. This diagram demonstrates how negative data are immediately processed, strengthening the core belief, while positive data are discounted (changed into negative data) or unnoticed.

Core beliefs are the most fundamental level of belief; they are global, rigid, and overgeneralized. *Automatic thoughts,* the actual words or images that go through a person's mind, are situation specific and may be considered the most superficial level of cognition. The following section describes the class of *intermediate beliefs* that exists between the two.

Attitudes, Rules, and Assumptions

Core beliefs influence the development of an intermediate class of beliefs, which consists of (often unarticulated) attitudes, rules, and assumptions. Reader E, for example, had the following intermediate beliefs:

> *Attitude*: "It's terrible to fail."
>
> *Rule*: "Give up if a challenge seems too great."
>
> *Assumptions*: "If I try to do something difficult, I'll fail. If I avoid doing it, I'll be okay."

These beliefs influence his view of a situation, which in turn influences how he thinks, feels, and behaves. The relationship of these intermediate beliefs to core beliefs and automatic thoughts is depicted below:

```
                    Core beliefs
                        ↓
                Intermediate beliefs
            (rules, attitudes, assumptions)
                        ↓
                 Automatic thoughts
```

How do core beliefs and intermediate beliefs arise? People try to make sense of their environment from their early developmental stages. They need to organize their experience in a coherent way in order to function adaptively (Rosen, 1988). Their interactions with the world and other people, influenced by their genetic predisposition, lead to certain understandings: their beliefs, which may vary in their accuracy and functionality. Of particular significance to the cognitive behavior therapist is that dysfunctional beliefs can be unlearned, and more reality-based and functional new beliefs can be developed and strengthened through treatment.

The quickest way to help patients feel better and behave more adaptively is to facilitate the direct modification of their core beliefs as soon as possible, because once they do so, patients will tend to interpret future situations or problems in a more constructive way. It is possible to undertake belief modification earlier in treatment with patients who have straightforward depression and who held reasonable and adaptive beliefs about themselves before the onset of their disorder. But when patients' beliefs are entrenched, you can lose credibility and endanger the therapeutic alliance if you question the validity of core beliefs too early.

The usual course of treatment in cognitive behavior therapy, therefore, involves an initial emphasis on identifying and modifying automatic thoughts that derive from the core beliefs (and on interventions that indirectly modify core beliefs). Therapists teach patients to identify these cognitions that are closest to conscious awareness, and to gain distance from them by learning:

- Just because they believe something doesn't necessarily mean it is true.
- Changing their thinking so it is more reality based and useful helps them feel better and progress toward their goals.

It is easier for patients to recognize the distortion in their specific thoughts than in their broad understandings of themselves, their worlds, and others. But through repeated experiences in which they gain relief by working at a more superficial level of cognition, patients become more open to evaluating the beliefs that underlie their dysfunctional thinking. Relevant intermediate-level beliefs and core beliefs are evaluated in various ways and subsequently modified so that patients' perceptions of and conclusions about events change. This deeper modification of more fundamental beliefs makes patients less likely to relapse (Evans et al., 1992; Hollon, DeRubeis, & Seligman, 1992).

RELATIONSHIP OF BEHAVIOR TO AUTOMATIC THOUGHTS

The hierarchy of cognition, as it has been explained to this point, can be illustrated as follows:

Core beliefs
↓
Intermediate beliefs (rules, attitudes, assumptions)
↓
Situation
↓
Automatic thoughts
↓
Reaction (emotional, behavioral, physiological)

In a specific situation, one's underlying beliefs influence one's perception, which is expressed by situation-specific automatic thoughts. These thoughts, in turn, influence one's emotional, behavioral, and physiological reaction. Figure 3.2 illustrates the cognitive conceptualization of Reader E in this particular situation, illustrating how his beliefs influence his thinking, which in turns influences his reaction.

Note that had Reader E been able to *evaluate* his thinking, his emotions, physiology, and behavior may have been positively affected. For example, he may have responded to his thoughts by saying, "Wait a minute. This may be hard, but it's not necessarily impossible. I've been able to understand this type of book before. If I keep at it, I'll probably understand it better." Had he responded in such a way, he might have reduced his sadness and kept reading.

To summarize, this reader felt discouraged because of his thoughts in a particular situation. Why did he have these thoughts when another reader did not? Unarticulated core beliefs about his incompetence influenced his perception of the situation.

Core belief: *"I'm incompetent."*
↓
Intermediate beliefs
Attitude: *"It's terrible to fail."*
Rule: *"I should give up if a challenge seems too great."*
Assumptions: *"If I try to do something difficult, I'll fail. If I avoid doing it, I'll be okay."*
↓
Situation: *Reading a new text*
↓
Automatic thoughts: *"This is just too hard. I'm so dumb. I'll never master this. I'll never make it as a therapist."*
↓
Reaction:
Emotional: *Discouragement*
Physiological: *Heaviness in body*
Behavioral: *Avoids task and watches television instead.*

FIGURE 3.2. Cognitive conceptualization of Reader E.

A More Complex Cognitive Model

It is important to note that the sequence of the perception of situations leading to automatic thoughts that then influence people's reactions is an oversimplification at times. Thinking, mood, behavior, physiology, and the environment all can affect one another. Triggering situations can be:

- Discrete events (such as getting a low mark on a paper).
- A stream of thoughts (such as thinking about doing schoolwork or intrusive thoughts).
- A memory (such as getting a poor grade in the past).
- An image (such as the disapproving face of a professor).
- An emotion (such as noticing how intense one's dysphoria is).
- A behavior (such as staying in bed).
- A physiological or mental experience (such as noticing one's rapid heartbeat or slowed-down thinking).

There may be a complex sequence of events with many different triggering situations, automatic thoughts, and reactions, as pictured in Figure 3.3.

As explained in the beginning of this chapter, it is essential for you to learn to conceptualize patients' difficulties in cognitive terms in order to determine how to proceed in therapy—when to work on a specific problem or goal, automatic thought, belief, or behavior; what techniques to choose; and how to improve the therapeutic relationship. The basic questions to ask yourself are:

"How did this patient end up here?"

"What vulnerabilities were significant?"

"How has the patient coped with her vulnerability?"

"Did certain life events (traumas, experiences, interactions) predispose her to her current difficulties?"

"What are the patient's automatic thoughts, and what beliefs did they spring from?"

It is important to put yourself in your patients' shoes, to develop empathy for what they are undergoing, to understand how they are feeling, and to perceive the world through their eyes. Given their history

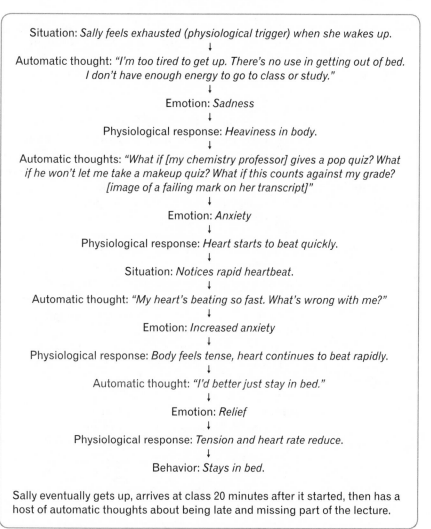

Situation: *Sally feels exhausted (physiological trigger) when she wakes up.*
↓
Automatic thought: *"I'm too tired to get up. There's no use in getting out of bed. I don't have enough energy to go to class or study."*
↓
Emotion: *Sadness*
↓
Physiological response: *Heaviness in body.*
↓
Automatic thoughts: *"What if [my chemistry professor] gives a pop quiz? What if he won't let me take a makeup quiz? What if this counts against my grade? [image of a failing mark on her transcript]"*
↓
Emotion: *Anxiety*
↓
Physiological response: *Heart starts to beat quickly.*
↓
Situation: *Notices rapid heartbeat.*
↓
Automatic thought: *"My heart's beating so fast. What's wrong with me?"*
↓
Emotion: *Increased anxiety*
↓
Physiological response: *Body feels tense, heart continues to beat rapidly.*
↓
Automatic thought: *"I'd better just stay in bed."*
↓
Emotion: *Relief*
↓
Physiological response: *Tension and heart rate reduce.*
↓
Behavior: *Stays in bed.*

Sally eventually gets up, arrives at class 20 minutes after it started, then has a host of automatic thoughts about being late and missing part of the lecture.

FIGURE 3.3. Complex cognitive model sequence.

and set of beliefs, their perceptions, thoughts, emotions, and behavior should make sense.

It is helpful to view therapy as a journey, and the conceptualization as the road map. You and the patient discuss the goals of therapy, the final destination. There are a number of ways to reach that destination: for example, by main highways or back roads. Sometimes detours change the original plan. As you become more experienced and better at conceptualization, you fill in the relevant details in the map, and your efficiency and effectiveness improve. At the beginning, however, it is reasonable to assume that you may not accomplish therapy in the most effective or efficient way. An accurate cognitive conceptualization aids you in determining what the main highways are and how best to travel.

Conceptualization begins at the first contact with patients and is refined at every subsequent contact. You make hypotheses about patients, based not just on the cognitive formulation of the case, but also on the specific data patients present. You confirm, disconfirm, or modify your hypotheses as patients present new data. The conceptualization, there-fore, is fluid. At strategic points, you will directly check your hypotheses and formulation with patients. Generally, if the conceptualization is on target, patients confirm that it "feels right"—they agree that the picture the therapist presents truly resonates with them.

Sally, for example, suffered from persistent sadness, anxiety, and loneliness. As part of her intake evaluation, I elicited a sampling of her automatic thoughts. I asked Sally when she generally was most dis-tressed—in which situations or times of day. Sally replied that she felt worst at bedtime, as she lay in bed, trying to fall asleep. Having ascer-tained that the previous night was a typical example, I asked the key question: "What was going through your mind last night, as you were lying in bed, trying to fall asleep?" Sally replied, "I'll never be able to finish my term paper. I'll probably flunk out of here. I'll never be able to make anything of myself." Sally also reported an image, an automatic thought in a pictorial form, which flashed through her mind. She saw herself, weighed down by a heavy backpack, trudging aimlessly down the street, looking quite downtrodden, directionless, and desperate. During the course of therapy, I rounded out my conceptualization. I organized my thinking through the use of a Cognitive Conceptualization Diagram (page 200) and a Cognitive Case Write-Up (Appendix A).

Sally's Core Beliefs

As a child, Sally tried to make sense of herself, others, and her world. She learned through her own experiences, through interactions with others, through direct observation, and through others' explicit and implicit messages to her. Her perceptions were also undoubtedly influ-enced by her genetic inheritance. Sally had a highly achieving older brother. As a young child, she perceived that she could not do anything as well as her brother and started to believe, although she did not put it into words, that she was incompetent and inferior. She kept comparing her performance to that of her brother and invariably came up lacking. She frequently had thoughts such as: "I can't draw like Robert can." "He rides his bike better than I do." "I'll never be as good a reader as he is. He does everything better than I do."

Not all children with older siblings develop these kinds of dysfunctional beliefs. But Sally's ideas were reinforced by her mother, who frequently criticized her: "You did a terrible job straightening up your room. Can't you do anything right?" "Your brother got a good report card. But you? You'll never amount to anything." Sally, like most children, placed enormous stock in her mother's words, believing that her mother was correct about nearly everything. So when her mother criticized her, implying or directly stating that Sally was incompetent, Sally believed her.

At school, Sally also compared herself to her peers. While she was an above-average student, she compared herself only to the best students, again coming up short. She had thoughts such as: "I'm not as good as they are." "I'll never be able to understand all this as well as they can." So the idea that she was incompetent and inferior was reinforced.

Without recognizing that she was doing so, Sally often screened out or discounted positive information that contradicted these ideas. When she got a high mark on a test, she would tell herself, "The test was easy." When she learned ballet and became one of the better dancers in the group, she thought, "I'll never be as good as my teacher." She usually made negative interpretations, thereby confirming her dysfunctional beliefs. For example, when her mother yelled at her for getting a B on a test, she thought, "Mom's right. I am stupid." She consistently interpreted negative events as demonstrating her shortcomings. In addition, when she experienced positive events such as winning an award, she often discounted them: "I was just lucky. It was a fluke."

This process led to Sally's developing a negative core belief about herself. Sally's negative beliefs were not rock solid, however. Her father, although he traveled for business and was home only intermittently, was generally encouraging and supportive. When he taught her to hit a baseball, for example, he would praise her efforts. "That's good … good swing … you're getting it … keep going." Some of Sally's teachers, too, praised her performance in school. Sally also had positive experiences with friends. She saw that if she tried hard, she could do some things better than her friends could—baseball, for example. So Sally also developed a counterbalancing positive belief that she was competent in at least some ways.

Sally's core beliefs about her world and about other people were, for the most part, positive and functional. She generally believed that other people were well-intentioned, and she perceived her world as being relatively safe, stable, and predictable.

Again, Sally's core beliefs about herself, others, and her world were her most basic beliefs, which she had never really articulated until she entered treatment. As a teenager, her more positive core beliefs were dominant until she became depressed, and then her highly negative core beliefs became activated.

Sally's Attitudes, Rules, and Assumptions

Somewhat more amenable to modification than her core beliefs were Sally's intermediate beliefs. These attitudes, rules, and assumptions developed in the same way as core beliefs, as Sally tried to make sense of her world, of others, and of herself. Mostly through interactions with her family and significant others, she developed the following attitudes and rules:

> "I should be great at everything I try."
> "I should always do my best."
> "It's terrible to waste your potential."

As was the case with her core beliefs, Sally had not fully articulated these intermediate beliefs. But the beliefs nevertheless influenced her thinking and guided her behavior. In high school, for example, she did not try out for the school newspaper (although it interested her) because she assumed she could not write well enough. She felt both anxious before exams, thinking that she might not do well, and guilty, thinking that she should have studied more.

When her more positive core beliefs predominated, however, she saw herself in a more positive light, although she never completely believed that she was competent. She developed the assumption "If I work hard, I can overcome my shortcomings and do well in school." When she became depressed, however, Sally did not really believe this assumption any longer and substituted the belief, "Because of my deficiencies, I'll never amount to anything."

Sally's Coping Strategies

The idea of being incompetent had always been quite painful to Sally, and she developed certain behavioral strategies to cope or compensate for what she saw as her shortcomings. As might be gleaned from her intermediate beliefs, Sally worked hard at school and at sports. She overprepared her assignments and studied quite hard for tests. She also became vigilant for signs of inadequacy and redoubled her efforts if she failed to master something at school. She rarely asked others for help for fear they would recognize her inadequacy.

Sally's Automatic Thoughts

While Sally did not articulate these core beliefs and intermediate beliefs (until therapy), she was at least somewhat aware of her automatic thoughts in specific situations. In high school, for example (during which time she was not depressed), she tried out for the girls' softball and hockey teams. She made the softball team and thought, "That's great. I'll get Dad to practice batting with me." When she failed to make the hockey team she was disappointed, but not particularly self-critical.

In college, however, Sally became depressed during her freshman year. Later, when she considered playing an informal softball game with students in her dorm, her depression influenced her thinking: "I'm no good. I probably won't even be able to hit the ball." Similarly, when she got a C on an English literature examination, she thought, "I'm so stupid. I'll probably fail the course. I'll never be able to make it through college."

To summarize, in her nondepressed high school years, Sally's more positive core beliefs were activated, and she had relatively more positive (and more realistic) thoughts. In her freshman year in college, however, her negative beliefs predominated during her depression, which led her to interpret situations quite negatively and to have predominantly negative (and unrealistic) thoughts. These distorted thoughts also led her to *behave* in self-defeating ways, which led to automatic thoughts about her behavior. Instead of interpreting her avoidance as a symptom of depression, she thought, "I'm a basket case," which then led to increased dysphoria and maladaptive behavior.

Sequence Leading to Sally's Depression

How did Sally became depressed? Depression is caused by a variety of biopsychological and psychosocial factors. Sally may have had a genetic predisposition toward developing depressogenic beliefs. Not all negative events, however, led her to feel dysphoric. She was able to get along until her innate vulnerability, influenced by the presence of negative beliefs, was challenged by a series of matching stressors (the "diathesis–stress" model; Beck, 1967).

When Sally began college, she had several experiences that she interpreted in a highly negative fashion. One such experience occurred the first week. She had a conversation with other freshmen in her dorm who were relating the number of advanced placement courses and exams they had taken that had exempted them from several basic freshman courses. Sally, who had no advanced placement credits, began to think how superior these students were to her. In her economics class, her professor outlined the course requirements and Sally immediately thought, "I won't be able to do the research paper." She had difficulty understanding the first chapter in her chemistry text and she thought, "If I can't even understand Chapter 1, how will I ever make it through the course?"

Sally's beliefs made her vulnerable to interpreting events in a negative way. She did not question her thoughts, but rather accepted them uncritically. As the weeks went on, Sally began to have more and more negative thoughts about herself and began to feel more and more discouraged and sad. She began to spend an inordinate amount of time studying, although she did not accomplish a great deal because of decreased concentration. She continued to be highly self-critical, and even had negative thoughts about her depressive symptoms: "What's wrong with me? I shouldn't feel this way. Why am I so down? I'm just hopeless." She withdrew somewhat from new friends at school and stopped calling her old friends for support. She discontinued running and swimming and other activities that had previously provided her with a sense of accomplishment. Thus she experienced a paucity of positive inputs. Eventually, her appetite decreased, her sleep became disturbed, and she became enervated and listless. Sally's perception of and behavior in the circumstances at the time facilitated the expression of a biological and psychological vulnerability to depression.

Conceptualizing a patient in cognitive terms is crucial to determining the most efficient and effective course of treatment. It also aids in developing empathy, an ingredient that is critical in establishing a good working relationship with the patient. In general, the questions to ask when conceptualizing patients are:

"How did the patient come to develop this disorder?"

"What were significant life events, experiences, and interactions?"

"What are the patient's most basic beliefs about himself, his world, and others?"

"What are the patient's assumptions, expectations, rules, and attitudes (intermediate beliefs)?"

"What strategies has the patient used throughout life to cope with these negative beliefs?"

"Which automatic thoughts, images, and behaviors help to maintain the disorder?"

"How did the patient's developing beliefs interact with life situations to make the patient vulnerable to the disorder?"

"What is happening in the patient's life right now and what are the patient's perceptions?"

Again, conceptualization begins at the first contact and is an ongoing process. You base your hypotheses on information you have collected from the patient, using the most parsimonious explanations and refraining from interpretations and inferences not clearly based on actual data. You will check out the conceptualization with patients at strategic points to ensure that it is accurate, as well as to help patients understand themselves and their difficulties. Your conceptualization is always subject to modification as you continually uncover new data that will lead you to confirm, refine, or discard your previous hypotheses. The ongoing process of conceptualization is emphasized throughout this book; Chapter 14 illustrates further how historical events shape patients' understanding of themselves and their worlds.

Chapter 4

THE EVALUATION SESSION

I n this chapter, you will learn about the goals and structure for this session. You will learn how to conduct the assessment, relate your tentative diagnosis, develop initial treatment goals, and shape the patient's expectations for treatment. You will also learn what to do following the evaluation session, including devising a tentative cognitive conceptualization of the patient.

Effective cognitive behavior therapy requires you to evaluate patients thoroughly, so you can accurately formulate the case, conceptualize the individual patient, and plan treatment. While there is overlap among treatments for various disorders, there are important variations as well, based on the key cognitions and behavioral strategies of a particular disorder. Attention to the patient's presenting problems, current functioning, symptoms, and history helps you develop an initial conceptualization and formulate a general therapy plan. Even if a patient has been evaluated by a different clinician, you will need to supplement the evaluation with additional data collection. There are a number of tasks to accomplish in your first contact with a patient, other than establishing the patient's diagnosis.

Assessment is not limited to this first meeting with a patient, however. You will continue to collect assessment data at each session to confirm, change, or add to your diagnosis and conceptualization. It is possible to miss a diagnosis at intake if patients deliberately withhold information (some patients with substance abuse problems or ego-syntonic eating disorders may do this) or inadvertently fail to report important data. Or you might erroneously attribute certain symptoms (e.g., social isolation) to a particular disorder (depression), when another disorder is also present (social phobia). When another clinician has performed the evaluation, you will undoubtedly need to collect additional information pertinent to the use of cognitive behavior therapy as the treatment modality.

GOALS OF THE ASSESSMENT SESSION

In addition to correctly diagnosing patients, the assessment helps you:

- Formulate the case and create an initial cognitive conceptualization of the patient.
- Determine whether you will be an appropriate therapist.
- Determine whether you can provide the appropriate "dose" of therapy (e.g., if you are able to provide only weekly therapy but the patient requires a day program).
- Determine whether adjunctive treatment or services (such as medication) may be indicated.
- Initiate a therapeutic alliance with the patient (and with family members, if relevant).
- Begin to socialize the patient into the structure and process of therapy.
- Identify important problems and set broad goals.

It is desirable to collect as much information as possible before you see the patient for the first time. Request that patients send, or arrange to have sent, relevant reports from current and previous clinicians, including both mental health and health professionals. The evaluation session itself will require less time if patients are able to fill out questionnaires and self-report forms beforehand. It is especially important that patients have had a recent medical checkup. Occasionally patients suffer from organic problems, not psychological ones. For example, hypothyroidism can be mistaken for depression.

Inform the patient during the initial phone call that it is often useful to have a family member, partner, or trusted friend accompany the patient to session to provide additional information and/or to learn how he or she can be helpful to the patient. Make sure patients understand that the evaluation will help you determine whether they are good candidates for cognitive behavior therapy and whether you believe you will be able to provide the needed treatment.

STRUCTURE OF THE ASSESSMENT SESSION

In this session, you will:

- Greet the patient.
- Collaboratively decide with the patient whether a family member should attend all, part, or none of the session.
- Set the agenda and convey appropriate expectations for the session.
- Conduct the assessment.
- Set initial broad goals.
- Elicit feedback from the patient.

STARTING THE EVALUATION SESSION

Before patients enter your office, review whatever records they have brought and the forms they have completed. It is usually desirable to meet with patients alone at first. Then you can discuss whether an accompanying family member (if there is one) should attend the session. It is often helpful to bring this person in at least toward the end of the session, as you convey your initial impressions, including tentative diagnosis, and review broad therapy goals. You can ask for the family member's perspective on the patient's problems and, if advisable, set the scene for the family member to return at some point to learn what he or she can do to be more helpful to the patient.

Next, let the patient know what to expect from this initial appointment.

THERAPIST: Sally, as I explained on the phone, this is our evaluation session. It's not a therapy session, so we won't work on solving your problems today. We'll start doing that next time. Today, I need to ask you a lot of questions [providing a rationale] so I can determine your diagnosis. Some of the questions will be relevant. A number won't be, but I need to ask them so I can rule in the problems you do have and rule out the problems you don't have. Is that okay?

PATIENT: Yes.

THERAPIST: I will probably need to interrupt you sometimes today, so I can get the information I need. If it bothers you, would you let me know?

PATIENT: Okay.

THERAPIST: Before we begin, I'd like to tell you what I expect to cover today. [setting the agenda] I'd like to find out a lot about symptoms you've been experiencing and how you've been functioning lately, and also about your history. Then I'll ask you to tell me anything else you think I should know. Then we'll set some broad goals for treatment. I'll tell you what my initial impressions are and what I think we should focus on in treatment. I'll ask you how that sounds. And at the end, I'll see whether you have any other questions or concerns. [being collaborative] Does that sound okay?

PATIENT: Yes.

THERAPIST: Anything else you want to cover today?

PATIENT: I was hoping you could help me figure out what to do about school. I'm so far behind.

THERAPIST: (*making a note*) Let me write that down. I don't know whether there will be time today, but we can definitely get to it next time, at our first treatment session.

THE ASSESSMENT PHASE

You will need to know about many areas of the patient's current and past experience to develop a sound treatment plan (across sessions), plan treatment within sessions, develop a good therapeutic relationship, guide the patient in setting goals, and generally carry out effective treatment. These areas include:

- Patient demographics.
- Chief complaints and current problems.
- History of present illness and precipitating events.
- Coping strategies (adaptive and maladaptive), current and historical.
- Psychiatric history, including kinds of psychosocial treatments (and perceived helpfulness of these treatments), hospitalizations, medication, suicide attempts, and current status.
- Substance use history and current status.
- Medical history and current status.
- Family psychiatric history and current status.
- Developmental history.

- General family history and current status.
- Social history and current status.
- Educational history and current status.
- Vocational history and current status.
- Religious/spiritual history and current status.
- Strengths, values, and adaptive coping strategies.

While a detailed account of assessment procedures and instruments are beyond the scope of this book, many sources can help, including Antony and Barlow (2010); Dobson and Dobson (2009); Kuyken and colleagues (2009); Lazarus and Lazarus (1991); Ledley, Marx, and Heimberg (2005). It is also critical to determine the degree to which patients might be suicidal. Wenzel, Brown, and Beck (2008) provide assessment and practice guidelines for suicidal patients.

Another important part of the evaluation is asking how patients spend their time. Asking patients to describe their typical day gives you additional insight into their daily experience and facilitates setting specific goals at the first treatment session. As they describe a typical day, look for:

- Variations in their mood.
- Whether and how they interact with family, friends, and people at work.
- How they are generally functioning at home, work, and elsewhere.
- How they spend their free time.

You will also probe for what they are *not* doing and what they are actively avoiding.

THERAPIST: Sally, I'd like to get an idea of what your daily routine is like. Can you tell me what you do from the time you wake up in the morning until the time you go to sleep at night?

PATIENT: Okay.

THERAPIST: What time do you wake up?

PATIENT: (*Sighs.*) Well, I usually wake up around 5 o'clock.

THERAPIST: Then what do you do?

PATIENT: Usually I toss and turn for a couple of hours at least.

THERAPIST: What time do you get out of bed for the day?

PATIENT: It depends. I usually stay in bed until the last minute. I have class at 9 o'clock 3 days a week, so I get up at 8:30, 8:40, something like that.

THERAPIST: And on the other days?

PATIENT: I don't have to get up that early. So I usually stay in bed till I get hungry for breakfast.

THERAPIST: So you have breakfast at ...?

PATIENT: Sometimes 10 o'clock. Sometimes noon.

THERAPIST: Is that a change from last semester?

PATIENT: Yeah, I used to get up by 9 at the latest.

THERAPIST: What do you do after breakfast?

PATIENT: I usually hang out in my dorm room. Watch television. Maybe try to do some reading for class. But I usually can't concentrate. So I stop doing it. Sometimes I fall asleep.

THERAPIST: What else do you do in the afternoon?

PATIENT: Most days I have class from 1 to 4.

THERAPIST: Do you go? Have you missed any classes?

PATIENT: No, I go. But it's really hard to sit there. Sometimes I just space out.

THERAPIST: What do you do after class?

PATIENT: Go back to my room.

THERAPIST: And then what?

PATIENT: It depends.

THERAPIST: What do you sometimes do?

PATIENT: Usually I try to study a little. But sometimes I end up surfing the Web or falling asleep or watching TV.

THERAPIST: What do you do for dinner?

PATIENT: I go to the cafeteria with someone from my dorm.

THERAPIST: What do you do after that?

PATIENT: It depends. Usually go back to my room. I try to do some work. Sometimes I can and sometimes I can't. I try for a little while and then I mostly watch TV.

THERAPIST: And then?

PATIENT: I get in bed around 11, 11:30.

THERAPIST: Do you fall asleep right away?

PATIENT: Not usually. It takes me about an hour.

THERAPIST: And then you sleep through until 5?

PATIENT: Yes.

This description helps me pinpoint difficulties we will probably need to address: difficulty sleeping, napping, irregular schedule, social isolation, limited opportunities for mastery (a sense of accomplishment), trouble concentrating, falling behind in schoolwork, too much TV watching. Because Sally, like most depressed patients, has focused on the problems she encounters, I also ask her about positive experiences and adaptive coping strategies. ("Sally, what are the better parts of the day for you?"; "It sounds like you were pretty tired. How did you get yourself to go to class?")

Collecting data in this way guides my thinking in developing an initial treatment plan. I'll also use the information in the first session when we set goals for treatment and do activity scheduling. In addition, I will ask Sally for a description of what she does on a typical weekend, when she doesn't have the structure of attending classes.

Throughout the assessment phase, you will be alert for indications that the patient is unsure about committing to treatment. For example, as Sally describes her current symptoms, she expresses hopeless thinking. I use her automatic thought to subtly relate the cognitive model, indicate how it will be a target of treatment in the future, and ensure that our tentative alliance hasn't suffered.

PATIENT: It feels like I've got so many problems. I don't think anything can help.

THERAPIST: Okay, that's an interesting thought: "I don't think anything can help." How does that thought make you feel? Sad? Hopeless?

PATIENT: Both.

THERAPIST: This is *exactly* the kind of depressed thought that we'll be talking about starting next week. We'll need to find out whether that thought is 100% true, 0% true, or someplace in the middle. Meanwhile, is there anything I said or did that makes you think I can't help, or this kind of treatment can't help?

It is important to structure the patient's responses to collect the data you need. Providing a guideline can help:

THERAPIST: For the next few questions, I just need you to [answer "yes," "no," or "I'm not sure"] or [answer in one or two sentences].

When patients start to provide unneeded details or go off on a tangent, it is important to gently interrupt:

THERAPIST: Sorry to interrupt, but I need to know ...

FINAL PART OF THE ASSESSMENT

Toward the end of the assessment, it is useful to ask patients whether there is anything else that is important for you to know. An important follow-up question is: "Is there anything you're reluctant to tell me? You don't have to tell me what it is. I just need to know whether there's more to tell, maybe at some point in the future."

INVOLVING A FAMILY MEMBER

If family members have accompanied patients to the office, you might now ask patients whether they would like to invite them into the session (unless, of course, they have been there from the beginning). Make sure there is nothing the patient wants you to refrain from saying to the family member. Elicit the patient's permission to:

- Inquire what the family member thinks is most important for you to know; if he or she focuses only on the negative, ask about the patients' positive qualities, strengths, and coping strategies.
- Go over your initial impressions.
- Present your tentative treatment plan.

RELATING YOUR IMPRESSIONS

Explain to patients that you will need time to review your notes, their forms, and previous reports to establish their diagnosis. For most cases of depression and anxiety, it is appropriate to give your initial impressions of their diagnosis and show them how you will confirm the diagnosis by using the DSM, a diagnostic manual listing psychiatric disorders and their symptoms. It may or may not help, at this initial encounter, to tell patients they have a severe mental illness or personality disorder. Instead, it may be more prudent to summarize the problems and symptoms the patient is experiencing.

SETTING INITIAL GOALS FOR TREATMENT
AND RELATING YOUR TREATMENT PLAN

Setting goals and relating a treatment plan help provide patients with hope.

THERAPIST: If it's okay, I'd like to spend a few minutes talking about your goals for treatment, and how I think treatment will go.

PATIENT: Okay.

THERAPIST: (*Writes "Goals" at the top of a sheet of paper.*) Goals are really just the flip side of problems. We'll set more specific goals next session, but very broadly, should we say: Reduce depression? Reduce anxiety? Do better at school? Get back to socializing?

PATIENT: Yes.

THERAPIST: (*Jots these down.*) Now I'd like to tell you how I think you're going to get better and then I want to hear how it sounds to you.

PATIENT: Okay.

THERAPIST: Starting next week, we're going to work toward your goals. At every session, I'll ask you what problems you want my help in solving. For example, next week you might say, "I'm still having trouble getting my schoolwork done," which relates to your goal of doing better at school. Then we'll do some problem solving. We might figure out ways to improve your concentration, to get yourself on a study schedule, and to get help from other people if you need it. (*pause*) Does that sound okay?

PATIENT: Yes.

THERAPIST: And we'll also look for depressed thinking that might get in the way. For example, earlier in the session you said, "I'm such a failure," and you told me how depressed you feel when you have thoughts like that. Do you see how that idea can sap your motivation to study? How it can make you feel terrible? How you might then curl up in bed instead of going to the library?

PATIENT: Yeah, that's what happens.

THERAPIST: So one thing we'll do together is evaluate thoughts like that. What's the evidence you're a failure? Any evidence that you're not a failure? Is there another way of looking at this situation, for example, that you're depressed and need some help in problem solving, but that doesn't mean you're a failure?

PATIENT: Hmm.

THERAPIST: So we'll help you change your depressed and anxious thinking to make it more realistic, and we'll come up with solutions to your problems that you can try out during the rest of the week. And you'll learn skills that you can use for the rest of your life, so you can continue solving your problems and think more realistically, and act in ways that can get you to your goals. [eliciting feedback] How does that sound?

PATIENT: It makes sense.

THERAPIST: Sally, that's how we find people get better, by making small changes in their thinking and behavior every day. [eliciting feedback] Now, was there anything I said that didn't sound good?

PATIENT: [expressing another automatic thought] I just don't know if it will work.

THERAPIST: Well, I don't have a crystal ball, so I can't give you a 100% guarantee. But there's nothing you've told me that makes me think it won't work. (*pause.*) Are you willing to give it a try? Do you want to come back next week?

PATIENT: Yes, I do.

Q: What if … patients express concern about the treatment plan?

A: First, positively reinforce them for expressing their skepticism or misgivings ("It's good you told me that"). Next, you will need to collect more data by asking, "What makes you think this treatment won't work?" and "What do you think would help more?" Based on the patient's answers, you will conceptualize the problem in cognitive terms and plan a strategy. For example, when patients believe your treatment won't help because past treatments have been ineffective, you can ask whether they felt they had a good therapeutic alliance with their previous therapists and whether, at every session, their therapists:

- Set agendas.
- Figured out with them what they could do to have a better week.
- Wrote down what patients wanted to remember to say to themselves when they had depressed thinking.
- Taught them specifically how to evaluate their thinking and change their behavior.
- Asked for feedback to make sure therapy was on the right track.

  Most patients have not experienced this kind of treatment, and you can say, "I'm glad to hear that, because it sounds as if our treatment here will be different. If it were exactly the same as your past experiences, I'd be less hopeful."

Q: What if ... patients reply that a previous therapist has engaged in all the above activities at every session?

A: In this case, you will need to spend more time finding out precisely what occurred, especially whether the therapist provided treatment individualized for the patient and his specific disorder(s), based on the latest research and practice guidelines. In any case, you can encourage the patient to give your treatment a try for a few sessions and indicate that you will then jointly review whether the treatment seems to be working.

EXPECTATIONS FOR TREATMENT

At this session, you will give patients a general sense of how long they should expect treatment to take. Usually it is best to suggest a range, 2–4 months for many patients with straightforward major depression, although some might be able to terminate sooner (or might have to, due to financial constraints or insurance limitations). Other patients, particularly those with chronic psychiatric disorders, or those who want to work on problems related to a personality disorder, may remain in treatment for a year or more. And patients with severe mental illness may need more intensive treatment when they are more highly symptomatic, and periodic booster sessions for a very long time (along with medication).

Most patients progress satisfactorily with weekly sessions unless they are severely depressed or anxious, suicidal, or clearly in need of more support. Toward the end of treatment, you may gradually space sessions further apart to give patients more opportunities to solve problems, make decisions, and use their therapy tools independently.

In the following transcript, I give Sally an idea of how I expect therapy will proceed.

THERAPIST: If it's okay with you, Sally, we'll plan to meet once a week until you're feeling significantly better, then we'll move to once every 2 weeks, then maybe once every 3 or 4 weeks. We'll decide how to space out therapy together. Even when we decide to end, I'll recommend that you come back for a "booster" session once every few months for a while. How does that sound?

PATIENT: Fine.

THERAPIST: It's hard to predict now how long you should be in therapy. My best guess is somewhere around 8 to 14 sessions. If we find that you have some long-standing problems that you want to work on, it could take longer. Again, we'll decide *together* what seems to be best. Okay?

Between the Evaluation and First Therapy Session

Before the first therapy session, you will write up your evaluation report and initial treatment plan. If you have obtained consent, you will contact the patient's previous mental health and health professionals to request reports, ask questions, and obtain additional information. You will also contact relevant current professionals to discuss your findings and coordinate care. Conversations by phone can reveal important information that had not been documented in writing. You will also start to devise a tentative cognitive conceptualization.

DEVISING AN INITIAL COGNITIVE CONCEPTUALIZATION AND TREATMENT PLAN

You will synthesize the information you gleaned from the evaluation to develop an initial cognitive conceptualization, informed by the cognitive formulation (the basic beliefs and behavioral patterns) associated with the patient's diagnosis. You will hypothesize about the development of the patient's disorder.

> "Were there important early life events that led to the development of negative core beliefs?"
>
> "What are the patient's core beliefs?"
>
> "What precipitated the disorder?"
>
> "Did the patient put an adverse construction on certain precipitating events?"
>
> "How do the patient's thinking and behavior contribute to the maintenance of the disorder?"

You will then use the conceptualization to develop a broad treatment plan.

Pulling together what I had learned from the evaluation, I hypothesized that Sally was vulnerable to seeing herself as incompetent (a belief that developed as a result of interactions with her parents, sibling, and some teachers). When she entered college, Sally began to perceive herself as unable to meet the new demands of school and independent living. She began to develop a generalized sense of incompetence; that is, a core belief of incompetence became activated. She began to have many automatic thoughts across situations about the likelihood that she would fail. These thoughts led her to feel sad, anxious, and hopeless. She was affected behaviorally, as well. She began to give up, spending too much time alone in her room. She failed to persist in doing assignments she viewed as difficult, and she began to fall behind in her schoolwork. She saw her difficulties as an innate flaw, and not as the result of depression. A paucity of pleasure and mastery activities increased her dysphoria (see Appendix A).

Understanding the cognitive model of depression and being familiar with the major treatment strategies for depression, I developed a more specific treatment plan than the simplified one I had presented to Sally. I hypothesized that I would initially need to focus on the following: helping her solve academic and daily living problems; encouraging her to become much more active; and teaching her to identify, evaluate, and modify her inaccurate or unhelpful negative thinking, especially thoughts associated with failure and incompetence (since she had expressed those ideas). I hypothesized that we would work more directly on her core belief of incompetence toward the middle of treatment, but I did not yet know whether it would be important to include a focus on the historic antecedents to her belief. I also did not know at this point whether Sally had dysfunctional beliefs associated with unlovability or worthlessness (see Chapter 14) that we would have to modify; she had not provided data to support the existence of these beliefs at the evaluation. I planned to emphasize relapse prevention in the final part of treatment. I continued to refine this basic treatment plan throughout therapy as I got to know Sally and the nature of her difficulties better.

Chapter 5

STRUCTURE OF THE FIRST THERAPY SESSION

In this chapter, you will learn how to structure the initial session, including how to:

- Discuss the patient's diagnosis.
- Do a mood check.
- Set goals.
- Start working on a problem.
- Set homework.
- Elicit feedback.

Most patients feel comfortable when you tell them how and why you would like to structure sessions. Doing so demystifies the process of therapy and keeps treatment on track. Chapter 6 focuses on an essential component for depressed patients: initiating behavioral activation. Chapter 7 describes the common structure for subsequent sessions, and Chapter 8 discusses problems in structuring sessions.

GOALS AND STRUCTURE OF THE INITIAL SESSION

Before the first session, you will review the patient's intake evaluation and you will keep your initial conceptualization and treatment plan in mind as you conduct the session, being prepared to change course if need be. Most standard cognitive behavior therapy sessions last for about 45–50 minutes, but the first one often takes an hour. Your goals for the first session are to:

- Establish rapport and trust with patients, normalize their difficulties, and instill hope.
- Socialize patients into treatment by educating them about their disorder(s), the cognitive model, and the process of therapy.
- Collect additional data to help you conceptualize the patient.
- Develop a goal list.
- Start solving a problem important to the patient (and/or get the patient behaviorally activated).

To accomplish these goals, you will use the following format:

Initial Part of Session 1
1. Set the agenda (and provide a rationale for doing so).
2. Do a mood check.
3. Obtain an update (since the evaluation).
4. Discuss the patient's diagnosis and do psychoeducation.

Middle Part of Session 1
5. Identify problems and set goals.
6. Educate the patient about the cognitive model.
7. Discuss a problem.

End of Session 1
8. Provide or elicit a summary.
9. Review homework assignment.
10. Elicit feedback.

SETTING THE AGENDA

As this is the first session, you will begin by greeting the patient and setting the agenda. Doing so frequently reduces patients' anxieties, as they quickly find out what to expect. You will provide a rationale and make sure the patient agrees with the topics you propose. (In future sessions, you will set the agenda sometime in the initial part of the session, but not necessarily at the very beginning.)

THERAPIST: Sally, I'm glad you came in today. Is it all right if we start off by deciding what we're going to talk about today? It's what we call "setting the agenda." We'll do this at the beginning of every session [providing a rationale] so we make sure we have time to cover what's most important to you. I have a list of things I'd like to go over today, and then [being collaborative] I'll ask you what you'd like to add. Is that okay?

PATIENT: Yes.

THERAPIST: Our first session will be a little different from future sessions, because we have a lot of ground to cover and we need to get to know each other better. Here's what I'd like to go over. First, in a couple of minutes [alerting Sally that I don't want to dive into a topic before setting a complete agenda], I'd like to check on how you've been feeling, find out what's happened since the evaluation, and talk a little about your diagnosis. (*pause*) Then I'd like to set some more specific goals. Does that sound okay?

PATIENT: Yes.

THERAPIST: Along the way, we might figure out some things for you to do before we meet again, [behavioral activation] especially making some changes in your schedule. And at the end, I'll ask you what you thought about the session. [eliciting feedback] How does that sound?

PATIENT: Fine.

THERAPIST: Is there anything you want to add to the agenda today?

PATIENT: Well, I know I should be doing more. But I'm so tired. It's just so hard to concentrate on my work and go out with friends. I end up spending a lot of time sleeping or watching TV and ...

THERAPIST: (*gently interrupting*) Is it okay if I interrupt you for a moment? How about if I put "doing more things" on our agenda, and we'll try to get to it today?

PATIENT: Okay.

THERAPIST: (*jotting down this agenda item*) You'll notice that I tend to write down a lot of things during our session. [providing a rationale] I want to make sure to remember what's important ... Okay, anything else even more important for the agenda today?

PATIENT: No, I don't think so.

THERAPIST: If you think of other important things as we go along, just let me know.

Ideally, setting the agenda is quick and to the point. Explaining the rationale for why you want to set an agenda makes the process of therapy more understandable to patients and elicits their active participation in a structured, productive way.

> **Q:** What if ... patients express a strong preference to spend therapy time in another way?
>
> **A:** Patients occasionally, *though infrequently*, balk at the agenda you present for this first session. This might happen for several reasons. You may have presented the agenda in too controlling a fashion, without being collaborative. There may be pressing issues on their mind for which they desperately want immediate help in the session. They might prefer to spend the session talking freely about whatever comes in their mind, without structure or interruption.
>
>   What do you do? Above all, you need to engage patients so they will return to treatment for the next session. If you judge that trying to persuade patients to adhere to your agenda will endanger their engagement, especially in this first session, you might offer to split the therapy time. If they demur, you can spend the session doing what they want. At the next session, you will find out whether doing so helped alleviate their suffering significantly during the week. If not, they may be more motivated to spend at least part of the session discussing what you think is important to help them feel better.

DOING A MOOD CHECK

Having set the agenda, you will next do a brief mood check. In addition to asking Sally for a brief narrative report of her mood since I saw her last, I quickly review the symptom checklists she filled out just prior to the session (see Appendix B for information about the Beck Depression Inventory, Anxiety Inventory, and Hopelessness Scale). Because I initially just want a brief overview of her mood, I cue her to provide me with an answer in just a few words.

THERAPIST: Okay, next. Can we start with how you've been doing this week? I'd like to see the forms you filled out. While I look them over, [providing a guideline] can you tell me in a sentence or two how you felt for most of the week?

PATIENT: I've been really depressed the whole time.

THERAPIST: (*looking over the forms*) It looks as if you've been feeling pretty anxious, too, is that right?

PATIENT: Yes.

THERAPIST: [being collaborative] If it's okay with you, I'd like you to come to every session a few minutes early so you can fill out these three forms. [providing a rationale] They help give me a quick idea of how you've been feeling in the past week, although I'll always want you to describe how you've been doing in your own words, too.

PATIENT: Okay.

In this first session, as in every session, I note the summed scores of the objective tests, comparing them to the scores from the evaluation. I also quickly scan individual items to determine whether the tests point out anything of particular importance. I especially note items related to hopelessness and suicidality on the Beck Depression Inventory–II. If these items are elevated, I will do a risk assessment (Wenzel et al., 2008) to determine whether we need to spend the next part of the session developing a plan to keep the patient safe.

Q: What if . . . patients cannot or will not fill out objective tests?

A: If you do not have access to symptom checklists, if they are inappropriate for patients (e.g., patients aren't sufficiently literate), or if they express reluctance about completing them, you can teach them, at this initial session or at the next session, to rate their mood on a 0–10 scale: "Can you think back over the past week? If 0 means not depressed at all, and 10 means the most depressed you've ever been, what has your depression been like for most of the week?" Or you can ask patients, "Can you tell me about your depression this week? Would you say it was mild, moderate, or severe? How did your mood compare to other weeks?" Other problems related to doing a mood check are discussed in Chapter 8.

OBTAINING AN UPDATE

In the next part of the session, you will question patients to discover whether there are any important problems or issues that they have not yet mentioned that might take priority in the session. Then you will probe for positive experiences the patient had during the week.

THERAPIST: Next, what happened between the evaluation and now that's important for me to know?

PATIENT: (*Thinks.*) Well, my parents have been putting pressure on me to figure out what I'm going to do this summer.

THERAPIST: [collecting data about the problem to establish whether it's of immediate importance and of high priority] Has this been really upsetting to you?

PATIENT: (*Sighs.*) Not that much. It's just one more thing.

THERAPIST: Is this something you want my help with?

PATIENT: Yes, I guess so.

THERAPIST: We don't have a lot of time today. Do you think we could postpone talking about it until another time?

PATIENT: That's okay.

THERAPIST: I'll put it at the bottom of my notes, and ask you next week how high a priority it is for you.

PATIENT: Okay.

THERAPIST: Was there anything else that was really important this week?

PATIENT: No, I guess not. It was pretty much the same as last week.

By asking these questions, I find out that there is not an important problem that needs to take priority over what is already on the agenda, so I can move ahead.

How do you decide which problems are pressing and which are not? You will establish how distressed the patient is by the problem and whether the patient really needs to solve it immediately (e.g., not solving it could put the patient or others in harm's way, or endanger the patient's livelihood or living situation). Discussion of most problems, especially chronic ones (such as difficulty functioning at home or arguments with family members), can usually be postponed to a future session so you can cover what you need to in this initial session.

Q: What if ... there had been a pressing agenda item?

A: There are several reasons for deviating from the usual structure in the first session.

1. If patients are at risk or they are putting others at risk.
2. If patients are so distressed by a problem that they cannot focus on the topics that you want to cover.
3. If you assess that patients will be so upset by not discuss-

ing the problem that the therapeutic relationship could be impaired, and/or that the patient is likely not to come back for another session.

When you ask patients for an update early in treatment, they invariably report only negative experiences. You then ask, "What positive things happened this week?" or "When were some times that you felt even a little bit better this week?" These questions help patients see reality more clearly, as the depression has undoubtedly led them to focus almost exclusively on the negative.

DISCUSSING THE DIAGNOSIS

In the next part of the session, you will briefly review patients' presenting problems and ask them to bring you up to date:

THERAPIST: Sally, I'd like to discuss what I found out in the evaluation session last week. Is it okay if we talk for a few moments about your diagnosis?

Most patients want to know their general diagnosis, and to establish that you don't think they are strange or abnormal. Usually it is preferable to avoid the label of a personality disorder diagnosis. Instead it is better to say something more general and jargon free, such as, "It looks as if you've been pretty depressed for the last year and you've had some long-standing problems with relationships and with work." It's also desirable to give patients some initial information about their condition so they can start attributing some of their problems to their disorder instead of to their character ("There's something wrong with me. I'm just no good.") The following transcript illustrates how to educate patients who are depressed.

THERAPIST: The evaluation shows that you have a moderate depression. I want you to know that it's a real illness. It's not the same as people saying, "Oh, I'm so depressed" when they're feeling down. You have a real depression.

PATIENT: (*Sighs.*)

THERAPIST: I know that because you have the symptoms in this diagnostic manual (*showing Sally the DSM*). For each mental health disorder, this manual lists the symptoms, just as a neurology diagnostic manual would list the symptoms of a migraine.

PATIENT: Oh, I didn't know that.

THERAPIST: [providing hope] Fortunately, cognitive behavior therapy is very effective in helping people overcome depression.

PATIENT: I was afraid you'd think I was crazy.

THERAPIST: Not at all. [normalizing] You have a fairly common condition, and it sounds as though you have a lot of the same problems as most of our patients here. But that's typical of how people with depression think. How do you feel now that you've found out I don't think you're crazy?

PATIENT: (*Sighs.*) Relieved.

THERAPIST: That's a lot of what we'll be doing in treatment. Identifying your depressed thinking and helping you see things more realistically.

PATIENT: Okay.

THERAPIST: [anticipating that Sally might blame herself for thinking in an unrealistic way] Now, it's not your fault that you have this kind of negative thinking. It's a primary symptom of depression. For everyone with depression, it's as if they're seeing themselves and their worlds and the future [the "cognitive triad" of depression] through eyeglasses covered with black paint. (*I pantomime painting an imaginary pair of glasses on my face.*) These dark glasses make *everything* look dark and hopeless. Part of what we'll do in therapy is to scrape off the black paint (*pantomiming*) so you can see things more realistically ... Is that clear? [Using an analogy often helps the patient to see her situation in a different way.]

PATIENT: Yeah. I understand.

THERAPIST: Okay, let's go over some of the other symptoms of depression that you have. I see from the evaluation that the depression is interfering with your sleep and your energy. It sounds as if it's also affecting your motivation to do things. [normalizing] Now, most depressed people start criticizing themselves for not being the same as they had been before. [eliciting specific incidents] Do you remember any recent times you've criticized yourself?

PATIENT: (*Sighs.*) Yeah. Lately I've been getting out of bed late and not getting my work done, and I think I'm lazy and no good.

THERAPIST: Now, if you had pneumonia, and had trouble getting out of bed and getting everything done, would you call yourself lazy and no good?

PATIENT: No, I guess not.

THERAPIST: Would it help this week if you answered back the thought, "I'm lazy and no good"?

PATIENT: Probably.

THERAPIST: What could you remind yourself? [Eliciting a response rather than just providing one fosters active participation and a degree of autonomy.]

PATIENT: I guess that I *am* depressed, and it's harder for me to do things.

THERAPIST: Good. It's going to be really important for you to remember that this week. Would you like me to write it down? Or would you like to?

PATIENT: You can.

THERAPIST: (*pulling out a piece of carbonless paper [see Figure 5.1]*) Okay, I'll date this paper at the top. Now what should we call this: your therapy homework? Your action plan?

PATIENT: Homework, I guess.

THERAPIST: Good. (*Writes "Homework" at the top.*) The first item is to read something about what we just discussed. I'll write down, "If I start thinking I'm lazy and no good, remind myself that I have a real illness, called depression, that makes it harder for me to do things." (*pausing and anticipating that this statement could lead to hopelessness*) Is it okay if I write down another reminder? "As the treatment starts to work, my depression will lift, and things will get easier."

Jan. 22

Homework:

Read this list twice a day; set an alarm to remember.

1. If I start thinking I'm lazy and no good, remind myself that I have a real illness, called depression, that makes it harder for me to do things. As the treatment starts to work, my depression will lift, and things will get easier.

2. Read goal list and add others, if I think of any.

3. When I notice my mood getting worse, ask myself, "What's going through my mind right now?" and jot down the thoughts. Remind myself that just because I think something, doesn't necessarily mean it's true.

4. Make plans with Allison and Joe. Remember, if they say no, it's likely that they'd like to hang out with me but they're too busy.

5. Read *Coping with Depression* booklet (optional).

FIGURE 5.1. Sally's first-session homework list.

Q: What if ... the patient negates the analogy?

A: Some patients say, "Yes, but pneumonia is a biological disease." A good reply to this includes the specific depressive symptoms the patient has been experiencing: "Depression is *biological*, too; it's a real disease with real symptoms. Now, just feeling sad or down is not an illness. But that's not just what you've been experiencing. You've been feeling sad and down and hopeless; you've been self-critical, hardly anything interests you any more, you've been withdrawing from activities; your sleep and energy have been affected. That's how I know you have a real illness, every bit as real as pneumonia."

Many patients benefit from another homework assignment: Reading a specific chapter in a cognitive behavior therapy book on depression for consumers (see *www.academyofct.org*), or a booklet such as *Coping with Depression* (see *www.beckinstitute.org*), will reinforce important ideas from this session. Ask patients to make mental or written notes about what they agree with, disagree with, or have questions about.

PROBLEM IDENTIFICATION AND GOAL SETTING

Next you will focus on identifying specific problems. As a logical extension, you will help patients turn these problems into goals to work on in treatment.

THERAPIST: Now, let's review the problems you've been having.

PATIENT: (*Sighs.*) Oh, I don't know. Everything is such a mess. I'm doing terribly at school. I'm way behind. I feel so tired and down all the time. I feel sometimes like I should just give up.

THERAPIST: (*questioning to make sure Sally is not actively suicidal*) Have you had any thoughts of harming yourself?

PATIENT: No, not really. I just wish all my problems would somehow go away.

THERAPIST: (*empathically*) It sounds like you're feeling overwhelmed?

PATIENT: Yes, I don't know what to do.

THERAPIST: [helping Sally to focus and to break down her problems into a more manageable size] Okay, it sounds like you have two major problems right now. One is that you're not doing well at school. The other is that you feel really tired and down. Are there any others?

PATIENT: Well, like I told you last week, I know I'm alone in my room too much. I should be spending more time with my friends.

THERAPIST: [getting Sally to participate more actively in the goal-setting process] Okay, let's turn these problems into goals. Would you like to write them down, or should I?

PATIENT: You can.

THERAPIST: Okay. (*writing as they go along*) Now, the first thing you mentioned was improving your schoolwork. Then you mentioned decreasing your worry about tests and grades and spending more time with friends. Good. Now what other goals do you have? How would you like to be different? Or how would you like your life to be different as a result of treatment?

PATIENT: (*pausing*) I'd like to be happier.

THERAPIST: [reinforcing the patient] That's a good goal.

This goal, however, is too broad. It's difficult to figure out how to help the patient become happier, so I ask Sally to specify in behavioral terms what being "happier" means to her.

THERAPIST: And if you were happier and not feeling depressed, what would you be doing?

PATIENT: I guess I would get involved in some activities at school, like I did last year ... I'd have some fun and not feel so depressed all the time.

THERAPIST: Good, I'll add these to the list: join school activities and do more fun activities.

Goal List—February 1

1. Improve schoolwork.
2. Decrease worrying about tests and grades.
3. Spend more time with friends.
4. Join school activities.
5. Do more fun activities.

THERAPIST: Now, for homework, could you read through this list and see whether you have any other goals to add?

PATIENT: Yes.

THERAPIST: (*Adds this assignment to the Homework List.*) Okay, now before we go on, can I quickly summarize what we've done so far? We've set the agenda, talked about your diagnosis, and started a goal list.

In this part of the session, I made sure that the goal list was recorded in writing. I also guided Sally in specifying a general goal ("I'd like to be happier") in behavioral terms. Rather than allowing a discussion of goals to dominate the session, I ask Sally to refine the list for homework. Finally, I summarized what we had discussed to that point. Doing so helps make the process of therapy more understandable and keeps us on track.

Q: What if ... a patient sets goals for someone else?

A: Occasionally patients state a goal over which they do not have direct control: "I'd like my partner to be nicer to me"; "I want my boss to stop putting so much pressure on me"; "I want my kids to listen to me." In this case, it is important to help them phrase the goal so that it is something they *do* have control over:

THERAPIST: I don't want to promise you that we can *directly* get Joe to be nicer to you. What do you think of phrasing it this way: "Learn new ways of talking to Joe." Maybe if you take control and change what *you're* doing, it will have some impact on Joe.

For a fuller discussion of what to do when patients set goals for others, see J. S. Beck (2005).

EDUCATING THE PATIENT
ABOUT THE COGNITIVE MODEL

An important feature of the initial session is helping patients understand how their thinking affects their reactions, preferably using their own examples. You can take advantage of patients' spontaneous utterances in session (e.g., "I can't do anything right. Nothing can help. I'll never feel better"). Or you can ask them, "What's going through your mind right now?" when you notice a shift in affect. It is probably easier, though, for the novice therapist to devote a portion of the first session providing psychoeducation about the relationship among triggering situations, automatic thoughts or images, and reactions (emotional, behavioral, and physiological).

THERAPIST: Can we talk for a few minutes about how your thinking affects your mood? Can you think of any time in the past few days when you noticed your mood change? When you were aware that you had become particularly upset?

PATIENT: I think so.

THERAPIST: Can you tell me a little about it?

PATIENT: I was having lunch with a couple of people from my English class, and I started to feel really bad. They were talking about something the professor had said in class that I didn't really understand.

THERAPIST: Do you remember what you were thinking?

PATIENT: Ummm, that they're much smarter than I am. That I'll probably flunk the course.

THERAPIST: (*using Sally's precise words*) So you had the thoughts "They're much smarter than I am. I'll probably flunk the course," and how did those thoughts make you feel emotionally? Happy, sad, worried, angry...?

PATIENT: Oh, sad, really sad.

THERAPIST: Okay, how about if we make a diagram? You just gave a good example of how, in a specific situation, your thoughts influence your emotion. (*Composes the diagram below and reviews it with Sally.*) Is it clear to you? That how you viewed this situation led to automatic thoughts that then then influenced how you felt?

PATIENT: I think so.

Situation: *At lunch with classmates*

↓

Automatic thoughts: *"They're much smarter than I am. I'll probably flunk the course."*

↓

Reaction (emotional): *Sad*

THERAPIST: Let's see if we can gather a couple more examples from the past few days. Is there another time when you were feeling particularly upset?

PATIENT: Well, just a few minutes ago, when I was waiting in the waiting room. I was feeling really down.

THERAPIST: And what was going through your mind at the time?

PATIENT: I don't remember exactly.

THERAPIST: [trying to make the experience more vivid in Sally's mind] Can you imagine yourself back in the waiting room right now? Can you imagine sitting there? Describe the scene for me as if it's happening right now.

PATIENT: Well, I'm sitting in the chair near the door, away from the receptionist. A woman comes in, she's smiling and talking to the receptionist. She looks kind of happy and ... normal.

THERAPIST: And how are you feeling as you look at her?

PATIENT: Kind of sad.

THERAPIST: What's going through your mind?

PATIENT: She's not like me. She's happy. I'll never be like that again.

THERAPIST: [reinforcing the cognitive model] Okay. That's another good example. The situation was that you saw a happy-looking woman in the reception area and you thought, "I'll never be like that again"—and that thought made you feel sad. Is this clear to you?

PATIENT: Yeah. I think so.

THERAPIST: [making sure Sally can verbalize her understanding of the cognitive model] Can you tell me in your own words about the connection between thoughts and feelings?

PATIENT: Well, it seems that my thoughts affect how I feel.

THERAPIST: Yes, that's right. [facilitating Sally's carrying through the work of the therapy session throughout the week] What I'd like you to do, if you agree, is to keep track this coming week of what's going through your mind when you notice your mood changing or getting worse. Okay?

PATIENT: Uh-huh.

THERAPIST: In fact, how about if I write it down on the Homework List: *When I notice my mood getting worse, ask, "What's going through my mind?" and jot down the thoughts.* When you come in next week, we can evaluate your thoughts to see whether they're 100% true, or 0% true, or someplace in the middle. Okay?

PATIENT: Yes.

THERAPIST: Lots of times, because you're depressed, I think you'll find that these thoughts *aren't* completely accurate. I'll write something down about that, too: *Just because I think something doesn't necessarily mean it's true.* When we find out your thoughts aren't true, or not completely true, I'll teach you how to look at the situation in a more realistic way. When you do that, I think you'll find that you feel better. For example, we might find that your classmates aren't much smarter than you, and that the reason you're struggling has nothing to do with your intelligence, but has everything to do with the fact that you're depressed. And we might then do some problem solving to help you with the course. For example, you might ask for help from a friend or a teaching assistant or a tutor.

PATIENT: That sounds hard.

THERAPIST: That's another good example of an automatic thought: "That sounds hard." Well, that's what I'm here for. We'll be working as a team, together, to help you solve your problems, and we'll go step by step. (*pause*) Can you see how changing your thinking and doing some problem solving might help improve your mood?

PATIENT: Yes.

THERAPIST: (*Using an encouraging tone of voice.*) And I think you'll find that you'll get good at it pretty soon. Meanwhile, can you try to write down other depressed thoughts like that so we can look at them next session?

PATIENT: Okay.

THERAPIST: [checking to see whether Sally anticipates difficulties that might require advance problem solving] Do you think you'll have any trouble doing that?

PATIENT: No. I think I'll be able to.

THERAPIST: Good. But even if you can't, that's okay. You'll come back next week and we'll work on it together.

PATIENT: Okay.

In this section, I explain, illustrate, and record the cognitive model *with the patient's own examples.* I try to limit my explanations to just a couple of sentences at a time; depressed patients, in particular, have difficulty concentrating. I also ask Sally to put what I've said in her own words so I can check on her understanding. Had Sally's cognitive abilities been impaired or limited, I might have used more concrete learning aids such as faces with various expressions to illustrate emotions, and cartoon characters with empty "thought bubbles" above their heads.

Q: What if ... patients have difficulty grasping the cognitive model in the first session?

A: You will decide whether to try other techniques (see Chapter 9), or whether to return to this task in the next session. Common sense dictates that you not push too hard, which could lead patients to have negative thoughts about their competence or about you. If you decide against further explication of the cognitive model at this point, take care to downplay the importance of the skill to reduce the probability that patients will blame themselves. ("Sometimes it's hard to figure out these thoughts. Usually they're so quick. It's no big deal, though. We'll come back to it another time.")

DISCUSSION OF PROBLEM
OR BEHAVIORAL ACTIVATION

If there is time in this first session, you will start discussing a specific problem of significant concern to the patient. Developing alternate ways of viewing the problem, or concrete steps patients can take to solve the problem, tends to increase their hopefulness that treatment will be effective. Unless patients express a problem of overriding importance, try to elicit their agreement to discuss the problem of inactivity—that is, if they have withdrawn from activities or are generally at least somewhat inactive. Overcoming depressive passivity and creating opportunities to experience pleasure and a sense of mastery is essential for most depressed patients. Behavioral activation is discussed in the next chapter.

END-OF-SESSION SUMMARY AND SETTING
OF HOMEWORK

The final summary ties together the threads of the session and reinforces important points. The summary also includes a review of what the patient has agreed to do for homework.

THERAPIST: Sally, our time is almost up. Can you tell me what you think is most important for you to remember this week? You can look at your notes [page 67].

PATIENT: Well, I guess that I'm not lazy. And I might have a lot of depressed thoughts that will make me feel bad, even if they're not true.

THERAPIST: Right. And how about the idea that getting more active might help improve your mood?

PATIENT: Yes.

THERAPIST: Can we go over the homework now? I want to make sure it's doable. (*pointing to the paper*) The first thing we wrote down is to remind yourself that you're depressed, so you won't start thinking that you're no good. Now, how will you remember to do that? Do you think you could read this sheet of paper when you get up every morning?

PATIENT: Yeah.

THERAPIST: How long do you think it will take you?

PATIENT: I don't know. Maybe 5 minutes?

THERAPIST: Actually, I think it will take less than a minute.

PATIENT: Yeah, that's probably right.

THERAPIST: How will you remember to do it?

PATIENT: (*Thinks.*) I'm not sure. I don't want to keep it out because my roommate could see it.

THERAPIST: [making specific suggestions] Could you keep the paper somewhere else, like in your backpack? Maybe you could set an alarm on your cell phone, so when it beeps, you'll remember to get it out and read it?

PATIENT: Yeah, that would work.

THERAPIST: It would also be good to read it at least once more every day. When do you think it would help most?

PATIENT: (*Thinks.*) Probably right after dinner.

THERAPIST: That sounds good. Do you want to set an alarm for then, also?

PATIENT: Okay.

THERAPIST: I'll write that plan at the top of the sheet.

Next, we add to the homework assignment sheet, noting aloud how long each task will probably take to accomplish. Many patients overestimate the difficulty and duration of tasks. Specifying time requirements help ease the perceived burden.

THERAPIST: Sally, we also talked earlier in the session about adding to your goal list this week. Do you think you could spend a minute or two on it this week?

PATIENT: Sure.

THERAPIST: And finally, I have a booklet here about depression [*Coping with Depression*; see Appendix B]. Should we make it optional?

PATIENT: (*Nods.*)

THERAPIST: I think it will take about 5 or 10 minutes to read. If you do read it, you can make mental notes or written notes on what you agree with and what you don't.

PATIENT: Okay.

In this part of the session, I want to maximize the chance that Sally will do the homework and feel successful. If you sense that the patient may not carry out any part of the assignment, you may offer to change it ("Do you think you'll have trouble jotting down your thoughts?" [If yes] "Do you think we should make it optional?"). Depressed patients can easily become overwhelmed and then self-critical if they do not complete their homework assignments. (See Chapter 17 for an extended discussion of homework.)

We also discussed when it would be helpful for Sally to read this sheet of paper. It is important to note that Sally, accustomed to doing homework for school, is less likely to be overwhelmed and more likely to follow through with these activities than another depressed patient might be. Some patients may decide to transfer this written list to their smartphone or other electronic device.

FEEDBACK

The final element of every therapy session, at least initially, is feedback. By the end of the first session, most patients feel positively about the therapist and the therapy. Eliciting feedback further strengthens rapport, providing the message that you care about what the patient thinks. It also gives patients a chance to express, and you to resolve, any misunderstandings. Patients may occasionally make an idiosyncratic interpretation of something you said or did. Asking them whether there was anything that bothered them gives them the opportunity to state and then to test their conclusions. In addition to verbal feedback, you may decide to have patients complete a written Therapy Report (see Figure 5.2).

THERAPIST: Now at the end of each session, I'm going to ask how you thought the session went. You actually get *two* chances—telling me directly or writing it on a Therapy Report, which you can fill out in the waiting room after our session. I'll read it over, and if there are any problems, we can put them on the agenda at our next session. Okay?

PATIENT: Okay.

THERAPIST: Now, what did you think of today's session? Was there anything about this session that bothered you or anything you thought I got wrong?

PATIENT: No, it was good.

THERAPIST: Anything you'd like us to do differently next session?

PATIENT: No, I don't think so.

THERAPIST: Okay then. It was a pleasure working with you today. Would you please fill out the Therapy Report in the waiting room now and the other forms I gave you just before our session next week? And you'll try to do the homework you wrote down on your homework sheet. Okay?

PATIENT: (*Nods.*) Okay. Thanks.

THERAPIST: See you next week.

1. What did we cover today that's important to you to remember?

2. How much did you feel you could trust your therapist today?

3. Was there anything that bothered you about therapy today? If so, what was it?

4. How much homework had you done for therapy today? How likely are you to do the new homework?

5. What do you want to make sure to cover at the next session?

FIGURE 5.2. Therapy Report. From J. S. Beck (2011). Copyight 2011 by Judith S. Beck. Reprinted by permission.

Reprinted by permission in *Cognitive Behavior Therapy: Basics and Beyond, Second Edition*, by Judith S. Beck (Guilford Press, 2011). Permission to photocopy this material is granted to purchasers of this book for personal use only (see copyright page for details). Purchasers may download a larger version of this material from *www.guilford.com/p/beck4*.

Q: What if ... patients have a negative reaction to the session?

A: You will try to specify the problem and establish its meaning to the patient, then intervene or mark the problem for intervention at the next session, as in the following example:

THERAPIST: Now, was there anything about this session that bothered you?

PATIENT: I don't know ... I'm not sure this therapy is for me.

THERAPIST: You don't think it'll help?

PATIENT: No, not really. You see, I've got real-life problems. It's *not* just my thinking.

THERAPIST: I'm glad you told me. This gives me the opportunity to say that I *do* believe that you have real-life problems. I didn't mean to imply that you don't. The problems with your boss and your neighbors and your feelings of loneliness ... Of course, those are all real problems; problems we'll work together to solve. I *don't* think that all we need to do is look at your thoughts. I'm sorry if I gave you that impression.

PATIENT: That's okay ... It's just, like ... well, I feel so overwhelmed. I don't know what to do.

THERAPIST: Are you willing to come back next week so we can work on the overwhelmed feelings together?

PATIENT: Yeah, I guess so.

THERAPIST: Is the homework contributing to the overwhelmed feeling, too?

PATIENT: (*pause*) Maybe.

THERAPIST: How would you like to leave it? We could make the homework optional, or some of it optional, if you want.

PATIENT: (*sigh of relief*) Yeah, that would be better.

THERAPIST: What seems hardest to do?

PATIENT: Trying to keep track of my thoughts.

THERAPIST: Okay, let's write "optional" next to that one. Or should I just cross it off?

PATIENT: No, you can write "optional."

THERAPIST: (*Does so.*) What else feels too hard?

PATIENT: Maybe calling my friends. I don't know if I'm up for that.

THERAPIST: Okay, should I write "optional" or cross it off?

PATIENT: Maybe cross it off.

THERAPIST: Okay. (*Does so.*) Now, was there anything else that bothered you about today's session?

Here the therapist recognizes the necessity for strengthening the therapeutic alliance. The therapist had either missed signs of the patient's dissatisfaction during the session or the patient was adept at concealing it. Had the therapist failed to ask for feedback about the session or been less adept at dealing with the negative feedback, it is possible that the patient would not have returned for another session. The therapist's flexibility about the homework assignment helps the patient reexamine his misgivings about the appropriateness of cognitive behavior therapy. By responding to feedback and making reasonable adjustments, the therapist demonstrates understanding of and empathy toward the patient, which facilitates collaboration and trust.

The therapist will make sure to express at the beginning of the next session how important it is that they work as a team to tailor the treatment and the homework so the patient finds them helpful. The therapist also uses this difficulty as an opportunity to refine the conceptualization of the patient. In the future, the therapist ensures that homework is set more collaboratively with the patient and that he does not feel overwhelmed.

The initial therapy session has several important goals: establishing rapport; refining the conceptualization; socializing patients to the process and structure of cognitive behavior therapy; educating patients about the cognitive model and about their disorder(s); and providing hope and some symptom relief. Developing a solid therapeutic alliance and encouraging patients to join with you to accomplish therapeutic goals are of primary importance in this session. Chapter 7 describes the structure of subsequent therapy sessions and Chapter 8 deals with difficulties in structuring sessions.

Chapter 6

BEHAVIORAL ACTIVATION

One of the most important initial goals for depressed patients is scheduling activities. Most have withdrawn from at least some activities that had previously given them a sense of achievement or pleasure and lifted their mood. And they frequently have increased certain behaviors (staying in bed, watching television, sitting around) that maintain or increase their current dysphoria. They often believe that they cannot change how they feel emotionally. Helping them to become more active and to give themselves credit for their efforts are essential parts of treatment, not only to improve their mood, but also to strengthen their sense of self-efficacy by demonstrating to themselves that they can take more control of their mood than they had previously believed.

CONCEPTUALIZATION OF INACTIVITY

When considering engaging in activities, patients' depressed automatic thoughts frequently get in their way.

Situation: *Thinking about initiating an activity*
↓
[Common] Automatic thoughts: *"I'm too tired. I won't enjoy it. My friends won't want to spend time with me. I won't be able to do it. Nothing can help me feel better."*

↓
[Common] Emotional reactions: *Sadness, anxiety, hopelessness*
↓
[Common] Behavior: *Remain inactive.*

Patients' relative inactivity then contributes to their low mood, as they have a paucity of opportunities to gain a sense of mastery or pleasure, which leads to more negative thinking, which leads to increased dysphoria and inactivity, in a vicious cycle.

CONCEPTUALIZATION OF LACK OF MASTERY OR PLEASURE

Even when patients do engage in various activities, they often derive low levels of satisfaction and pleasure because of their self-critical automatic thoughts.

Situation: *Engaging in an activity*
↓
[Common] Automatic thoughts: *"I'm doing a terrible job. I should have done this long ago. There's still so much left to do. I can't do this as well as I used to. This used to be more fun. I don't deserve to be doing this."*
↓
[Common] Emotional reactions: *Sadness, guilt, anger at self*
↓
[Common] Behaviors: *Stop the activity. Push self beyond a reasonable point. Fail to repeat this activity in the future.*

Self-critical thoughts may arise as patients engage in activities or afterward, as they reflect on the results. When scheduling activities, it is important to anticipate automatic thoughts that could interfere with patients' initiation of activities, as well as thoughts that could diminish patients' sense of pleasure or achievement during or after an activity.

When you are treating relatively "easy" patients like Sally, you will facilitate the identification of activities that could potentially help them feel better, address interfering thoughts, and assist them in putting pleasurable or productive activities in their schedule. You may need to help more severely depressed patients develop an hourly schedule of activities for the week to counteract their extensive passivity and inactivity. It may also be useful for some patients to rate their sense of pleasure and achievement following their activities, to examine whether becoming more active and responding to their dysfunctional thinking does improve their mood.

Perhaps the easiest and quickest way to get patients behaviorally activated is to review their typical daily schedule (pages 50–52). The following questions can guide your discussion.

- Which activities are patients doing too little of, thus depriving themselves of obtaining a sense of achievement (mastery), a sense of pleasure, or both? These might be activities related to work or school, family, friends, their neighborhood, volunteering, sports, hobbies, physical exercise, their household, nature, spirituality, or sensual, intellectual, or cultural pursuits.

- Do patients have a good balance of mastery and pleasure experiences? For example, are patients driving themselves too hard, and so have a dearth of pleasure? Are they avoiding activities they predict will be challenging, and so have little opportunity to obtain a sense of mastery?

- Which activities are lowest in mastery and/or pleasure? Are these activities inherently dysphoric, such as ruminating in bed, and so should their frequency be reduced? Or are patients feeling dysphoric during potentially rewarding activities because of their depressed thinking?

In the following transcripts, I review Sally's schedule with her, reinforce her conclusions about how she might better plan her time, encourage her to commit to specific changes, elicit the thoughts that might impede instituting the changes, label her thoughts as predictions that can be tested, give her the choice of a follow-up homework assignment, and teach her to give herself credit.

THERAPIST: Thinking about your schedule, what do you notice? How are your activities different from say, a year ago, when you weren't depressed?

PATIENT: Well, I'm spending a lot of time in bed.

THERAPIST: Does staying in bed make you feel much better? Do you get out of bed feeling refreshed and energetic?

PATIENT: (*Thinks.*) No ... I guess not. I usually feel groggy and down when I get up.

THERAPIST: Well, that's valuable information. [providing psychoedu-cation] It seems most people who are depressed think they'll feel better if they stay in bed. But they usually find that doing almost *anything* else is better ... What else is different?

PATIENT: Last semester, I used to go out more with friends or just hang around with them. Now I just go from my dorm room, to class, to the library, to the cafeteria, and back to my room.

THERAPIST: Does that give you an idea of what you might like to change this coming week?

PATIENT: Yes, well, I'd like to spend more time with other people, but I just don't seem to have any energy.

THERAPIST: So you end up staying in bed?

PATIENT: Yes.

THERAPIST: Well, that's an interesting idea you have: "I don't have the energy to spend time with people." Let's write that down. [inquir-ing about setting up a behavioral experiment] Now, how could we test this idea to see if it's true?

PATIENT: I guess I could plan to spend some time with my friends and see if I could do it.

THERAPIST: [trying to motivate Sally to do so] Would there be an advantage to doing that?

PATIENT: I guess I might feel better.

I infer from Sally's tone of voice that she might be reluctant to do the experiment. I conceptualize that automatic thoughts might be interfering.

Situation: *Discussing spending time with friends*
↓
Automatic thought: *??*
↓
Emotional reaction: *Unspecified negative emotion*

To discover Sally's automatic thought, I ask her directly:

THERAPIST: What's going through your mind right now?

PATIENT: I don't know.

THERAPIST: [providing Sally with the *opposite* of what I actually believed she was thinking] Were you thinking what a good time you'd have with your friends?

PATIENT: No, I guess I'm worried that my friends won't want to hang out with me.

THERAPIST: Okay. [reinforcing the cognitive model] Can you see how that thought might stop you from approaching them?

I mentally hypothesize the following scenario:

Situation: *Thinking of hanging out with friends*
↓
Automatic thought: *"They won't want to hang out with me."*
↓
Emotional reaction: *Sadness?*
↓
Likely behavioral reaction (if she doesn't respond to the automatic thought): *Stay in her room.*

Next, I determine whether Sally can devise her own response. When she cannot, I help her evaluate the validity of her thought and devise a behavioral experiment.

THERAPIST: How can you answer that thought?

PATIENT: ... I don't know.

THERAPIST: Do you have any evidence that they won't want to hang out with you?

PATIENT: No, not really, not unless they're busy ... Except I'm not much fun these days.

THERAPIST: Have they said something?

PATIENT: No ...

THERAPIST: Do you have any evidence on the other side—that maybe they would want to spend time with you?

PATIENT: (*Thinks.*) Well, Emily asked me to go to lunch with her today, but I couldn't.

THERAPIST: Okay, that sounds pretty good. So how could you find out for sure whether Emily or others would want to hang out?

PATIENT: I guess I could ask them if they want to have dinner or something.

Next I ask a series of questions to set up the behavioral experiment in a way that maximizes the chance of a positive outcome.

THERAPIST: Who would be easiest for you to ask? Emily?

PATIENT: No, Allison and Joe, I guess.

THERAPIST: Good. Then you can test two of your predictions. One, that your friends won't want to hang out, and two, that you're too tired to spend time with them. Does that sound right?

PATIENT: Yes.

THERAPIST: [trying to increase the likelihood that Sally will follow through] How likely are you to approach Allison and Joe or someone else?

PATIENT: (*in an affirmative tone of voice*) I'll do it.

THERAPIST: [recognizing that Sally is more likely to do it if she does it immediately] Do you think you could do it today?

PATIENT: I guess I could. I could text them after the session.

THERAPIST: [giving positive reinforcement] That's great. Then if it turns out okay, could you keep trying to get together for friends for the rest of the week? What do you think?

PATIENT: Yeah, okay.

THERAPIST: [hypothesizing that Sally might turn her friends off if she is too down] Do you want to talk about what to say to your friends about your depression? Or how to balance talking about it with some more upbeat things?

PATIENT: No, I don't need to. They already know I've been down. They're pretty supportive.

THERAPIST: Good ... [predicting that Sally could feel worse if she's turned down] Now, if it turns out that friends say no, do you think it will be important to remember that it might be because they're busy, not because they don't want to spend time with you?

PATIENT: Yeah.

THERAPIST: Should I write that down?

PATIENT: (*Nods.*)

THERAPIST: (*writing*) "If they say no, it's likely that they'd like to hang out with me but they're too busy." (*pause*) Good. Now, can we go back to your schedule? Anything you think you need to change?

PATIENT: I guess I'm watching too much TV.

THERAPIST: Anything you'd like to try to replace it with this week?

PATIENT: I really don't know.

THERAPIST: I notice you don't seem to be spending much time doing physical activities—is that right?

PATIENT: Yeah. I used to run most mornings or swim.

THERAPIST: What's gotten in the way of your doing these things lately?

PATIENT: Same thing as before, I guess. I've felt really tired. And I didn't think I'd enjoy it.

Situation: *Thinking about getting exercise*
↓
Automatic thoughts: *"I'm too tired. I won't enjoy it."*
↓
Emotional reaction: *Dysphoria*
↓
Behavioral reaction: *Stays in bed.*

THERAPIST: Would you like to plan more exercise, say, going for a short run or swim a few times this week?

PATIENT: Okay.

THERAPIST: How likely is it that you'll make plans to see friends and swim or run—maybe at least three times?

PATIENT: Oh, I will.

THERAPIST: Should we write these things on an activity chart [see Figure 6.1] so you'll be more likely to commit to them?

PATIENT: No, I don't need to. I'll do them.

THERAPIST: One more thing. Do you think you could give yourself credit every time you do one of these things? You could just say, "Good. I did it."

PATIENT: (*Looking quizzical.*) You mean you want me to give myself credit for making plans with my friends?

THERAPIST: Absolutely. [providing psychoeducation] When people are depressed, it's often difficult for them to do things that they used to do easily. Doing things like calling a friend or going for just a short run are really important in starting to get yourself over the depression. And they do take more energy than lying in bed. So of course you deserve credit.

PATIENT: But those things used to be easy.

THERAPIST: When you're over the depression, you don't have to give yourself credit. But if they're even a little bit difficult to do now, you *do* deserve credit. And reminding yourself of that will help you recognize that you're doing something productive to get better.

	MON.	TUE.	WED.	THU.	FRI.	SAT.	SUN.
6–7							
7–8							
8–9							
9–10							
10–11							
11–12							
12–1							
1–2							
2–3							

Morning / Afternoon

(cont.)

FIGURE 6.1. Activity Chart. From J. S. Beck (2011). Copyright 2011 by Judith S. Beck. Adapted by permission.

Reprinted by permission in *Cognitive Behavior Therapy: Basics and Beyond, Second Edition*, by Judith S. Beck (Guilford Press, 2011). Permission to photocopy this material is granted to purchasers of this book for personal use only (see copyright page for details). Purchasers may download a larger version of this material from *www.guilford.com/p/beck4*.

	MON.	TUE.	WED.	THU.	FRI.	SAT.	SUN.
3–4							
4–5							
5–6							
6–7							
7–8							
8–9							
9–10							
10–11							
11–12							
12–1							

Afternoon / Evening

FIGURE 6.1. *(cont.)*

PATIENT: Okay.

THERAPIST: In fact, I'd like you to give yourself credit whenever you do something active—that is, whenever you're not napping or watching TV or surfing the Web. [See pages 274–276 for a further description of giving oneself credit.]

In this segment, I lead Sally to draw conclusions from a review of her typical day. Some patients need more guidance than others to do this (e.g., "Do you notice how much time you spend in bed? What is your mood like when you get up—do you feel much better? What changes do you think you might like to try this week?"). I guide Sally to commit to implementing specific changes and identify automatic thoughts that might interfere, proposing behavioral experiments to test the validity of her negative predictions. I also ask her to give herself credit whenever she is active.

Q: What if ... patients believe they are incapable of becoming more active, or that becoming more active will not improve their mood?

A: You will provide education, set up behavioral experiments to help patients test their thoughts, and use an activity chart, as below.

THERAPIST: [summarizing a review of the patient's typical day] Okay, so it seems as if your activities changed a lot when you got depressed.

PATIENT: Yes, I just don't have much energy. I just lie around the house most of the time.

THERAPIST: And what's your mood been like?

PATIENT: Pretty bad. I'm depressed all the time.

THERAPIST: And what do you think will happen if you keep lying around the house?

PATIENT: I don't know. Nothing, I guess.

THERAPIST: So you'll keep being depressed?

PATIENT: I guess so.

THERAPIST: What would you think about trying to make a better schedule for yourself, planning some things to do that could give you a sense of pleasure or achievement, like calling friends or going for walks?

PATIENT: I don't think it would help. And I'm so tired all the time. I think I should wait until I'm feeling better.

THERAPIST: You know, that's exactly what most people with depression say. But research shows us that it's actually the opposite. The way people get over their depression is to get more active first—then they start to feel better.

PATIENT: Oh.

THERAPIST: Would you be willing to do an experiment this week— to see whether you're too tired, and to see what happens to your mood if you do try to do more things?

PATIENT: I guess so.

THERAPIST: Let's see. [providing a contrast among energy required for various activities] What are some things you know for sure would be too hard? Running? Doing errands for an entire day? Cleaning up your whole apartment?

PATIENT: Yeah, I couldn't do those things.

THERAPIST: So what's something on the other side, something that takes just a little energy?

PATIENT: (Sighs.) I could go to the library. Return my overdue book and maybe get some DVDs.

THERAPIST: [providing positive reinforcement] Good idea! What else could you do?

PATIENT: I'm not sure.

THERAPIST: Do you think you could do a few tasks a day—if they were only for 10 minutes each?

PATIENT: I guess I could.

THERAPIST: Good.

The therapist helps the patient specify these tasks and continues to elicit additional activities, then requests that the patient use an activity chart.

THERAPIST: These are all good activities. (*pulling out the Activity Chart in Figure 6.2*) I'd like to figure out with you when you might do these things. Is it okay if we write them down on this chart?

PATIENT: Okay.

THERAPIST: (*looking at the description of the patient's typical day*) So, it looks as if you usually get up around 11:00 or 11:30. What would you think about getting up by 10:00 and 10:30 in the morning?

	MON.	TUE.	WED.	THU.	FRI.	SAT.	SUN.
6–7	Sleep						
7–8	Sleep						
8–9	Sleep						
9–10	Sleep						
10–11	Get up/shower/ dress						
11–12	Breakfast Kitchen cleanup—10 min						
12–1	TV Newspaper						
1–2	Errand or window-shopping						
2–3	Rest						

Morning / Afternoon

FIGURE 6.2. Initial (partial) Activity Chart for a more severely depressed patient. From J. S. Beck (2011). Copyright 2011 by Judith S. Beck. Adapted by permission.

(cont.)

		MON.	TUE.	WED.	THU.	FRI.	SAT.	SUN.
Afternoon	3–4	TV Lunch Kitchen cleanup—10 min						
	4–5	Call sister Laundry—10 min						
	5–6	TV Walk						
	6–7	Rest Laundry—10 min						
	7–8	Dinner Kitchen cleanup—10 min						
Evening	8–9	Call Jonathan E-mail						
	9–10	YouTube Surf Web						
	10–11	Read						
	11–12	Get in bed Sleep						
	12–1	Sleep						

FIGURE 6.2. *(cont.)*

PATIENT: I could do that.

THERAPIST: What would be good to do next?

PATIENT: Take a shower, I guess. Get dressed. Have breakfast.

THERAPIST: So that's a change from what you usually do?

PATIENT: Yeah, sometimes I don't get dressed all day.

THERAPIST: How about if you write down, in the 10 o'clock space, "Get up, shower, get dressed." And then write "Have breakfast" in the 11 o'clock space." [See Figure 6.2.]

PATIENT: Okay. (*Does so.*)

THERAPIST: Now, what do want to do after breakfast? Wash your breakfast dishes?

PATIENT: I should. I've been letting dishes pile up in the sink. The kitchen is kind of a mess.

THERAPIST: So, how about doing dishes or cleaning up the kitchen for 10 minutes? You don't have to finish everything at once.

PATIENT: (*sigh of relief*) Okay.

THERAPIST: And then after the dishes? Do you want to take a break, watch TV or read the newspaper or surf the Web like you usually do?

PATIENT: Yeah, that would be good.

THERAPIST: Okay, so in the 11 o'clock space, let's put "clean kitchen for 10 minutes," and in the 12 o'clock space put "TV or newspaper or surf the Web."

The therapist and patient continue in this vein until they have made a schedule for the next day. Because the patient has been so inactive, the therapist takes care not to overwhelm him by creating too busy a schedule. She builds in short periods of activity with longer periods of leisure activity or rest. She also asks the patient to give himself credit every time he follows the schedule. Next she asks the patient if he is willing to try to follow the same basic schedule every day. They make lists of potential tasks the patient could do at home, people he could call, and places he could go.

At the following session, the therapist reviews this homework assignment of following the schedule. She asks the patient about his previous predictions: that he would be too tired to do activities and that they would not help. Discovering that his automatic thoughts were inaccurate can motivate the patient to get up earlier and engage in a greater number of productive or pleasurable activities.

Q: What if ... patients can't come up with any pleasurable activities?

A: There are many lists from which patients can choose activities. See, for example, Frisch (2005) or a list described in MacPhillamy and Lewinsohn (1982), which can be accessed at: *www.healthnet-solutions.com/dsp/PleasantEventsSchedule.pdf.* It is useful to give a forced choice when reviewing a list with a patient: "Which five or 10 activities from the list do you think could be most enjoyable?" If patients are reluctant, it is useful to help them recognize that staying in bed maintains or increases their dysphoria. Then ask them whether they think engaging in a given activity from the list is likely to make their mood worse than staying in bed. If they reply no, ask them whether they are willing to schedule the activity. If they say yes, ask them whether they are willing to do a behavioral experiment to see if they are right.

Q: What if ... patients are already fully scheduled or overscheduled?

A: If patients already have a good balance of activities, they may not need to change their schedule. If the balance is not good, they may need to build in some rest time and/or increase the number of pleasurable and/or mastery activities. If they are *over*scheduled, they may need to decrease their activity level. (They also need to give themselves credit for making any of these changes.) In any case, if they do not gain a sense of pleasure and mastery from their activities, they may need your help in responding to the dysfunctional cognitions they are experiencing. They may also need to respond to automatic thoughts that interfere with changing their activities.

Q: What if ... patients report that changing their activities has no impact on their mood?

A: Except in the most severe cases of depression, it is unlikely that patients experience no fluctuations in how they feel. But the fluctuations may be small, and patients may not remember them. For these patients, it is helpful to teach them to rate their sense of achievement and mastery on 10-point scales and to rate their mood immediately following their activities, as below.

THERAPIST: [summarizing a review of the patient's homework] So you did a lot of things this week that we predicted could lift your mood, but you found that nothing helped? Your mood was the same, no matter what you did?

PATIENT: Yeah.

THERAPIST: I have two theories. One, you had interfering automatic thoughts. And/or two, maybe you did experience slight mood changes, but you either didn't notice them or don't remember them.

PATIENT: I don't know.

The therapist then elicits the cognitions the patient had when engaging in various activities and helps him respond to them, in anticipation of their re-occurrence in the coming week. The therapist also ascertains that the patient had neglected to give himself credit. Next they decide to have the patient rate the sense of mastery and pleasure he gets.

THERAPIST: Suppose we make up a pleasure scale first so you'll have a guideline to rate your activities [see Figure 6.3]. Now on a scale from 0 to 10, what activity would you call a 10? An activity that has given you great pleasure or that you could imagine giving you great pleasure?

PATIENT: Oh, I guess that would be when I went to the championship game [of his home football team].

THERAPIST: Okay, next to "10" write "At football game" on the chart.

PATIENT: (*Does so.*)

THERAPIST: Now, what would you call a 0? An activity that gives you absolutely no pleasure?

PATIENT: That would be arguing with my partner.

THERAPIST: All right, write that next to 0.

PATIENT: (*Does so.*)

THERAPIST: And what would be something midway in between?

	Pleasure	**Mastery**
10	At football game	Building the deck
5	Dinner with brother	Raking leaves last year
0	Arguing with partner	Bouncing a check

FIGURE 6.3. Pleasure and Mastery Rating Scale.

PATIENT: I guess … having dinner with my brother.

THERAPIST: Good, write that.

If the patient can easily match activities with numbers, these three anchor points are usually sufficient, although the patient can add more points if desired. If the patient has difficulty with numbers, you can change the anchor points to "low," "medium," and "high." After completing the pleasure scale, the patient fills out the accomplishment scale in the same way. Next the therapist asks the patient to use his scales to rate today's activities.

THERAPIST: That's good. Now let's have you fill in a little of today's schedule. Here—it's the 11 o'clock block—write "therapy" and under that, "A = _____" and "P = _____." Now how much of a sense of accomplishment or mastery have you felt during therapy today?

PATIENT: About a 3.

THERAPIST: And pleasure?

PATIENT: About a 2. (*Fills in the blocks.*)

THERAPIST: And what did you do in the hour right before therapy today?

PATIENT: I went to the bookstore.

THERAPIST: Okay. Write "bookstore" in the 10 o'clock block. Now, look at the scale. How much of a sense of accomplishment did you get during that hour?

PATIENT: Maybe 2 or 3. (*Writes it down.*) I found the book I wanted.

THERAPIST: And pleasure?

PATIENT: None, really.

THERAPIST: So being at the bookstore was like arguing with your partner?

PATIENT: No, I guess it was about a 2.

THERAPIST: But isn't that interesting? Your first reaction was that you got no pleasure at all. The depression probably interferes with recognizing, or maybe remembering, pleasurable activities. That's why I think it's worth your keeping this activity chart this week, to find out whether some activities are better than others. (*pause*) Do you think you're straight on what to do?

PATIENT: Yeah.

THERAPIST: Could you tell me why it might be worth the effort to do all this?

PATIENT: Well, it sounds like you're saying that maybe my mood does change some, based on what I'm doing.

THERAPIST: What do *you* think?

PATIENT: I guess that could be right.

THERAPIST: If that's true, we can try to schedule more activities that do make you feel better next week. Now, the ideal thing would be to have you fill this out as close to the time you finish an activity as you can—so you won't forget what you did, and so your ratings will be more accurate. If that's impossible, could you try to fill this out at lunch, dinner, and bedtime?

PATIENT: Yeah, it shouldn't be a problem.

THERAPIST: And if you can fill it out every day, that would give us the most information. But even if you just do a couple of days, that would give us some. Now one last thing. How about if you look over the activity chart the day before our next session? See if there are any patterns, or anything you can learn from it. You can write down your conclusions on the back if you want. Okay?

PATIENT: Okay.

USING THE ACTIVITY CHART TO ASSESS THE ACCURACY OF PREDICTIONS

When patients are skeptical that scheduling activities can help, you can ask them to *predict* levels of mastery and pleasure or mood on one activity chart and then record *actual* ratings on another. These comparisons can be a useful source of data.

THERAPIST: Let's take a look now at your predictions on the first activity chart and what actually *happened* on the second one.

PATIENT: (*Nods.*)

THERAPIST: Let's see … it looks as if you predicted very low scores, mostly 0's to 3's, for these three times you scheduled to meet your friends. What *did* happen?

PATIENT: Actually, I had a better time than I'd thought—my pleasure scores were 3's to 5's.

THERAPIST: What does that tell you?

PATIENT: I guess I'm not a good predictor. I thought I wouldn't enjoy myself, but I did, at least some.

THERAPIST: Would you like to schedule more social activities for this coming week?

PATIENT: Yes, I should.

THERAPIST: Good. Do you see what could have happened—and, in fact, what was happening before you came to therapy? You kept predicting that you'd have a lousy time with your friends so you didn't make any plans; in fact, you turned down their invitations. It sounds as if this therapy homework helped you test your ideas; you found it was wrong that you'd have a lousy time, and now it sounds as if you're more willing to schedule more. Is that right?

PATIENT: Yes. But that reminds me, I wanted to talk about one prediction that actually turned out worse.

THERAPIST: Okay, when was that?

PATIENT: I predicted that I'd get 4's in accomplishment and pleasure when I went running over the weekend. But both were 1's.

THERAPIST: Do you have any idea why?

PATIENT: Not really.

THERAPIST: How were you feeling when you were running?

PATIENT: Mostly frustrated.

THERAPIST: And what was going through your mind?

PATIENT: I don't know. I wasn't feeling very good. I got winded real easily. I couldn't believe how hard it was.

THERAPIST: Did you have thoughts like that—"I don't feel very good," "I'm winded," "This is hard"?

PATIENT: Yeah, I think so.

THERAPIST: Anything else go through your mind?

PATIENT: I remembered how it used to be. I could go 2 or 3 miles without getting too winded.

THERAPIST: Did you have a memory, an image of how it used to be?

PATIENT: Yeah. It was easy. I'm in really bad shape now. It's going to be so hard to get back in shape. I'm not sure I'll *ever* be able to get back in shape.

THERAPIST: Okay, let me see if I understand. [summarizing] Here in my office you thought you'd get a moderate sense of accomplishment and pleasure when you went running. But instead, you got very little. It sounds as if you had a memory of how it used to be and you also had thoughts that interfered, such as, "This is hard," "I'm real winded," "I used to do this easily," "I'm in such bad shape now," "Maybe I'll never be able to get back in shape." And these thoughts made you feel frustrated. Does that sound right?

PATIENT: Yeah.

In this last part, the therapist uses the activity chart as a vehicle for identifying a number of automatic thoughts that were undermining the patient's enjoyment of an activity. In the next part, the therapist will:

1. Help him evaluate a key cognition, "Maybe I'll never be able to get back in shape."
2. Teach him to compare himself to how he was at his worst point instead of his best point, so he can feel good about running instead of being so self-critical.

Behavioral activation is essential for most depressed patients. Many patients need only to be provided with a rationale, guidance in selecting and scheduling activities, and responses to predicted automatic thoughts that might interfere with implementing the activities or with gaining a sense of pleasure or mastery from them. Therapists often need to be gently persistent in helping patients become more active. Patients who are quite inactive initially benefit from learning how to create and adhere to a daily schedule with increasing degrees of activity. Patients who are skeptical about scheduling activities may benefit from doing behavioral experiments to test their ideas, and/or checking the accuracy of their automatic thoughts by comparing their predictions to what actually occurs.

Chapter 7

SESSION 2 AND BEYOND: STRUCTURE AND FORMAT

S ession 2 uses a format that is repeated in every subsequent session. This chapter presents the format and describes the general course of therapy from Session 2 to near termination. The final phase of treatment is described in Chapter 18, and typical problems that arise in socializing the patient during early sessions are presented in Chapter 8.

The typical agenda for the second session and beyond is as follows:

Initial Part of Session
1. Do a mood check.
2. Set the agenda.
3. Obtain an update.
4. Review homework.
5. Prioritize the agenda.

Middle Part of Session
6. Work on a specific problem and teach cognitive behavior therapy skills in that context.

---

7. Follow-up discussion with relevant, collaboratively set homework assignment(s).
8. Work on second problem.

End of Session
9. Provide or elicit a summary.
10. Review new homework assignments.
11. Elicit feedback.

If you are new to this format, you can make a copy of this chart to keep with you. You can show it (or a simplified version) to patients so they can get a better idea of what treatment will be like, and so the two of you can keep track of where you are in the session.

Your goals during this second session are to help patients identify important problems on which to work and, in the context of problem solving, you will teach patients relevant skills, especially identifying and responding to automatic thoughts and, for most depressed patients, scheduling activities. You will continue to socialize patients into cognitive behavior therapy: following the session format, working collaboratively, providing feedback, and starting to view their past and ongoing experience in light of the cognitive model. If the patient is feeling somewhat better, you will also start relapse prevention work (see Chapter 18). Above all, you are concerned with building the therapeutic alliance and providing symptom relief.

THE FIRST PART OF THE SESSION

The specific goals of the introductory part of the session, described below, are to:

- Reestablish rapport.
- Elicit the names of problems patients want help in solving.
- Collect data that may indicate other important problem areas to discuss.
- Review homework.
- Prioritize the problems on the agenda.

The achievement of these goals is facilitated when patients review the Preparing for Therapy Worksheet (Figure 7.1) prior to the session (either mentally or in writing).

1. What did we talk about last session that was important? What do my therapy notes say?
2. What has my mood been like, compared to other weeks?
3. What happened (positive and negative) this week that my therapist should know?
4. What problems do I want help in solving? What is a short name for each of these problems?
5. What homework did I do? (If I didn't do it, what got in the way?) What did I learn?

FIGURE 7.1. Preparing for Therapy Worksheet.

Mood (and Medication) Check

The mood check is usually brief. It helps you and patients keep track of how they are progressing. If patients complete symptom checklists, you will examine them to determine whether patients have additional problems that they may not report verbally, such as suicidal ideation, difficulties sleeping, feeling worthless or punished, fearing the worst will happen, increased irritability, and so on. It may be important to address one or more of these problems during the session.

You will also elicit a subjective description from patients and match it with objective test scores. If there is a discrepancy between the test scores and the self-report, question the patient (e.g., "So you've been feeling worse, but your depression inventory is actually lower than last week. What do you make of that?"). You will also make a quick comparison between the objective scores of the previous session and the present objective scores (e.g., "Your anxiety score is lower this week than last. *Have* you been feeling less anxious?"). You should also confirm that patients are not reporting how they feel just that day, but instead are providing an overview of their mood for the past week. A typical second session begins as follows:

THERAPIST: Hi, Sally. How have you been feeling?

PATIENT: About the same, I guess. I'm still feeling pretty depressed. And a lot more worried.

THERAPIST: Can I take a look at your forms? When you filled them out, were you thinking about the week as a whole—or just today?

PATIENT: The whole week.

THERAPIST: Good. Okay, yes, it sure looks like you were much more anxious this week. Should we put "anxiety" on the agenda to talk about in a few minutes?

PATIENT: (*Nods.*)

THERAPIST: (*indicating the Beck Depression Inventory*) It looks like your depression score is down a little this week, compared to last week. Did it feel that way to you?

PATIENT: Yeah, I think so.

THERAPIST: Okay, that's good.

> **Q:** What if ... patients elaborate at length about their mood?
>
> **A:** You will socialize them to give a concise description. For example:
>
> "Sally, can I interrupt you for a moment? Can you tell me in just a couple of sentences how your depression and anxiety have been this week compared to last week? Have you been feeling more depressed, about the same, or less depressed?"

Having gained an overall sense of Sally's mood in the past week, I elicit her attribution for the change. I want her to recognize the positive actions she took and the adaptive changes in her thinking.

THERAPIST: Why do you think you're a little less depressed?

PATIENT: I guess I've been feeling a little more hopeful, like maybe therapy might help.

THERAPIST: [subtly reinforcing the cognitive model] So you had thoughts like, "Therapy might help," and those thoughts made you feel more hopeful, less depressed?

PATIENT: Yes ... and Lisa—she's in my chemistry class—asked me to study with her. We spent a couple of hours yesterday going over some formulas. That made me feel better, too.

THERAPIST: What went through your mind when you were studying with her yesterday?

PATIENT: That I was glad she asked me to study with her ... I understand it more now.

THERAPIST: So we have two good examples of why you felt better this week. One, you had hopeful thoughts about therapy. And two, you *did* something different—studying with Lisa—and got at least a small sense of achievement.

PATIENT: Yeah.

THERAPIST: Can you see how your thinking and what you did affected how you felt—in a positive way?

To build a sense of self-efficacy and to encourage further cognitive and behavioral change, I positively reinforce Sally for the adaptive changes she made:

THERAPIST: It's great that you were having these hopeful thoughts about therapy and that you made the effort to study with Lisa.

If patients have been feeling better but are unsure why, ask, "Have you noticed any changes in your thinking or in what you've been doing?"

Q: What if … patients attribute positive changes in their mood to external factors?

A: Patients often say, "I felt better because the medication started working/my boss was out sick/my partner was nicer to me." You might then suggest, "I'm sure that helped, but did you also find yourself *thinking* differently or *doing* anything different?"

Likewise, you will seek patients' attributions if their mood has worsened: "Why do you think you're feeling worse this week? Could it have anything to do with your thinking, or with the things you did or didn't do?" In this way, you subtly reinforce the cognitive model and imply that patients can take some control over how they feel.

Q: What if … patients state that *nothing* can improve their mood?

A: For some patients who persist in this belief, it might be helpful to put "Things that can help me feel better and things that can help me feel worse" on the agenda to discuss later in session. A chart such as the one in Figure 7.2 can help reinforce the notion that patients can take at least minimal control of their mood. Through guided discovery, you can help them see that avoidance, isolation,

Things that make me feel better	Things that make me feel worse
Riding my bike	Staying in bed
Getting through my e-mails	Taking long naps
Going on Facebook	Watching too much TV
Meeting up with friends	Sitting around
Working on the car	

FIGURE 7.2. A better/worse list.

and inactivity generally increase their dysphoria (or at least does not improve it), while engagement in certain activities (usually that involve interpersonal interaction or that have the potential for pleasure or mastery) can lead to an improvement in their mood, even if initially it is small.

The brief mood check creates several opportunities:

- You demonstrate your concern for how patients have been feeling in the past week.
- You and they can monitor how they have been progressing over the course of treatment.
- You can identify (and then reinforce or modify) their explanation for progress or lack thereof.
- You can also reinforce the cognitive model; namely, how patients have been viewing situations and how they have been behaving have influenced their mood.

When reviewing objective measures, make sure to review individual items to look for important positive or negative changes (e.g., changes in suicidal ideation or hopelessness). According to patients' diagnoses and symptomatology, you might also ask for additional information not specifically covered in the tests (e.g., number and severity of panic attacks, binges, substance use, angry outbursts, self-harm, destructive behavior).

If patients are taking medication for their psychological difficulties, you will briefly check on adherence, problems, side effects, or questions. It is important to phrase the adherence question in terms of frequency—not "Did you take your medicine this week," but rather, "*How many times this week* were you able to take your medicine the way [the provider] prescribed?" (See, e.g., J. S. Beck, 2001, for suggestions on how to increase medication adherence.)

If you are not the prescribing healthcare provider, you will obtain patients' permission and then periodically contact the provider to exchange information. You will not recommend changes in medication, but you might help patients respond to cognitions that interfere with their taking medication (or, if applicable, reducing medication). If they have concerns about issues such as side effects, dosage, addiction to medications, or alternative medications or supplements, you will help patients write down specific questions to ask their provider. If patients are not taking medication but you believe a pharmacological intervention is indicated, you might suggest a medical or psychiatric consultation.

Setting an Initial Agenda

The purpose of this *brief* segment is to set an initial agenda. You socialize patients into bringing up the *names of problems* they want help in
solving. Rather than asking, "What do you want to talk about today?" or
"What do you want to put on the agenda?"(which can lead to less productive discussions), you phrase the question in a problem-solving way
(until patients are socialized to setting the agenda in this way):

THERAPIST: Okay, Sally, what problem or problems do you want my help
in solving today? Can you just tell me the *names* of the problems?

PATIENT: Well, I've got this economics exam coming up and I just don't
understand the material. I've been so worried. I just can't concentrate. I don't know what to do. I keep reading ...

THERAPIST: (*gently interrupting*) [socializing the patient into briefly
specifying a problem to be discussed later in the session] Should
we put the exam on the agenda?

PATIENT: Yes, definitely.

Rather than having Sally provide a full description of the problem
at this point, I gently interrupt her, name the problem, and ask to put it
on the agenda to discuss in a few minutes. Had I allowed her to launch
into a lengthier description of the problem, *I would have deprived her of
the opportunity to reflect on and prioritize what she most wanted to talk about
during the session*, which may or may not have been the first problem she
brought up. Next I probe for additional important agenda topics:

THERAPIST: Are there any other problems you want help with?

PATIENT: Well, things aren't going too well with my roommate. We keep
such different hours. She ...

THERAPIST: (*gently interrupting*) Should we call that, "problem with your
roommate"?

PATIENT: Yes.

THERAPIST: Anything else?

PATIENT: I'm not sure.

THERAPIST: [probing for other problems that might be even more
important to address during the session than these first two] When
did you feel the worst this week?

PATIENT: (*Thinks.*) I guess when I was trying to study for the exam. And
in class.

THERAPIST: Any other times that were particularly bad?

PATIENT: No, those were the worst.

THERAPIST: Should we put "studying and class" on the agenda?
PATIENT: Yes, that would be good.

I then ascertain whether the patient anticipates the occurrence of other important difficulties before I see her again:

THERAPIST: And are there any other problems you think are likely to come up this week?
PATIENT: No, I don't think so.

> **Q:** What if ... patients have difficulty coming up with agenda items?
>
> **A:** Often patients need a little encouragement initially to suggest agenda items. They may not be clearly cognizant of what has been bothering them, and/or they may be unsure of what is appropriate to bring up. Chapter 8 describes what to do with patients who display this difficulty.

Update of Week

The next part of the session helps you make a bridge between the previous session and the current one. It includes a brief update of the patient's week, during which you will remain alert for potential problems that could be important for the agenda. First you seek to get the general gist of how the patient's week went.

THERAPIST: Did anything else happen this week that's important for me to know?
PATIENT: (*Thinks.*) Ummm. (*sigh*) Yeah, I overslept and missed a class.
THERAPIST: [probing to see whether it is important enough to add to the agenda] Is that a problem we need to talk about today?
PATIENT: No, I don't think so. I just forgot to set my alarm.
THERAPIST: Okay, anything else?
PATIENT: No, not that I can think of.

Next you will elicit positive experiences:

THERAPIST: All right. Now, can you tell me what happened this week that was positive? Or situations in which maybe you felt a little bit better?
PATIENT: (*Thinks.*) Umm, I think running helped. I also felt better when I talked to my mom on the phone.
THERAPIST: Okay, that's good. Were there any other good things that happened?

Asking for positive experiences helps patients realize that they did not feel the same unrelenting severity of distress for the entire week. You should note the positive data, which you may use later in the session or in future sessions, especially when planning positive activities for patients to engage in or when helping them evaluate relevant automatic thoughts and beliefs. Uncovering positive data may also put patients in a better frame of mind, making them more receptive to upcoming problem solving. You may decide to engage patients conversationally about these items (usually briefly), either at the time or later, to brighten their mood or to demonstrate your interest in them, thereby strengthening the therapeutic alliance.

Homework Review

Next you will find out what the patient accomplished for homework. (Chapter 17 provides a more extensive description of this part of the session.) Reviewing the patient's homework is critical. If you do not, patients invariably stop doing it. Sometimes the review of homework is relatively brief; at other times, however, it may become the major part of the session, if it is related to the problems on the agenda. Part of the art of therapy is determining how much time to spend reviewing homework versus discussing other problems the patient wants help in solving.

Generally you ask patients to read aloud the assignments from their Homework List (see, e.g., page 67). You ask them to rate how much they currently believe the adaptive statements, the responses to their automatic thoughts and beliefs you discussed in the previous sessions(s). You find out which behavioral assignments they did and what they learned from them. And you discuss which assignments would be helpful for them to continue in the coming week. If any homework items require a lengthy discussion (or if there are any assignments they failed to do), you can collaboratively decide to discuss them later in the session, so you can quickly review the rest of the assignments.

THERAPIST: Next, can we talk about your homework? Do you have the notes from last week?

PATIENT: Yes (*Pulls out list* [Figure 5.1, page 67]; *therapist pulls out her copy, too.*)

THERAPIST: Good. Okay if we go through it?

PATIENT: Sure.

THERAPIST: So how did you do with reading this twice a day?

PATIENT: Pretty good. I think I only missed one or two days.

THERAPIST: Can you read the first item?

PATIENT: (*Reads aloud.*) "If I start thinking I'm lazy and no good, remind myself that I have a real illness, called depression, that makes it harder for me to do things. As the treatment starts to work, my depression will lift, and things will get easier."

THERAPIST: How much do you believe that right now?

PATIENT: I guess I do believe it.

THERAPIST: Good. (*going on to second item on list*) Did you think of any other goals?

PATIENT: No.

THERAPIST: Okay. If you do, let me know. (*Moving on to third item*) Were you able to catch your automatic thoughts when you noticed your mood changing?

PATIENT: I tried, but I don't think I always know what I'm thinking.

THERAPIST: That's okay. We'll be talking about automatic thoughts at every session. Were you able to identify *any* automatic thoughts when your mood changed?

PATIENT: Yeah, I think so, but I didn't write them down.

THERAPIST: What was the situation?

PATIENT: I was sitting in class, and all of a sudden I got really nervous.

THERAPIST: What was going through your mind?

PATIENT: I was thinking the exam was coming up, and there's no way I'll be ready for it.

THERAPIST: Good. Let me jot that down. Can we get back to this thought in a few minutes when we talk about the exam?

PATIENT: Yeah.

THERAPIST: Any other automatic thoughts you were aware of this week?

PATIENT: Not really.

THERAPIST: So you didn't get much of an opportunity to remind yourself that just because you think something doesn't necessarily mean it's true?

PATIENT: (*Shakes her head.*)

THERAPIST: What do you think of that idea now?

PATIENT: I guess it's true. Like the *Coping with Depression* booklet says.

THERAPIST: Did you get together with Allison or Joe or other people this week?

Sally and I quickly review this assignment. We collaboratively agree that she will continue to look for her automatic thoughts and make social plans in the coming week. Then we briefly discuss key concepts in the *Coping with Depression* booklet.

Prioritizing the Agenda

Now that you have set an initial agenda and possibly added more topics as you collected data about the patient's week and homework, you will summarize the topics. If there are too many agenda items, you and the patient will collaboratively prioritize items and agree to move the discussion of less important problems to a future session. You may also find out whether patients want to spend about an equal amount of time on each item.

THERAPIST: Okay, can we prioritize the agenda now [providing a rationale] so we can figure out how to spend our time this session? You mentioned your exam, a problem with your roommate, and feeling particularly worse when you were studying and in class. (*pause*) Is there any other problem that is even more important than those?

PATIENT: Well, I've been feeling bad about not calling my cousin.

THERAPIST: Okay. (*jotting it down and then adding my own items to the agenda*) I'd also like to talk about how you can expect your mood to improve and some more about automatic thoughts. Does that sound okay?

PATIENT: Yes, that's fine.

THERAPIST: Anything else for the agenda?

PATIENT: I don't think so.

THERAPIST: I don't know if we'll get to everything. [helping Sally prioritize her problems] If we run out of time, are there some things we can put off until next week?

PATIENT: Ummm ... I guess the problem with my roommate. It'll probably just blow over. And my cousin. That can wait.

THERAPIST: Okay, let's put those last on our list, and we'll see if we get to them.

Alternatively, you can ask:

THERAPIST: If we only have time to talk about one or two of these problems, which would be the most important?

It is important to note that you need not always adhere to the agenda. Indeed, under some circumstances, you *should not* follow the agenda. When deviating from the agenda, however, you should explicitly note the change and elicit the patient's agreement.

THERAPIST: Sally, I can see that you're still worried about your exam, but we're running out of time. Would you like to spend the rest of the session on it and postpone our other agenda items to next week? Or we could try to spend just 5 more minutes on it, so we'll still have time to talk about feeling bad when you're studying or in class.

PATIENT: I guess we should try to get to those things, too.

THERAPIST: Okay, let's both keep an eye on the clock.

You might suggest a change in how you and a patient spend time during a session for a number of reasons. For example, as in the previous transcript, the patient is quite upset about a particular issue and needs more time to discuss it. Or a new topic arises that seems especially important. Or the patient's mood changes (for the worse) during the session.

Q: What if ... patients start talking about a whole new topic that is not on the agenda?

A: When patients drift into a new topic, you gently interrupt them, calling attention to the change and allowing the patient to make a conscious choice of which issue to pursue. Patients frequently introduce new topics without quite realizing they are doing so.

PATIENT: Then another time I was trying to study in the library and I got so distracted when I saw this girl from my high school, Julia. I just started to obsess over whether I should go talk to her. When we were in 10th grade, Julia was pretty friendly, and then something happened, I'm not sure what it was. I think she may have ...

THERAPIST: Can I just interrupt you for a moment? We started off talking about the trouble you've been having studying for your exam, and now it sounds as if the focus is Julia. Is it more important to you to go back to talking about the exam, or is Julia more important to talk about?

PATIENT: Oh, the exam. Julia's not that important.

THERAPIST: Okay, so you were saying that it's generally hard for you to get to work at the library?

You steer patients away from peripheral issues that were not on the original agenda, and which hold little promise for helping them progress during the session. A notable exception occurs when you deliberately (though usually briefly) engage patients in more casual conversation to achieve a specific goal. For example, you might ask about their family, movies, or social events they have recently attended to brighten their mood, facilitate the alliance, or assess their cognitive functioning or social skills.

THE MIDDLE PART OF THE SESSION

Next you will list the names of the problems on the prioritized agenda and ask patients which problem they want to work on first. Doing so affords them the opportunity to be active and take responsibility. At times, though, you may take the lead in suggesting an agenda item with which to start, especially when you judge that a *particular* problem is the most important. ("Is it okay with you if we start with the problem of finding a part-time job?")

You will collect data about the problem, conceptualize the patients' difficulties according to the cognitive model, and collaboratively decide on which part of the cognitive model you will begin working (solving the problem situation, evaluating automatic thoughts, reducing patients' immediate distress (if the patients' affect is so high they cannot focus on problem solving, evaluating thoughts, or behavioral change), suggesting behavioral changes (and teaching behavioral skills if needed), or decreasing patients' physiological arousal (if it is interfering with an important discussion). In the context of discussing problems on the agenda, you will be teaching patients skills and setting new homework. You will also make periodic summaries, if needed, to help you and the patient recall what you have been doing in this part of the session.

In discussing the first problem (and subsequent problems), you will interweave your therapy goals as appropriate. In this second session, I seek not only to help Sally do some problem solving, but also to:

- Reinforce the cognitive model.
- Continue teaching Sally to identify her automatic thoughts.
- Provide some symptom relief through helping Sally respond to her anxious thoughts.
- As always, maintain and build rapport through accurate understanding.

Agenda Item No. 1

THERAPIST: Okay, let's take a look at the agenda. Where do you think we should start? We could talk about your exam, your mood when you're studying or when you're in the library, or the course of improvement.

PATIENT: My economics exam, I guess, I'm really worried about it.

THERAPIST: [collecting data] Okay, can you give me an overview of what happened this week? How much did you study? What happened with your concentration?

PATIENT: Well, I meant to study all the time. But every time I sat down, I just got so nervous. Sometimes I didn't realize that my mind had wandered, and I had to keep rereading the same page.

THERAPIST: [continuing to collect data so I can help problem-solve and identify possible distortions in Sally's thinking] When is the exam, and how many chapters does it cover?

PATIENT: It's in 2 weeks, and I think it covers the first five chapters.

THERAPIST: And how many chapters have you read at least once?

PATIENT: About three.

THERAPIST: And there are still some things in these first three chapters that you don't understand?

PATIENT: A lot of things.

THERAPIST: Okay. So, in a nutshell, you have an exam in 2 weeks, and you're worried that you won't understand the material well enough?

PATIENT: Right.

In this first part, I seek an overview of the problem. I subtly model how to express this problem succinctly. Next, I help Sally identify her automatic thoughts by having her recall a *specific* situation.

THERAPIST: Can you remember a time this week when you thought about studying or tried to study, and the anxiety got really bad?

PATIENT: Yes, sure … last night.

THERAPIST: What time was it? Where were you?

PATIENT: It was about 7:30. I was walking to the library.

THERAPIST: Can you picture it in your head now? It's 7:30, you're walking to the library.… What goes through your mind?

PATIENT: What if I flunk the exam? What if I flunk the course? How will I ever make it through the semester?

THERAPIST: Okay, so you were able to identify your automatic thoughts. And how did these thoughts make you feel? Anxious?

PATIENT: Very.

THERAPIST: Let me tell you a little more about these automatic thoughts. We call them *automatic* because they seem just to pop into your mind. Most of the time, you're probably not even aware of them; you're probably much more aware of how you're feeling emotionally. Even if you *are* aware of them, you probably don't think to evaluate how accurate your thoughts are. You just accept them as true.

PATIENT: Hmmm.

THERAPIST: What you'll learn to do here in therapy is first to identify your thoughts, and then judge for yourself whether they're completely true, partially true, or not true at all. (*pause*) Can we look at the first thought together? [starting the process of evaluating the automatic thought] What evidence do you have that you'll flunk the exam?

PATIENT: Well, I don't understand everything.

THERAPIST: Anything else?

PATIENT: No ... just that I'm running out of time.

THERAPIST: Okay. Any evidence that you might *not* flunk?

PATIENT: Well, I did do okay on the first quiz.

THERAPIST: Anything else?

PATIENT: I guess I understand the first two chapters better than the third one. The third one is the one I'm *really* having trouble with.

THERAPIST: [starting problem solving; having Sally take the lead] What could you do to learn the third chapter better?

PATIENT: I could read it again. I could look through my lecture notes.

THERAPIST: Anything else?

PATIENT: (*Hesitates.*) I can't think of anything.

THERAPIST: Anyone else you could ask for help?

PATIENT: Well, I suppose I could ask Sean; he's the teaching assistant. Or maybe Ross, the guy down the hall who took this course last year.

THERAPIST: That sounds good. Did you think of asking either of them for help this week? Did any automatic thoughts get in the way?

PATIENT: No, I guess I just didn't even think of it.

THERAPIST: Whom do you think would be better to ask?

PATIENT: Sean, I guess.

THERAPIST: How likely are you to ask him?

PATIENT: I will. He has office hours tomorrow morning.

THERAPIST: Okay, assuming you get help this week, what do you think of your prediction that you might flunk?

PATIENT: Well, I guess I do know some of the stuff. Maybe I *could* get help with the rest.

THERAPIST: And how do you feel now?

PATIENT: A little less worried, I guess.

THERAPIST: Okay, to summarize, you had a lot of automatic thoughts this week that made you feel anxious. But when you stop to evaluate these thoughts, it seems likely that there are some things you *can* do to pass. When you really look at the evidence and answer the thoughts, you feel better ... Is that right?

PATIENT: Yeah, that's true.

THERAPIST: For homework this week, I'd like you to look for these automatic thoughts again when you notice your mood changing. These thoughts may have a grain of truth, but often I think you'll find that they're not necessarily completely true. Next week we'll look for evidence together to figure out whether the thoughts you wrote down for homework are completely accurate. Okay?

PATIENT: Okay.

THERAPIST: Now, identifying and evaluating thoughts is a skill for you to learn, like learning to drive or type. You may not be very good at it at first, but with practice you'll get better and better. And I'll teach you more about this in future sessions. See what you can do this week just to identify some thoughts, but don't expect yourself to be good at it yet. Okay?

PATIENT: Yeah.

THERAPIST: One more word about this. When you write down some thoughts this week, remind yourself again that the thoughts *may or may not be true.* Otherwise, writing them down before you've learned to evaluate them could make you feel a little worse.

PATIENT: Okay.

THERAPIST: Let's write this assignment down. And while we're at it, let's see if there's anything else you want to do to get ready for the test. [See Figure 7.3.]

Jan. 29

Read this list twice a day

1. When I notice my mood changing, ask myself, "What's going through my mind right now?" and jot down my automatic thoughts (which may or may not be completely true). Try to do this at least once a day.

2. If I can't figure out my automatic thoughts, jot down just the situation. Remember, learning to identify my thinking is a skill I'll get better at, like typing.

3. Ask Sean for help with Chapter 3 of Econ book.

4. Read over therapy notes.

5. Continue running/swimming.

6. Plan 3 social activities.

7. Daily: Add to credit list

FIGURE 7.3. Sally's homework (Session 2).

In this section, I accomplish many things at once. I address a problem from the agenda that is of concern to Sally; I teach her more about automatic thoughts; I help her identify, evaluate, and respond to a specific distressing thought; I facilitate symptom relief by decreasing her anxiety; and I set up a homework assignment and advise Sally to have realistic expectations about learning the new skill. Chapters 9–12 describe in greater detail the process of teaching patients to identify and evaluate their automatic thoughts.

Q: What if ... I don't know how to help patients solve a particular problem?

A: There are several things you can do:

- Find out how they have already tried to solve the problem and why it didn't work. You may be able to modify the solution or modify thoughts that got in the way of the solution working.

- Use yourself as a model. Ask yourself, "If I had this problem, what would I do?"

- Ask the patient to name another person (usually a friend or family member) who could conceivably have the same kind of problem. What advice would the patient give him or her? See whether that advice could apply to the patient.

- If you're stuck, postpone the discussion: "I'd like to think more about the problem this week. Could we put it on the agenda to talk more about next week?"

Also, see pages 256–258 for a further description of problem solving.

Agenda Item No. 2

In the next section of the therapy session, I provide Sally with some information about the course of improvement. Having just finished a segment of the session, I briefly summarize first:

THERAPIST: Okay, we just finished talking about your exam and how your automatic thoughts really made you feel anxious and interfered with problem solving. Next, I'd like to talk about the course of getting better, if that's okay.

PATIENT: Sure.

THERAPIST: I'm glad you're feeling a little less depressed today, and I hope you continue to feel better. But probably you won't just feel a little bit better every single week until you're back to your old self. You should expect to have your ups and downs. Now I'm telling you this for a reason. Can you imagine what you might think if you expected to keep feeling better and better and then one day you felt a lot worse?

PATIENT: I'd probably think I would never get better.

THERAPIST: That's right. So I want you to remember that we predicted a possible setback, that setbacks are a normal part of getting better. Do you want to get down something in writing about that?

See Chapter 18 for a more extensive discussion of relapse prevention and a pictorial representation of the normal course of therapy.

Periodic Summaries

Three kinds of summarizing are important throughout sessions. The first summarizes content. Patients often describe a problem with many details. You will summarize what they have said in the form of the cognitive model to ensure that you have correctly identified what is most troublesome to patients, and to present it in a way that is more concise and clear. You use patients' own words as much as possible, both to convey accurate understanding and to keep the key difficulty activated in their mind:

THERAPIST: Let me make sure I understand. You were considering getting a part-time job again, but then you thought, "I'll never be able to handle it," and the thought made you so sad that you turned off your computer and went back to bed and cried for half an hour. Is that right?

Had I paraphrased the patient's ideas and failed to use her own words ("Sounds like you weren't sure if you could do well if you got a part-time job"), I might have lessened the intensity of the automatic thought and emotion, and our subsequent evaluation of the thought might then have been less effective. Summaries that substitute the *therapist's* words may also lead to patients' believing that they have not been accurately understood:

PATIENT: No, it's not that I thought I might not do well; I'm afraid I might not be able to handle it *at all*.

You will often ask patients to make a second kind of summary after you have evaluated an automatic thought or belief:

"Can you summarize what we just talked about?"
Or
"What do you think the main message is here?"
Or
"What do you think would be important for you to remember?"

If patients do a good job of summarizing, you or they should write down this summary so they can read it for homework. If their summary misses the mark, you might say, "Well, that's close, but I wonder if it would be more helpful if you remembered it this way ..." If the patient agrees, the latter summary is recorded in their notes.

The third is a brief summary when a section of a session has been completed, so both therapist and patient have a clear understanding of what they have just accomplished and what they will do next:

THERAPIST: Okay, so we've finished talking about the course of treatment. Next, should we talk about the problem with your cousin?

FINAL SUMMARY AND FEEDBACK

The goal of the final summary is to focus the patient's attention on the most important points of the session in a positive way. In early sessions, you will generally summarize.

THERAPIST: Well, we have just a few minutes left. Let me summarize what we covered today, and then I'll ask you for your reaction to the session.

PATIENT: Okay.

THERAPIST: It sounds like when you had more hopeful thoughts this week, you felt less depressed. But then your anxiety increased because you had all these negative thoughts about your exam. When we looked at the evidence that you'll flunk, though, it seemed unconvincing. And you came up with a couple of good strategies to help your studying, some of which you'll try between now and our next session. We also discussed what you should remind yourself if you have a setback. Finally, we talked about having you continue to go running. And we went over identifying and evaluating your automatic thoughts, which is a skill we'll keep practicing in therapy. (*pause*) Do you think that about covers it?

PATIENT: Yes.

As the patient progresses, the therapist may ask the patient to summarize the most important points. Summarizing is much more easily accomplished if the patient has taken good notes during the session:

THERAPIST: Okay, Sally, we just have a few minutes left. What do you think is going to be most important for you to remember this week? You can look at your notes.

Following the final summary, the therapist elicits feedback about the session from the patient.

THERAPIST: Okay, Sally, what did you think about the session today? Was there anything I said that bothered you? Anything you think I got wrong?

PATIENT: I am a little bit worried that I could have a setback.

THERAPIST: Well, a setback is possible, and if you do find yourself feeling significantly worse before our next session, I'd like you to call me and we can discuss whether you should come in sooner. On the other hand, you may very well have another better week.

PATIENT: I hope so.

THERAPIST: Should we put the topic "setbacks" on the agenda again next week?

PATIENT: Yes, I think so.

THERAPIST: Anything else about the session? Anything you want us to do differently next time?

PATIENT: No, I don't think so.

THERAPIST: Okay. See you next week.

If you sense that patients have not fully expressed their reaction to the session, you may ask them to complete a therapy report (see Figure 5.2). When patients do express negative feedback, you will positively reinforce them and then try to solve the problem. If there is insufficient time to do so, you may apologize and tell patients that you would like to discuss their negative reaction at the very beginning of the following session. Negative feedback usually indicates difficulty in the therapeutic alliance (discussed more fully in J. S. Beck, 2005).

SESSION 3 AND BEYOND

Later therapy sessions maintain the same basic format. The content varies according to the patient's problems and goals, and your therapeutic goals. In this section, I outline the flow of therapy across sessions. A more detailed description of treatment planning can be found in Chapter 19.

As mentioned previously, you initially take the lead in helping patients identify and modify automatic thoughts, devising homework assignments, and summarizing the session. As therapy progresses, there is a gradual shift in responsibility. Toward the end of therapy, patients themselves tend to identify their distorted thinking, devise their own homework assignments, and summarize the session.

Another gradual shift is from an emphasis on automatic thoughts to a focus on both automatic thoughts and underlying beliefs (see Chapters 13 and 14). As therapy moves into the final phase, there is another shift: preparing the patient for termination and relapse prevention (see Chapter 18).

When planning an individual session, you are mindful of the stage of therapy and you continue to use your conceptualization of the patient to guide treatment, noting potential agenda items before a session. As patients report on their mood, briefly review the week, and specify agenda topics, you formulate in your own mind a specific goal or goals for the session. For example, in Session 3, my goals for Sally (though not necessarily for all depressed patients) are to begin teaching her in a structured way to evaluate her automatic thoughts and to continue to schedule pleasurable activities. In Session 4, I aim to help Sally do some problem solving about finding a part-time job and continue to respond to her dysfunctional thoughts. I continually seek to integrate my goals with Sally's agenda items. Thus I teach her problem-solving and cognitive restructuring skills in the context of situations she brings to therapy. This combination of solving problems and helping patients respond to their thoughts generally allows the novice therapist sufficient time to discuss in depth only about two problematic situations from the agenda during a given therapy session. Experienced therapists can often cover more.

To refine your conceptualization, to keep track of what is being covered in a therapy session, and to plan future sessions, you take notes during the session (see Figure 7.4) and keep a copy of notes the patient takes. It is useful to note the problem(s) discussed, dysfunctional thoughts and beliefs written verbatim (and the degree to which the patient initially believed them), interventions made in session, newly restructured thoughts and beliefs (and the degree of belief in them), the assigned homework, and topics for the agendas of future sessions. Even experienced therapists have difficulty remembering all these important items without written notes.

Therapy Notes

Patient's name: Sally   **Date:** 3/15   **Session no.:** 7

Objective scores: Beck Depression Inventory = 18, Beck Anxiety Inventory = 7, Hopelessness Scale = 9

Patient's agenda:

Problem with English paper

Problem with roommate

Therapist's objectives:

Continue to modify perfectionist thinking.

Decrease anxiety and avoidance around participating in class.

Session highlights:

1. Feeling less depressed and anxious this week.

2. Situation/problem   Automatic thought   Emotion

English paper due tomorrow → It's not good enough. → Anxious

Intervention—Thought Record (attached)
Outcome—Anxiety (reduced)

(cont.)

FIGURE 7.4. Therapy notes.

3. Old belief: If I don't get an A, it means I don't have what it takes to be
                      a success.   90% [strength of belief]

Intervention: Advice to Rebecca (friend)

Outcome: 80% [rerating strength of belief]

Intervention 2:   Intellectual–emotional role play

Outcome: 60% [rerating strength of belief]

New belief: I don't need all A's to succeed now or in the future. 80%

4. Coping card about asking questions after class (attached).

5. Roommate problem—too noisy at night

   Intervention—role-played how to approach roommate

Homework: [If written on a separate piece of paper, attach instead.]

Thought Record and credit list.
Read therapy notes and think about old and new beliefs about success.
Read coping cards in the morning and as needed
Ask 1 or 2 questions after class.
Spend one more hour to edit English paper.
Ask roommate to be quieter at night.

Future sessions:

See how perfectionism affects other parts of life.

FIGURE 7.4. *(cont.)*

As you take notes, you maintain eye contact as much as possible. It is important at times, especially when patients are revealing emotionally painful material, *not* to take notes so you can be more fully present with the patient.

This chapter outlined the structure and format of a typical early therapy session and briefly described therapy across sessions. The following chapter discusses problems in following the prescribed format, while Chapter 19 describes in detail how to plan treatment before individual sessions, within sessions, and across sessions.

Chapter 8

PROBLEMS WITH STRUCTURING THE THERAPY SESSION

Problems invariably arise in structuring sessions. When you become aware of a problem, you will specify it, conceptualize why the problem arose, and devise a solution. If you have correctly diagnosed the patient and developed a sound treatment plan but still have difficulties in structuring sessions, you should check on the following:

* Have you failed to gently interrupt the patient to direct the session?
* Have you failed to socialize the patient into treatment?
* Have you failed to sufficiently engage the patient in treatment or to develop a strong therapeutic alliance?

These difficulties are described in this chapter. Then problems and remedies for each segment of a typical session are offered.

THERAPIST COGNITIONS

If you are a novice therapist or a therapist experienced in a less directive modality, you may have interfering cognitions about structure, interrupting patients, and implementing the standard structure.

Automatic Thoughts

"I can't structure the session."

"[My patient] won't like the structure."

"She can't express herself succinctly."

"He'll get mad if I'm too directive."

"I shouldn't interrupt her."

"He won't do homework."

"She'll feel invalidated if I evaluate her thinking."

You should monitor your own level of discomfort and identify your automatic thoughts during and between sessions. You can then identify a problem, evaluate and respond to your thoughts, and problem-solve to make it easier for you to experiment with implementing the standard structure at the next session.

INTERRUPTING THE PATIENT

To structure sessions effectively so therapy can proceed most efficiently, you need to use gentle interruption. In the following transcript, the therapist finds himself feeling slightly overwhelmed by the patient's outpouring of problems. He uses his own emotional reaction as a cue to interrupt and structure the patient.

PATIENT: And then, I couldn't believe it, but my sister told me—told me!—that I had to go help out Mom. She knows that I can't do that. I mean, my mother and I have never gotten along. If I go over, she'll just bombard me with stuff to do. And she'll criticize me. I just can't take any more criticism. I get it all day at work and ...

THERAPIST: Can I interrupt you for a minute? I want to make sure I get what's been going on. We started talking about holiday plans and what you should do and then you described a few more problems. Which do you think would be most important to work on? Holiday plans, your sister, mom, or work?

Q: What if ... patients get upset when you interrupt?

A: If they do not spontaneously tell you that your interruptions were distressing, ask them what was just going through their minds when you notice a negative affect shift. If they fail to identify their automatic thoughts, you can offer your hypothesis: "I was wondering whether you thought I was interrupting you too much?" Once you ascertain that interrupting has been a problem, positively reinforce them: "It's good you told me that." Next, apologize; simply say, "I'm sorry." (An apology is in order because you have apparently misgauged how much interruption they could tolerate.) Then solve the problem, for example, by asking patients if they would like to talk without interruption for the next 5 or 10 minutes, at the end of which time you will summarize what they said, "Because it's important to me that I really understand what's going on with you."

SOCIALIZING THE PATIENT

A second common difficulty in maintaining the prescribed structure can arise if you do not adequately socialize patients. Patients who are new to cognitive behavior therapy do not know in advance that you would like them to report on the week, describe their mood, and set the agenda in a succinct way. They do not know that you will ask them to summarize discussions of important problems, provide feedback, remember session content, and consistently do daily homework. In addition, you are essentially teaching patients certain skills and also a new way of relating to you (for those who have been in another type of therapy), or a new way of relating to their difficulties so that they can adopt a more objective, problem-solving orientation. Therefore, you must often describe, provide a rationale, and monitor with gentle, corrective feedback each of the session elements.

ENGAGING THE PATIENT

A third common difficulty arises when patients have dysfunctional beliefs that interfere with their ability to commit to working in treatment. They may not have clear goals (described in Chapter 5) that they really want to achieve. They may have unrealistic hopes that they will somehow get better without doing the work of therapy. They may feel hopeless about their ability to solve problems, affect their life, or change. They may even fear that if they get better, their life will get worse in some way (e.g., they will lose you as a therapist, or have to return to work). You need to be alert for the possibility of these kinds of interfering cognitions and help patients respond to them so they will be more amenable to the structure and tasks of treatment.

STRENGTHENING THE THERAPEUTIC ALLIANCE

A fourth common difficulty involves patients' unwillingness to conform to the prescribed structure because of their perceptions of and dysfunctional beliefs about themselves, about therapy, or about you. If you believe it will not interfere with the alliance, you may acknowledge patients' discomfort, but encourage them to comply as an experiment. At the other end of the spectrum, you may allow the patient to dominate and control the flow of the session—initially. With most patients, however, you will negotiate a compromise satisfactory to both of you, and you will try, over time, to move the patient toward the standard structure.

How do you determine whether the difficulty in adherence to session structure is due to faulty socialization or reluctance in complying? You first intervene by further socializing patients to the cognitive behavior therapy model and by monitoring their verbal and nonverbal responses. If it is simply a problem in socialization, patients' responses are fairly neutral (or perhaps slightly self-critical), and subsequent compliance is good.

THERAPIST: Can I interrupt for a moment? Can we get back to what happened when you called your friend?

PATIENT: Oh, sure.

When patients react negatively, they have undoubtedly perceived your request in a negative way, and you need to switch gears.

PATIENT: (*irritably*) But this thing with my mother is really upsetting.

THERAPIST: Oh, should we spend a few minutes on your mom, then? We may not have time, though, to get back to talking about David. Is that okay?

Problems can also arise if you impose structure in a controlling or demanding fashion. If patients are reluctant to provide you with honest feedback about how overbearing you are, you may not know you have made this mistake. It will be important for you to review a recording of the session, or better yet, have a peer, colleague, or supervisor review it. Then you can model apologizing, and remedy the problem at the next session: "I think I came across as too heavy-handed last week. I'm sorry, I do want to make sure that you agree with how the session goes."

Typical problems with each stage of the therapy session, excluding significant mistakes therapists make, are presented below.

MOOD CHECK

Common problems involve patients' failure to fill out forms, annoyance with forms, or difficulty in subjectively expressing (in a concise manner) their general mood during the week. If the difficulty is simply faulty socialization relating to completing the forms, you can ask patients whether they remember and agree with the rationale for filling them out, and determine whether there's a practical difficulty that needs to be resolved (e.g., insufficient time, forgetting, or a problem in literacy).

When patients are annoyed by the request to fill out the forms, you can ask for their automatic thoughts when thinking about or actually filling them out, or you can ask for the significance of the situation: "What's the worst part about them?" Or "What does it *mean* that I've asked you to fill out these forms?" You can then empathically respond to patients' concerns, help them evaluate relevant thoughts and beliefs, and/or do problem solving. These responses are provided in the three examples below.

PATIENT: These forms don't really seem to apply to me. Half of the questions are irrelevant.

THERAPIST: Yes, I know. But actually they're helpful to me—I can look at them quickly and get the overall picture, and not bother you with dozens of questions. Would you be willing to fill them out again next week, and we can talk more about them then if they still bother you?

In the next example, the patient clearly expresses his annoyance through his choice of words, tone of voice, and body language.

PATIENT: These forms are a waste of time. Half the questions are irrelevant.

THERAPIST: What's the worst part about filling them out?

PATIENT: I'm busy. I have a lot to do. If my life fills up with meaningless tasks, I'll never get anything done.

THERAPIST: I can see you feel pretty irritated. How long does it take to fill out these forms?

PATIENT: ... I don't know. A few minutes, I guess.

THERAPIST: I know some of the items don't apply, but actually they save us time in the therapy session because I don't have to ask you lots of questions myself. Could we try to problem-solve and see where you could fit in the time to do them?

PATIENT: I guess it's not that big a deal. I'll do them. I'll just leave work a little earlier next time.

Here I avoided directly evaluating the accuracy of the patient's automatic thoughts, because he is annoyed and I sense that he will perceive such questioning in a negative way. Instead I provide a rationale and help the patient realize that the task is not as time consuming as he has perceived it to be.

In a third case, I judge that further persuasion to fill out forms will negatively affect a tenuous therapeutic alliance.

PATIENT: (*in an angry voice*) I hate these forms. They don't apply to me. I know *you* want me to fill them out, but I'm telling you, they're worthless.

THERAPIST: Let's skip them, then, at least for the time being. I *would* like to get a clear idea of how you've been feeling during the week, though. Maybe you could just rate your emotions on a 0 to 100 or 0 to 10 scale.

A different problem involves patients' difficulty in subjectively expressing their mood, either because they do not do so concisely, or because they have difficulty labeling their moods. You might gently interrupt, and either ask specific questions or demonstrate to them how to respond.

THERAPIST: Can I interrupt for a moment? Can you tell me in just a sentence how your mood has been this week as compared to last week? I *do* want to hear more about the problem with your brother in a few minutes, but first I just need to know whether you've generally felt better, worse, or the same compared to last week.

PATIENT: A little worse, I think.

THERAPIST: More anxious? More sad? More angry?

PATIENT: Maybe a little more anxious. About the same amount of sad. Not angry really.

When patients have difficulty labeling their moods, you might respond differently:

THERAPIST: It sounds like it's hard to pin down how you've been feeling. Maybe we should put on the agenda "identifying feelings."

During the session, you might use the techniques described in Chapter 10 to teach patients to specify their mood.

BRIEF UPDATE

A common difficulty arises when patients provide too detailed an account of or unfocused rambling about their week. After several such sentences, you should gently jump in:

THERAPIST: Can I interrupt you for a moment? Right now, I just need to get the big picture of how you've been feeling. Could you just tell me about your week in two or three sentences? Was it generally a good week? A bad week? Or did it have its ups and downs?

If patients continue to offer details instead of the broader picture, you might demonstrate what you are looking for:

THERAPIST: It sounds to me like you're saying, "I had a pretty hard week. I had a fight with a friend, and I was really anxious about going out, and I had trouble concentrating on my work." Is that right?

Some patients do understand and are capable of providing a concise review, but do not *choose* to do so. If you have data to suggest that questioning patients about their reluctance to comply could damage the alliance, you may initially allow them to control the update portion of the session. (Such data might include patients' verbal and/or nonverbal reactions to your prior attempts at structuring, their direct statements of strong preferences in the therapeutic process, or their reports of a strong reaction in the past when they have perceived others as controlling or dominating.)

Extreme reactions to structuring are not common, however. Usually you can matter-of-factly elicit reasons for patients' reluctance, and then problem-solve. After asking patients to review their week more concisely and noting a negative shift in affect, you might ask, "When I just asked you to give me the big picture, what went through your mind?" Having identified patients' automatic thoughts, you might then (1) help them evaluate the validity of their thoughts, (2) use the downward arrow technique (see pages 206–208) to uncover the meaning of their thoughts, and/or (3) make an empathic statement and move straight to problem solving, as below:

THERAPIST: I'm sorry you felt I cut you off again. I can see you have a lot on your mind, and I *would* like to hear it. Do you want to continue with the update now, or should we put "update of week" on the agenda? I just want to make sure I know all the problems you want to talk about today.

This latter choice is usually better than helping patients evaluate their thoughts at the moment if they are particularly annoyed. By expressing your concern and willingness to compromise, you can often modify patients' perception that you are being too controlling.

BRIDGE BETWEEN SESSIONS

A problem arises when patients provide too much or too little information. For example, when asked to relate important events in the preceding week, patients can give too detailed an account, necessitating gentle interruption by the therapist. Or they may shrug or say that they cannot think of anything, and you either need to ask a more pointed question ("What happened when you went to see the professor?") or return to this question a little later on, if you have not collected the data you need. Patients may also have difficulty recalling the important points from the previous session, particularly if you neglected to send them home with therapy notes, or if they failed to read their notes for homework.

Typical difficulties in setting the agenda arise when patients fail to contribute to the agenda, ramble when setting the agenda, or are hopeless about discussing problems on the agenda. Patients who fail to contribute to the agenda may be inadequately socialized (or too confused to name specific problems), or they may put a special negative *meaning* on contributing. These two cases are illustrated below.

THERAPIST: What problem or problems do you want my help in solving today?

PATIENT: ... I don't know.

THERAPIST: What problems came up for you this past week? Or what problems do you expect might come up this week?

PATIENT: I don't know. Things are status quo, I guess.

THERAPIST: When did you feel worst this week?

PATIENT: (*Thinks.*) I don't know. The whole week was terrible.

THERAPIST: Do you think you felt worst during the day, when you were at work? Or in the evenings?

PATIENT: In the evenings, I guess.

THERAPIST: Okay, can we put "evenings" on the agenda to see if there's anything we can do to make them a little better?

PATIENT: All right.

At the end of the session, I will ask the patient to add a homework assignment to his list, to think about what problems he wants help in solving at the next session. If he fails to contribute to the agenda the following week, even in the face of an update that suggests he did experience some difficulties, I might elicit his automatic thoughts about and/or the meaning of my request.

THERAPIST: Were you able to think about problems you want help with?

PATIENT: (*in a slightly annoyed tone*) I thought about it. But I didn't come up with anything.

THERAPIST: How were you feeling when you were thinking about it? Annoyed?

PATIENT: Maybe a little.

THERAPIST: What was going through your mind?

PATIENT: I'm just not sure that this therapy is right for me.

THERAPIST: It's good you told me that. Do you have a sense of what might help you more?

PATIENT: My last therapist just let me talk about whatever I wanted. He didn't make me decide at the beginning.

THERAPIST: So when I ask you to name problems you want help with, do you feel kind of hemmed in?

PATIENT: Yeah, I guess it does.

THERAPIST: So let's figure out together how to make it better. Would you like to skip setting the agenda at the very beginning of our sessions? How would it be if you came in and talked about whatever you want for the first 10 minutes? Then I'd like to summarize what you said so I can make sure I really understood you. Then maybe we could pick something out from what you've said to focus on for the next part of the session. (*pause*) How does that sound?

PATIENT: It sounds better.

THERAPIST: Is there anything else that bothers you about this therapy?

PATIENT: No, I don't think so.

THERAPIST: Could you be sure to let me know if you think of something?

PATIENT: Okay.

This patient's response was unusual. Most patients are much more easily socialized into agenda setting. But in this case, I recognized that pushing the patient further might alienate him, so I demonstrated my desire to collaboratively "fix" the problem. He needed more flexibility in session structure initially, but I moved him toward a more standard structure as soon as I could.

Patients who ramble during agenda setting or launch into a detailed account of a problem instead of naming it usually just require further instruction.

THERAPIST: (*gently interrupting*) Can I interrupt you for a moment? Should we call this "problem with boss"?

PATIENT: Yes.

THERAPIST: Good. Can you tell me the name of any other problem you'd like my help in solving?

Patients who persist in the next session in describing problems rather than just naming them during agenda setting can be asked to jot down their agenda topics for homework (see Figure 7.1, page 102).

A third problem in agenda setting arises when patients feel hopeless about discussing their problems. Here I try to get the patient into a problem-solving mode.

THERAPIST: Okay. So on the agenda so far, we've got the problems of tiredness, organizing your finances, and balancing your checkbook. Anything else?

PATIENT: (*sighs*) No ... Yes ... I don't know ... I'm so overwhelmed. I don't think any of this is going to help.

THERAPIST: You don't think talking about your problems in here will help?

PATIENT: No. What's the use? I mean, you can't fix the fact that I owe too much money and I'm so tired I can't even get out of bed most mornings—not to mention the fact that I'm making so many mistakes at work that I'll probably get fired.

THERAPIST: Well, it's true that we can't fix everything at once. And you do have real problems that we need to work on together. Now, if we just have time to work on *one* thing today, which do you think will help more than the others?

PATIENT: I don't know ... the tiredness, maybe. If I could sleep better, maybe I could get more done.

In this case, I give the patient the message that his problems are real, that they can be worked on one by one, and that he need not work on them alone. Asking him to make a forced choice *does* help him focus on selecting a problem, and seems to help him get oriented toward problem solving. Had the patient refused to make a choice, I might have tried a different tactic:

THERAPIST: It sounds like you're feeling pretty hopeless. I don't know for sure that working together we can make a difference, but I'd like to try. Would you be willing to try? Could we talk about the tiredness for a few minutes and see what happens?

Acknowledging his hopelessness and my inability to guarantee success increased the patient's willingness to experiment with problem solving.

REVIEW OF HOMEWORK

A typical problem arises when therapists, in their haste to get to patients' agenda issues, fail to ask patients about the homework they did over the past week. You are more likely to remember to ask about homework if you keep it as a standard agenda item and if you review your therapy notes from the previous session before patients enter your office. The opposite problem sometimes arises when the therapist reviews homework (unrelated to the patient's distress that day) in too much detail before turning to the patient's agenda topics. Other homework problems are discussed in detail in Chapter 17.

DISCUSSION OF AGENDA ITEMS

Typical problems here include hopelessness, unfocused or tangential discussion, inefficient pacing, and the failure to make a therapeutic intervention. *Unfocused discussion* usually results when you fail to structure the discussion appropriately through gentle interruptions (guiding the patient back to the issue at hand); when you fail to emphasize *key* automatic thoughts, emotions, beliefs, and behaviors; and when you fail to summarize frequently. In the following transcript, I summarize several minutes of the patient's description in just a few words and redirect the patient to identify her automatic thoughts.

THERAPIST: Let me just make sure I understand. You had a fight with your sister yesterday. This reminded you of previous fights, and you began to get more and more angry. Last night you called her again, and she began to criticize you for not helping out with your mother. Is that right?

PATIENT: Yeah.

THERAPIST: What went through your mind as she said, "You're the black sheep of the family"?

Pacing is often a problem when you overestimate how many issues can be discussed during one therapy session. It is preferable to prioritize and then to specify two problems (or possibly a third) to be discussed during a session, especially if you are a novice cognitive behavior therapist. Together you and the patient should keep track of the time, and collaboratively decide what to do if time is running short. In practical terms, it is advisable to have two clocks (one for each of you to easily see) so you can encourage patients to monitor the passage of time along with you:

THERAPIST: We only have 10 minutes left before we have to start finishing up the session. Would you like to continue talking about this problem with your neighbor, or finish up in the next minute or two so we have time to discuss the problem with your coworker?

A third problem with discussion of problems is the *therapist's failure to make a therapeutic intervention*. Much of the time, merely describing a problem or identifying dysfunctional thoughts or beliefs related to the problem will *not* result in the patient's feeling better. You should be conscious of your goal to help patients (during the session itself) respond to their dysfunctional cognitions, solve or partially solve a problem, and set up homework assignments designed to ameliorate the problem or help them feel less distressed. Throughout the session, you should ask yourself:

> "How can I help the patient feel better by the end of the session?"
> "How can I help the patient have a better week?"

SETTING NEW HOMEWORK

Patients are less likely to do homework when the therapist:

> • Suggests an assignment that is too difficult or is unrelated to the patient's concerns.
> • Fails to provide a good rationale.

- Forgets to review homework assigned during previous sessions.
- Does not stress the importance of daily homework in general and of specific assignments.
- Does not explicitly teach the patient how to do the assignment.
- Does not start the assignment in session, do covert rehearsal (pages 303–305), or ask standard questions about potential obstacles that might get in the way.
- Does not have the patient write down the homework assignment.
- Noncollaboratively sets a homework assignment that the patient does not want to do.

If none of the above is true, you will try to ascertain whether patients hold dysfunctional beliefs about homework (e.g., "I should feel better without working hard"; "My therapist should cure me without my having to change things"; "I'm too incompetent to do homework"; "Homework is trivial and won't get me better"). You then help patients specify and test their dysfunctional ideas about homework. Homework is discussed more extensively in Chapter 17.

FINAL SUMMARY

You will periodically make summaries throughout the session to make sure you understand what patients have been expressing. If you have followed standard procedure and you have made sure the important points of the session are recorded as you go along, then the end summary can consist of a quick review of these notes and a verbal summary of any other topics that were discussed and of the homework assignments. Without therapy notes to refer to, patients usually experience difficulty summarizing the session and remembering the important conclusions they drew.

FEEDBACK

Problems arise when patients are distressed at the end of a session and you have not left sufficient time to resolve their distress, or when patients are upset but fail to relate their distress to you. A practical solution to avoid running out of time is to start closing down the session 5–10 minutes before the end. You can then more effectively review homework already assigned, discuss whether any other assignments might be helpful, summarize the session or ask patients to do so, and elicit and respond to feedback. A sample response to negative feedback follows:

THERAPIST: What did you think about today's session? Was there anything I got wrong? Or did I say anything that bothered you?

PATIENT: I don't think you realize how hard it is for me to get things done. I have so many responsibilities and so many problems. It's easy for *you* to say I should just concentrate on my work and forget all about what's happening with my boss.

THERAPIST: Oh, it's good you told me—and I'm sorry you got that impression. What I *meant* to get across was that I realize you are very distressed by the problem with your boss. I wish we had time to talk about that problem now. (*pause*) But meanwhile, was there something I said or did that made you think I was suggesting that you just forget all about the problem with your boss?

Next, I clarified the misunderstanding, and we agreed to put the problem on the agenda at our next session.

Therapists at all levels of experience encounter difficulties in structuring with particular patients. Careful review of your session tapes can be invaluable in identifying and then solving these problems. A more extensive account of how to conceptualize and modify problems patients present in session can be found in J. S. Beck (2005).

Chapter 9

IDENTIFYING AUTOMATIC THOUGHTS

The cognitive model states that the interpretation of a situation (rather than the situation itself), often expressed in automatic thoughts, influences one's subsequent emotion, behavior, and physiological response. Of course, certain events are almost universally upsetting: for example, a personal assault or rejection. People with psychological disorders, however, often misconstrue neutral or even positive situations, and thus their automatic thoughts are biased. By critically examining their thoughts and correcting thinking errors, they often feel better.

This chapter describes the characteristics of automatic thoughts. Then it describes how to:

> - Explain automatic thoughts to patients.
> - Elicit and specify automatic thoughts.
> - Teach patients to identify automatic thoughts.

CHARACTERISTICS OF AUTOMATIC THOUGHTS

Automatic thoughts are a stream of thinking that coexists with a more manifest stream of thought (Beck, 1964). These thoughts are not peculiar to people with psychological distress; they are an experience common to us all. Most of the time we are barely aware of these thoughts, although with just a little training we can easily bring these thoughts into consciousness. When we become aware of our thoughts, we may automatically do a reality check if we are not suffering from psychological dysfunction.

A reader of this text, for example, while focusing on the content of this chapter, may have the automatic thought, "I don't understand this," and feel slightly anxious. He may, however, spontaneously (i.e., without conscious awareness) respond to the thought in a productive way: "I *do* understand *some* of it; let me just reread this section."

This kind of automatic reality testing and responding to negative thoughts is a common experience. People who are in distress, however, may not engage in this kind of critical examination. Cognitive behavior therapy teaches them tools to evaluate their thoughts in a conscious, structured way, especially when they are upset.

Sally, for example, when she is reading an Economics chapter, has the same thought as the reader above: "I don't understand this." Her thinking becomes more extreme, however: "And I'll *never* understand it." She accepts these thoughts as correct and feels quite sad. After learning tools of cognitive behavior therapy, however, she is able to use her negative emotion as a cue to look for, identify, and evaluate her thoughts, and develop an adaptive response: "Wait a minute, it's not necessarily true that I'll never understand this. I am having some trouble now. But if I reread it or come back to it when I'm fresher, I may understand it more. Anyway, understanding it isn't crucial to my survival, and I can ask someone else to explain it to me if need be."

Although automatic thoughts seem to pop up spontaneously, they become fairly predictable once the patient's underlying beliefs are identified. You are concerned with identifying those thoughts that are dysfunctional—that is, those that distort reality, are emotionally distressing, and/or interfere with patients' ability to reach their goals. Dysfunctional automatic thoughts are almost always negative unless the patient is manic or hypomanic, has a narcissistic personality, or is a substance abuser.

Automatic thoughts are usually quite brief, and patients are often more aware of the *emotion* they feel as a result of their thoughts than of the thoughts themselves. Sitting in session, for example, patients may be somewhat aware of feeling anxious, sad, irritated, or embarrassed, but unaware of their automatic thoughts until their therapist questions them.

The emotions patients feel are logically connected to the content of their automatic thoughts. For example, a patient thinks, "I'm such a dope. I don't really understand what everyone [at the meeting] is saying," and feels sad. Another time he thinks, "She [my wife] doesn't appreciate me," and feels angry. When he has the thoughts, "What if my loan doesn't go through? What will I do next?" the patient feels anxious.

Automatic thoughts are often in "shorthand" form, but can be easily spelled out when you ask for the *meaning* of the thought. For example, when a patient had the thought, "Oh, no!" the meaning was, "[My boss] is going to give me too much work." "Damn!" for another patient was the expression of the idea, "I was stupid to leave my cell phone at home."

Automatic thoughts may be in verbal form, visual form (images), or both. In addition to his verbal automatic thought ("Oh, no!"), the patient above had an image of himself, alone at his desk late at night, toiling over taxes (see Chapter 16 for a description of automatic thoughts in imaginal form).

Automatic thoughts can be evaluated according to their *validity* and their *utility*. The most common type of automatic thought is distorted in some way and occurs despite objective evidence to the contrary. A second type of automatic thought is accurate, but the *conclusion* the patient draws may be distorted. For example, "I didn't do what I promised [a friend]" is a valid thought, but the conclusion, "Therefore I'm a bad person," is not.

A third type of automatic thought is also valid, but decidedly dysfunctional. For example, Sally was studying for an exam and thought, "It's going to take me hours to finish this. I'll be up until 3:00 A.M." This thought was undoubtedly accurate, but it increased her anxiety and decreased her concentration and motivation. A reasonable response to this thought would address its *utility*: "It's true it will take a long time to finish this, but I can do it; I've done it before. Dwelling on how long it will take makes me feel miserable, and I won't concentrate as well. It'll probably take even longer to finish. It would be better to concentrate on finishing one part at a time and giving myself credit for having finished it." Evaluating the validity and/or utility of automatic thoughts and adaptively responding to them generally produces a positive shift in affect.

To summarize, automatic thoughts coexist with a more manifest stream of thoughts, arise spontaneously, and are not based on reflection or deliberation. People are usually more aware of the associated emotion but, with a little training, they can become aware of their thinking. The thoughts relevant to personal problems are associated with *specific* emotions, depending on their content and meaning. They are often brief and fleeting, in shorthand form, and may occur in verbal and/or imaginal form. People usually accept their automatic thoughts as true, without reflection or evaluation. Identifying, evaluating, and responding to automatic thoughts (in a more adaptive way) usually produces a positive shift in affect.

EXPLAINING AUTOMATIC THOUGHTS TO PATIENTS

It is desirable to explain automatic thoughts by using the patient's own examples. In the context of discussing a specific problem with a patient, you will elicit the automatic thoughts associated with the problem.

THERAPIST: [moving to the first agenda topic] Should we talk about how upset you were at the park yesterday?

PATIENT: Yes.

THERAPIST: How were you feeling emotionally: Sad? Anxious? Angry?

PATIENT: Sad.

THERAPIST: What was going through your mind?

PATIENT: [further describing the situation instead of relating her automatic thoughts] I was looking at the people in the park, hanging out, playing Frisbee, things like that.

THERAPIST: What was going through your mind when you saw them?

PATIENT: I'll never be like them.

THERAPIST: Okay. [providing psychoeducation] You just identified what we call an *automatic thought*. Everyone has them. They are thoughts that just seem to pop into our heads. We're not deliberately trying to think about them; that's why we call them automatic. Most of the time, they're very quick and we're much more aware of the emotion—in this case, sadness—than we are of the thoughts. Lots of times the thoughts are distorted in some way. But we react *as if* they're true.

PATIENT: Hmmm.

THERAPIST: What we'll do is teach you to identify your automatic thoughts, and then evaluate them to see just how accurate they are. For example, in a minute we'll evaluate the thought, "I'll never be like them." What do you think would happen to your emotions if you discovered that your thought wasn't true—that when your depression lifts you'll realize that you *are* like the people in the park?

PATIENT: I'd feel better.

Here I suggest an alternative scenario in order to illustrate the cognitive model. Later in the session, I use Socratic questioning (see Chapter

11) to examine the thought with the patient so she can develop her own adaptive response. In the next part, I write down the automatic thought, emphasizing the cognitive model.

```
Situation: Looking at people at the park
                        ↓
Automatic thought: "I'll never be like them."
                        ↓
            Emotion: Sad
```

THERAPIST: Let's get that down on paper. When you have the thought, "I'll never be like them," you feel sad. Do you see how what you're thinking influences how you feel?

PATIENT: Uh-huh.

THERAPIST: That's what we call the *cognitive model*. What we'll do in therapy is teach you to identify your automatic thoughts when you notice your mood changing. That's the first step. We'll keep practicing it until it's easy. Then you'll learn how to evaluate your thoughts and change your thinking if it's not completely right. Is that clear?

PATIENT: I think so.

THERAPIST: [checking on the patient's understanding] Could you tell me in your own words about the relationship between thoughts and feelings?

PATIENT: Sometimes I have thoughts that are wrong and these thoughts make me feel bad ... But what if the thoughts are right?

THERAPIST: Good point. Then we'll do some problem solving or find out what's so bad about it if they *are* right. My guess, though, is that we'll find a lot of mistakes in your thinking because you *are* depressed. Unrealistically negative thinking is always part of depression. In any case, we'll figure out together whether your thoughts are right or wrong.

At the end of this session, I check again to ascertain how well the patient seems to understand the cognitive model.

THERAPIST: To review a bit, could you tell me what you now understand about the relationship between thoughts and feelings?

PATIENT: Well, sometimes automatic thoughts just pop into my head and I accept them as true. And then I feel ... whatever: sad, worried ...

THERAPIST: Good. How about for homework this week if you look for some of these automatic thoughts?

PATIENT: Okay.

THERAPIST: Why do you think I'm suggesting this?

PATIENT: Because sometimes my thoughts aren't true, and if I can figure out what I'm thinking, I can change it around and feel better.

THERAPIST: That's right. Okay, let's write this assignment down: Whenever I notice a change in mood or my mood is getting worse, ask myself ... Do you remember the question?

PATIENT: What was just going through my mind?

THERAPIST: Good! Get that down.

ELICITING AUTOMATIC THOUGHTS

The skill of learning to identify automatic thoughts is analogous to learning any other skill. Some patients (and therapists) catch on quite easily and quickly. Others need much more guidance and practice to identify automatic thoughts and images. The basic question you will ask is:

> **"What was going through your mind?"**

You will ask this question:

- When patients describe a problematic situation that arose, usually since your previous session together, or
- When you notice a shift to, or intensification of, negative affect during a session.

This latter situation is often important and it is vital to be alert to both verbal and nonverbal cues from the patient, so as to be able to elicit their "hot cognitions"—that is, important automatic thoughts and images that arise in the therapy session itself, and are associated with a change or increase in emotion. These hot cognitions may be about the patient herself ("I'm such a failure"), the therapist ("She doesn't understand me"), or the subject under discussion ("It's not fair that I have so much to do") and may undermine the patient's motivation or sense of adequacy or worth. They may interfere with the patient's concentration in session. Finally, they may interfere with the therapeutic relationship. Identifying automatic thoughts on the spot gives the patient the opportunity to test and respond to the thoughts immediately, so as to facilitate the work in the rest of the session.

How do you know when patients have experienced an affect shift? You are on the alert for nonverbal cues such as changes in facial expression, tightening of muscles, shifts in posture, or hand gestures. Verbal cues include change in tone, pitch, volume, or pace. Having noticed a change, you infer an affect shift and check it out by asking patients what just went through their mind.

Difficulties in Eliciting Automatic Thoughts

If patients are unable to answer the question "What was just going through your mind?" you can:

1. Ask them how they are/were feeling and where in their body they experienced the emotion.
2. Elicit a detailed description of the problematic situation.
3. Request that the patient visualize the distressing situation.
4. Suggest that the patient role-play the specific interaction with you (if the distressing situation was interpersonal).
5. Elicit an image.
6. Supply thoughts opposite to the ones you hypothesize actually went through their minds.
7. Ask for the meaning of the situation.
8. Phrase the question differently.

These techniques are illustrated in the transcripts below.

Heightening the Emotional and Physiological Response

THERAPIST: Sally, when you were thinking about volunteering in class, what was just going through your mind?

PATIENT: I'm not sure.

THERAPIST: How were you feeling?

PATIENT: Anxious, I think.

THERAPIST: Where did you feel the anxiety?

PATIENT: Here (*pointing to her abdomen*). In the pit of my stomach.

THERAPIST: Can you feel the same feeling now?

PATIENT: (*Nods.*)

THERAPIST: So you're sitting in class, thinking about volunteering, and you feel that anxiety in the pit of your stomach ... What's going through your mind?

PATIENT: If I say something, it won't come out right. People will judge me.

Eliciting a Detailed Description

THERAPIST: So, you were alone in your room last night and you began feeling really upset?

PATIENT: Yes.

THERAPIST: What was going through your mind?

PATIENT: I don't know. I was just feeling so down, sad.

THERAPIST: Can you describe the scene for me? What time was it? Were you alone? What were you doing? What else was going on?

PATIENT: It was about 6:15. I had just gotten back from dinner. The dorm was pretty empty because I ate early. I was about to get my books out of my backpack so I could do my Chem homework ...

THERAPIST: So you were about to do your homework and you were thinking ...

PATIENT: [expressing her automatic thoughts] This is just too hard. I'll never understand it.

THERAPIST: And then what happened?

PATIENT: I just lay down on my bed.

THERAPIST: And as you were lying there, what was going through your mind?

PATIENT: I don't want to do this. I don't want to be here.

Visualizing the Situation

THERAPIST: Sally, can you imagine that you're back in the class *right now*, the professor is talking, the student next to you is whispering, you're feeling nervous ... Can you visualize it, as if it's happening right now? How big is the class? Where are you sitting? What is the professor saying? What are you doing? And so on.

PATIENT: I'm in my Economics class. The professor is standing in front of the class. Let's see, [shifting to past tense, which makes the experience less immediate and decreases the emotional response] I was sitting about three-quarters of the way back, I was listening pretty hard ...

THERAPIST: [guiding the patient to speak as if it's happening right at the moment] So, "I'm sitting three-quarters of the way back, I'm listening pretty hard ..."

PATIENT: She's saying something about what topics we can choose, a macroeconomic view of the economy or ... something, and then this guy on my left leans over and whispers, "When's the paper due?"

THERAPIST: And what's going through your mind right now?

PATIENT: What did she say? What did I miss? Now I won't know what to do.

Re-Creating an Interpersonal Situation through Role Play

Patients describe who said what verbally, then patients play themselves while you play the other person in the interaction.

THERAPIST: So, you were feeling down as you were talking to your classmate about the assignment?

PATIENT: Yes.

THERAPIST: What was going through your mind as you were talking to her?

PATIENT: (*Pauses.*) ... I don't know. I was just really down.

THERAPIST: Can you tell me what you said to her and what she said to you?

PATIENT: (*Describes verbal exchange.*)

THERAPIST: How about if we try a role play? I'll be the classmate and you be you.

PATIENT: Okay.

THERAPIST: While we're recreating the situation, see if you can figure out what's going through your mind.

PATIENT: (*Nods.*)

THERAPIST: Okay, you start. What do you say first?

PATIENT: Lisa, can I ask you a question?

THERAPIST: Sure, but can you call me later? I've got to run to my next class.

PATIENT: It's fast. I just missed part of what Dr. Smith said about our paper.

THERAPIST: I'm really in a hurry now. Call me after 7 o'clock, okay? Bye ... Okay, out of role play. Were you aware of what was going through your mind?

PATIENT: Yeah. I was thinking that she was too busy for me, that she didn't really want to help me, and I wouldn't know what to do.

THERAPIST: You had the thoughts, "She's too busy for me," "She doesn't really want to help me," "I won't know what to do."

PATIENT: Yes.

THERAPIST: And those thoughts made you feel sad?

PATIENT: Yes.

Eliciting an Image

THERAPIST: So, when I asked, "How's school going?" you felt sad. What was going through your mind?

PATIENT: I think I was thinking about my Economics class, getting my paper back.

THERAPIST: Did you imagine that? Did you have an image in your mind?

PATIENT: Yeah. I pictured a "C" at the top, in red ink.

Suggesting an Opposite Thought

THERAPIST: So when you were sitting alone in your room, were you thinking how *great* everything is going?

PATIENT: No, not at all! I was thinking that I don't know whether I belong here.

Uncovering the Meaning of the Situation

THERAPIST: What did it mean to you that you got a B– on your paper?

PATIENT: That I'm not smart enough. I don't have what it takes.

Phrasing the Question Differently

THERAPIST: So when your mom didn't call you back, what were you thinking? Were you making a prediction? Were you remembering something?

It is also possible, though usually less desirable, to ask patients, "What do you guess what you were thinking?" or "Could you have been thinking about _____ or _____?" because patients may speculate inaccurately. Sometimes, however, these two questions are effective.

You will try one or more of the techniques above when patients have difficulty identifying their automatic thoughts. But if they still experience difficulty, you might collaboratively decide to change the subject, to avoid patients' feeling that they are being interrogated, or to reduce the possibility of their viewing themselves as a failure:

THERAPIST: Well, sometimes these thoughts are hard to catch. No big deal. How about if we move on to _____.

Identifying Additional Automatic Thoughts

It is important to continue questioning patients even after they report an initial automatic thought. Additional questioning may bring to light other important thoughts.

THERAPIST: So when you got the test back, you thought, "I should have done better. I should have studied harder." What else went through your mind?
PATIENT: Everyone else probably did better than I did.
THERAPIST: Then what?
PATIENT: I was thinking, "I shouldn't even be here. I'm such a failure."

You should be aware that patients may, in addition, have other automatic thoughts not about the same situation itself, but about their *reaction* to that situation. They may perceive their emotion, behavior, or physiological reaction in a negative way.

THERAPIST: So you had the thought, "I might embarrass myself," and you felt anxious? Then what happened?
PATIENT: My heart started beating real fast and I thought, "What's wrong with me?"
THERAPIST: And you felt...?
PATIENT: More anxious.
THERAPIST: And then?
PATIENT: I thought, "I'll never feel okay."
THERAPIST: And you felt...?
PATIENT: Sad and hopeless.
THERAPIST: And then...?
PATIENT: I felt so bad I thought I wouldn't be much fun at lunch with Allison so I told her I wasn't feeling well and just went back to my room.

Note that the patient first had automatic thoughts about a specific situation (volunteering in class). Then she had thoughts about her anxiety and her bodily reaction. In many cases, these secondary emotional reactions can be quite distressing, and significantly compound an already upsetting situation. Then Sally made a negative prediction that affected her behavior.

To work most efficiently, it is important to determine at which point patients were *most* distressed (before, during, or after a given incident), and what their automatic thoughts were at that point. Patients may have had distressing automatic thoughts:

- *Before* a situation, in anticipation of what might happen ("What if she yells at me?"),
- *During* a situation ("She thinks I'm stupid"), and/or
- *After* a situation, reflecting on what had happened ("I can't do anything right; I never should have tried").

Identifying the Problematic Situation

Sometimes, in addition to being unable to identify automatic thoughts associated with a given emotion, patients have difficulty even identifying a particular situation or issue that is most troublesome to them (or which part is the most upsetting). When this happens, you can help them pinpoint the most problematic situation by proposing a number of upsetting problems, asking them to hypothetically eliminate one problem, and determining how much relief the patient feels. Once a specific situation has been identified, the automatic thoughts are more easily uncovered.

THERAPIST: [summarizing] So, you've been very upset for the past few days and you're not sure why, and you're having trouble identifying your thoughts—you just feel upset most of the time. Is that right?

PATIENT: Yes. I just don't know why I've been so upset all the time.

THERAPIST: What kinds of things have you been thinking about?

PATIENT: Well, school for one. And I'm not getting along well with my roommate. And then I tried to get hold of my mother again and I couldn't reach her, and, I don't know, just everything.

THERAPIST: So, there is a problem with school, with your roommate, with reaching your mom ... anything else?

PATIENT: Yeah. I haven't been feeling too well. I'm afraid I might be getting sick.

THERAPIST: Which of these situations bothers you the most—school, roommate, reaching your mom, feeling sick?

PATIENT: Oh, I don't know. I'm worried about all of them.

THERAPIST: Let's jot these four things down. Now let's say hypothetically we could completely eliminate the feeling sick problem. Let's say you now feel physically fine, how anxious are you now?

PATIENT: About the same.

THERAPIST: Okay. Say, hypothetically, you do reach your mom right away after therapy, and everything's fine with her. How do you feel now?

PATIENT: A little bit better. Not that much.

THERAPIST: Okay. Let's say the school problem—what is the school problem?

PATIENT: I have a paper due next week.

THERAPIST: Okay, let's say you've just handed the paper in early, and you're feeling good about it. Now how do you feel?

PATIENT: That would be a great relief, if that paper were done and I thought I'd done well.

THERAPIST: So it sounds as if it's the paper that is the most distressing situation.

PATIENT: Yeah. I think so.

THERAPIST: Now, just to make sure ... If you still had the paper to do, but the roommate problem disappeared, how would you feel?

PATIENT: Not that good. I think it *is* the paper that's bothering me the most.

THERAPIST: In a moment, we'll focus on the school problem, but first I'd like to review how we figured it out, so you'll be able to do it yourself in the future.

PATIENT: Well, you had me list all the things I was worried about, and pretend to solve them one by one.

THERAPIST: And then you were able to see which one would give you the most relief if it had been resolved.

PATIENT: Yeah.

We then focus on the school problem, identifying and responding to automatic thoughts and doing some problem solving.

The same process can be used in helping the patient to determine which *part* of a seemingly overwhelming problem is most distressing.

THERAPIST: So you've been pretty upset about your roommate. What *specifically* has been bothering you?

PATIENT: Oh, I don't know. Everything.

THERAPIST: Can you name some things?

PATIENT: Well, she's been taking my food and not replacing it. Not in a malicious way, but it still bothers me. And she's got a boyfriend, and whenever she talks about him, it reminds me that I don't have one. And she's messy; she leaves stuff all around ... And she's kind of inconsiderate. Sometimes she talks really loudly on her cell phone.

THERAPIST: Anything else?

PATIENT: Those are the major things.

THERAPIST: Okay, we've done this before. Let me read these back to you so you can figure out which one bothers you the most. If you can't, we'll hypothetically eliminate them one by one, and see which one makes the biggest difference in how you feel. Okay?

Differentiating between Automatic Thoughts and Interpretations

When you ask for patients' automatic thoughts, you are seeking the *actual* words or images that have gone through their mind. Until they have learned to recognize these thoughts, many patients report *interpretations*, which may or may not reflect their actual thoughts. In the following transcript, I guide a patient in reporting her thoughts.

THERAPIST: When you saw that woman in the cafeteria, what went through your mind?

PATIENT: I think I was denying my real feelings.

THERAPIST: What were you actually thinking?

PATIENT: I'm not sure what you mean.

In this exchange, the patient reported an *interpretation* of what she was feeling and thinking. Below, I try again, by focusing on and heightening her emotion.

THERAPIST: When you saw her, what emotion did you feel?

PATIENT: I think I was just denying my feelings.

THERAPIST: Uh-huh. What feelings were you denying?

PATIENT: I'm not sure.

THERAPIST: [supplying an emotion opposite to the expected one to jog her recall] When you saw her, did you feel happy? Excited?

PATIENT: No, not at all.

THERAPIST: Can you remember walking into the cafeteria and seeing her? Can you picture that in your mind?

PATIENT: Uh-huh.

THERAPIST: What are you feeling?

PATIENT: Sad, I think.

THERAPIST: As you look at her, what goes through your mind?

PATIENT: [reporting an emotion and a physiological reaction, instead of an automatic thought] I feel really sad, an emptiness in the pit of my stomach.

THERAPIST: What's going through your mind now?

PATIENT: She's really smart. [automatic thought] I'm nothing compared to her.

THERAPIST: Okay. Anything else?

PATIENT: No. I just walked over to the table and started talking to my friend.

Specifying Automatic Thoughts Embedded in Discourse

Patients need to learn to specify the actual words that go through their minds in order to evaluate them effectively. Following are some examples of embedded thoughts versus actual words:

Embedded expressions	Actual automatic thoughts
I guess I was wondering if he likes me.	Does he like me?
I don't know if going to the professor would be a waste of time.	It'll probably be a waste of time if I go.
I couldn't get myself to start reading.	I can't do this.

You gently lead patients to identify the *actual* words that went through their mind.

THERAPIST: So when you turned bright red in class, what went through your mind?

PATIENT: I guess I was wondering if he thought I was strange.

THERAPIST: Can you recall the exact words you were thinking?

PATIENT: (*puzzled*) I'm not sure what you mean.

THERAPIST: Were you thinking, "I guess I was wondering if he thought I was strange," or were you thinking, "Does he think I'm strange?"

PATIENT: Oh, I see, the second one. Or actually I think it was, "He probably thinks I'm strange."

Changing the Form of Telegraphic or Question Thoughts

Patients often report thoughts that are not fully spelled out. As it is difficult to evaluate such a telegraphic thought, you guide the patient to express the thought more fully.

THERAPIST: What went through your mind when the paper was announced?

PATIENT: "Uh-oh." I just thought, "Uh-oh."

THERAPIST: Can you spell the thought out? "Uh-oh" means ...

PATIENT: I'll never get the work done in time. I have too much to do.

If patients are unable to spell out their thought, you might try supplying an opposite thought: "Did 'Uh-oh' mean, 'That's really good'?"

Automatic thoughts are sometimes expressed in the form of a question, making evaluation difficult. Therefore, you guide patients in expressing their thoughts in a statement form prior to helping them evaluate it.

THERAPIST: So you felt anxious? What was going through your mind right then?

PATIENT: I was thinking, "Will I pass the test?"

THERAPIST: Okay. Were you thinking you probably would or wouldn't pass the test?

PATIENT: That I wouldn't.

THERAPIST: Okay. So can we rephrase your thought as, "I might not pass the test"?

Another example follows:

THERAPIST: So you had the thought, "What will happen to me [if I get more and more nervous]?" What are you *afraid* could happen?

PATIENT: I don't know ... lose control, I guess.

THERAPIST: Okay, let's look at that thought, "I could lose control."

Here I lead the patient into revealing precisely what she fears. In the next example, the patient initially has difficulty identifying the fear behind her automatic thought. I try several different questions.

THERAPIST: So you thought, "What next?" What did you think would happen next?

PATIENT: I don't know.

THERAPIST: Were you afraid something specific might happen?

PATIENT: I'm not sure.

THERAPIST: What's the worst thing that *could* happen in this situation?

PATIENT: Ummm ... that I'd get kicked out of school.

THERAPIST: Do you think that was what you were afraid would happen?

Other examples of how questions can be restated in order to be evaluated more effectively are presented below:

Question	Statement
"Will I be able to cope?"	"I won't be able to cope."
"Can I stand it if she leaves?"	"I won't be able to stand it if she leaves."
"What if I can't do it?"	"I'll lose my job if I can't do it."
"What if she gets mad at me?"	"She'll hurt me if she gets mad at me."
"How will I get through it?"	"I won't be able to get through it."
"What if I can't change?"	"I'll be miserable forever if I can't change."
"Why did this happen to me?"	"This shouldn't have happened to me."

Recognizing Situations That Can Evoke Automatic Thoughts

Up to this point, most of the examples of automatic thoughts provided in this chapter have been associated with external events (e.g., talking to a friend) or a stream of thoughts (e.g., thinking about an upcoming exam). But a wide range of both external stimuli and internal experiences can give rise to automatic thoughts. As illustrated in Figure 9.1,

Situation/Stimulus	Example	Automatic Thoughts
External event (or series of events)	Mother keeps hanging up the phone.	"How dare she treat me like this!"
Stream of thoughts	Thinking about the exam	"I'll never learn this stuff."
Cognition: thought, image, belief, daydream, dream, memory, flashback	Becomes aware of a violent image.	"I must be crazy."
	Has a flashback of a traumatic event	"I'll never get over this. I'll always be plagued by these terrible flashbacks."
Emotion	Anger	"I shouldn't be angry at him. I'm such a bad person."
Behavior	Binge eats	"I'm so weak. I just can't get my eating under control."
Physiological or mental experience	Rapid heartbeat	"What if there's something seriously wrong with me?"
	Sense of unreality	"I must be going crazy."

FIGURE 9.1. Situations that evoke automatic thoughts.

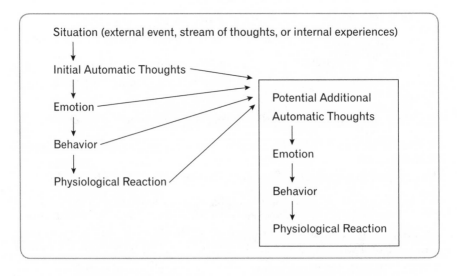

FIGURE 9.2. Initial and secondary thoughts and reactions.

patients may have automatic thoughts in other categories, too. They can have thoughts about their cognitions (thoughts, images, beliefs, day-dreams, dreams, memories, or flashbacks), their emotions, their behavior, or their physiological or mental experiences. Any of these stimuli may engender an initial automatic thought (or series of automatic thoughts), followed by an initial emotional, behavioral, and/or physiological reaction. Patients may then have additional thoughts about any part of the cognitive model, leading to an additional associated emotional, behavioral, and/or physiological reaction (Figure 9.2).

TEACHING PATIENTS TO IDENTIFY AUTOMATIC THOUGHTS

As described in Chapter 5, you can begin teaching patients the skill of identifying automatic thoughts even during the first session. Here I have just demonstrated the cognitive model, using Sally's own examples.

THERAPIST: Sally, when you notice your mood changing or getting worse in the next week, could you stop and ask yourself, "What is going through my mind right now?"

PATIENT: Yeah.

THERAPIST: Maybe you could jot down a few of these thoughts on a piece of paper?

PATIENT: Sure.

In later sessions, you might also explicitly teach the patient other techniques if the basic question ("What's going through your mind right now?") is not effective.

THERAPIST: Sometimes you may not be able to tell what you were thinking. So either at the time or later, you can try what we just did here in session. Replay the scene as vividly as you can in your imagination, as if it's happening again, and concentrate on how you're feeling. Then ask yourself, "What's going through my mind?" Do you think you could do that? Or should we practice it again?

PATIENT: I'll give it a try.

Again, if asking the basic questions and trying the imagery technique are not sufficient, you might explicitly teach the patient to hypothesize about her thoughts. This method is less desirable because it is more likely the patient will report a later interpretation instead of her actual thoughts at the time.

THERAPIST: If you still have trouble figuring out what was going through your mind, here are some other questions [see Figure 9.3 you can ask yourself.

PATIENT: Okay.

THERAPIST: First question: If I had to, what would I guess I was thinking about? Or could I have been thinking about _____ or _____? Or, was I imagining something or remembering something? Or, finally, what does this situation mean to me? Or you might try to figure out what the opposite thought might be to jog your memory.

PATIENT: Okay.

TECHNIQUES TO ELICIT AUTOMATIC THOUGHTS

Basic question:

What was going through your mind just then?

To identify automatic thoughts:

1. Ask this question when you notice a shift in (or intensification of) affect during a session.

2. Have the patient describe a problematic situation or a time during which she experienced an affect shift and ask the above question.

3. If needed, have the patient use imagery to describe the specific situation or time in detail (as if it is happening now) and then ask the above question.

4. If needed or desired, have the patient role-play a specific interaction with you and then ask the above question.

Other questions to elicit automatic thoughts:

1. What do you guess you were thinking about?

2. Do you think you could have been thinking about _____ or _____? (Therapist provides a couple of plausible possibilities.)

3. Were you imagining something that might happen or remembering something that did?

4. What did this situation mean to you? (Or say about you?)

5. Were you thinking _____? (Therapist provides a thought opposite to the expected response.)

FIGURE 9.3. Summary of techniques to identify automatic thoughts. From J. S. Beck (2011). Copyright 2011 by Judith S. Beck. Reprinted by permission.

THERAPIST: How about trying out these questions this week if you have trouble identifying your automatic thoughts, and if imagining the situation again doesn't help?

PATIENT: Fine.

To summarize, people with psychological disorders make predictable errors in their thinking. You teach patients to identify their dysfunctional thinking, then to evaluate and modify it. The process starts with the recognition of specific automatic thoughts in specific situations. Identifying automatic thoughts is a skill that comes easily and naturally to some patients and is more difficult for others. You need to listen closely to ensure that patients report actual thoughts, and you may need to vary your questioning if patients do not readily identify their thoughts. The next chapter clarifies, among other things, the difference between automatic thoughts and emotions.

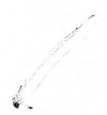

Chapter 10

● ● ○

IDENTIFYING EMOTIONS

E motions are of primary importance in cognitive behavior therapy. After all, the major goals of treatment are symptom relief (especially a reduction in the patient's level of distress) and a remission of the patient's disorder.

Intense negative emotion is painful and may be dysfunctional if it interferes with a patient's capacity to think clearly, solve problems, act effectively, or gain satisfaction. Patients with a psychiatric disorder often experience an intensity of emotion that can seem excessive or inappropriate to the situation. Sally, for example, felt enormous guilt and then sadness when she had to cancel a minor social event with her roommate. She was also extremely anxious about going to a professor for help. Yet the intensity and quality of patients' emotions make sense when you recognize the strength of their automatic thoughts and the beliefs (which are usually quite painful) that have become activated.

It is important to acknowledge and empathize with how patients feel and refrain from challenging or disputing their emotions. Evaluate the thoughts and beliefs that underlie patients' distress to reduce their dysphoria; do not evaluate their emotions.

You won't discuss *all* situations in which patients feel dysphoric, though—you will use your conceptualization of the patient to decide which problems are most important. Typically, the most important problems are those associated with high levels of distress. Problems in which patients seem to be having a "normal" level of distress are usually less important. The aim of cognitive behavior therapy is not to get rid of all distress; negative emotions are as much a part of the richness of life as positive emotions and serve as important a function as does physical pain, often alerting us to potential problems that may need to be addressed.

In addition, you will seek to increase patients' *positive* emotions through discussion (usually relatively brief) of their interests, positive events that occurred during the week, and positive memories. You will often suggest homework assignments aimed at increasing the number of activities in which the patient is likely to experience mastery and pleasure (see Chapter 6).

This chapter explains how to:

> - Differentiate automatic thoughts from emotions.
> - Distinguish among emotions.
> - Label emotions.
> - Rate the intensity of emotions.

DISTINGUISHING AUTOMATIC THOUGHTS FROM EMOTIONS

Many patients do not clearly understand the difference between their thoughts and their emotions. You will endeavor to make sense of the patients' experience and share your understanding with them. You will continually and subtly help patients view their experiences through the cognitive model.

You will organize the material patients present into the categories of the cognitive model: situation, automatic thought, and reaction (i.e., emotion, behavior, and physiological response). Be alert to occasions when patients confuse their thoughts and emotions. At these times, based on the flow of the session, their goals, and the strength of the collaboration, you may decide to:

> - Ignore the confusion,
> - Address it at the time (either subtly or explicitly), or
> - Address it later.

Most of the time, mislabeling a thought as a feeling is relatively unimportant in a given context, and you can make a subtle correction.

THERAPIST: You mentioned when we set the agenda that you wanted to talk about the phone call you had with your brother?

PATIENT: Yeah. I called him a couple of nights ago and he sounded kind of distant.

THERAPIST: And how were you feeling emotionally?

PATIENT: I felt like he really didn't want to talk, like he didn't really care whether I had called or not.

THERAPIST: So when you had the thoughts, "He doesn't really want to talk. He doesn't really care that I called," how did you feel emotionally? Sad? Angry? Something else?

In another session, I viewed the confusion as important because I wanted to teach Sally how to evaluate her thinking, using the Thought Record (page 195). I deliberately decided to distinguish the two, judging that it was important to do so at the time, and that the flow of the session would not be unduly interrupted and that important data would not be forgotten.

THERAPIST: Were there any times this week when you thought about going out for a walk?

PATIENT: Yeah, a few times.

THERAPIST: Can you remember one time specifically?

PATIENT: Last night after dinner, I was cleaning up ... I don't know.

THERAPIST: How were you feeling emotionally?

PATIENT: [expressing thoughts] Oh, I was feeling like it's no use, that it probably wouldn't help.

THERAPIST: Those are important thoughts. We'll get back to evaluating them in a minute, but first I'd like to review the difference between thoughts and feelings. Okay?

PATIENT: Sure.

THERAPIST: Feelings are what you feel *emotionally*—usually they're one word, such as sadness, anger, anxiety, and so on. (*pause*) Thoughts are *ideas* that you have; you think them either in words or in pictures or images. (*pause*) Do you see what I mean?

PATIENT: I think so.

THERAPIST: So let's get back to the time last night when you thought about going out for a walk. What emotion were you feeling?

PATIENT: Sad, I think.

THERAPIST: And your thoughts were, "This is no use. I'll never get better"?

PATIENT: Yes.

In the examples above, Sally initially labeled thoughts as feelings. At times, patients do the reverse: that is, they label an emotion as a thought.

THERAPIST: As you walked into your empty dorm room, Sally, what went through your mind?

PATIENT: I was sad, lonely, real down.

THERAPIST: So you felt sad and lonely and down. What thought or image made you feel that way?

Importance of Distinguishing among Emotions

You continuously conceptualize patients' problems, trying to understand their experience and point of view and how their underlying beliefs give rise to specific automatic thoughts in a specific situation, influencing their emotions and behavior. The connection among patients' thoughts, emotion, and behavior should make sense. You will investigate further when patients report an emotion *that does not seem to match* the content of their automatic thoughts, as in the transcript below.

THERAPIST: How did you feel when your mother didn't call you back right away?

PATIENT: I was sad.

THERAPIST: What was going through your mind?

PATIENT: I was thinking, "What if something happened to her? Maybe there's something wrong."

THERAPIST: And you felt sad?

PATIENT: Yes.

THERAPIST: I'm a little confused because those sound more like *anxious* thoughts. Was there anything else going through your mind?

PATIENT: I'm not sure.

THERAPIST: How about if we have you imagine the scene? [helping the patient vividly recall the scene in imagery form] You said you were sitting by the phone, waiting for her call?

PATIENT: And then I thought, "What if something happened? Maybe there's something wrong."

THERAPIST: What happens next?

PATIENT: I'm looking at the phone, and I get teary.

THERAPIST: What's going through your mind?

PATIENT: If anything happened to Mom, there would be no one left who cares.

THERAPIST: "There would be no one left who cares." How does that thought make you feel?

PATIENT: Sad. Real sad.

This interchange started with a discrepancy. I was alert and so was able to pick up an inconsistency between the *content* of the automatic thought and the *emotion* associated with it. I was then able to help Sally retrieve a key automatic thought by using imaginal recall. Had I chosen to focus on the anxious thoughts, I may have missed Sally's central concern. Although it may have been helpful to focus on a less central thought, finding and working with *key* automatic thoughts usually speeds up therapy.

DIFFICULTY IN LABELING EMOTIONS

Most patients easily and correctly label their emotions. Some, however, display a relatively impoverished vocabulary for emotions; others understand emotional labels intellectually but have difficulty labeling their own specific emotions. In either of these two cases, it is useful to have patients link their emotional reactions in specific situations to their labels. Devising an "Emotion Chart" such as the one in Figure 10.1 helps patients learn to label their emotions more effectively. Patients can list current or previous situations in which they felt a particular emotion and refer back to it whenever they are having difficulty naming how they felt.

THERAPIST: I'd like to spend a few minutes talking about different emotions so we can both understand better how you feel in different situations. Okay?

Angry	Sad	Anxious
1. Brother cancels plans with me.	1. Mom doesn't return phone call.	1. Seeing how low my bank account is.
2. Friend doesn't return my gym bag.	2. Not enough money to go away on vacation.	2. Hearing that we might have a tornado.
3. Carpool driver plays music too loudly.	3. Nothing to do on Saturday.	3. Finding a bump on my neck.

FIGURE 10.1. Sample Emotion Chart.

PATIENT: Sure.

THERAPIST: Can you remember a time when you felt angry?

PATIENT: Uh, yeah ... When my brother cancelled plans to see this movie; I forget which one, but I really wanted to go. Anyway, he told me he was going out with his friends instead ...

THERAPIST: And what was going through your mind?

PATIENT: Who does he think he is? I wouldn't do that to him. He should treat me better.

THERAPIST: And you felt—

PATIENT: Mad.

Here I had the patient recall a *specific* event in which he felt a given emotion. From his description, it sounded as if he had correctly identified his emotion. Because I wanted to make sure, I asked him to identify his automatic thoughts. The content of the automatic thoughts did match his stated emotion.

Next, I asked the patient to recall other occasions when he felt angry, sad, and anxious. Again I asked for his specific automatic thoughts in these situations to ensure he was accurately labeling his emotions. We then created the Emotion Chart (Figure 10.1). I asked the patient to refer to it in session and at home whenever he was having difficulty labeling what he was feeling.

It is not necessary to use this technique to differentiate emotions with most patients. Others may benefit from a quick discussion along the above lines. A few might profit from a list of negative emotions (see Figure 10.2) and a brief discussion.

Sad, down, lonely, unhappy

Anxious, worried, fearful, scared, tense

Angry, mad, irritated, annoyed

Ashamed, embarrassed, humiliated

Disappointed

Jealous, envious

Guilty

Hurt

Suspicious

FIGURE 10.2. Negative emotions.

RATING DEGREES OF EMOTION

It is sometimes important for patients not only to *identify* their emotions, but also to quantify the *degree* of emotion they are experiencing. Some have dysfunctional beliefs about experiencing emotion (Greenberg, 2002; Holland, 2003; Leahy, 2003)—for example, believing that if they feel a small amount of distress, it will increase and become intolerable. Learning to rate the intensity of emotions aids patients in testing this belief.

In addition, you will assess whether questioning and adaptively responding to a thought or belief have been effective, so you can judge whether a cognition requires further intervention. Failure to do so may sometimes lead you to inaccurately conclude that an intervention has succeeded, and you may proceed to the next thought or problem prematurely. Or the opposite may happen—you may continue discussing an automatic thought or belief, not realizing that the patient is no longer significantly distressed by it.

Finally, gauging the intensity of an emotion in a given situation helps you and the patient determine whether that situation warrants closer scrutiny. A situation that is relatively less emotionally laden may be less valuable to discuss than one that is more distressing to the patient, where important beliefs may have been activated.

Most patients learn to judge the intensity of an emotion fairly easily.

THERAPIST: How did you feel when your friend said, "Sorry, I don't have time now"?

PATIENT: Pretty sad, I guess.

THERAPIST: If 100% is the saddest you ever felt or could imagine feeling, and 0% is completely *not* sad, how sad did you feel right when he said, "Sorry, I don't have time now"?

PATIENT: About 75%.

Some patients have difficulty with or don't like putting a specific number to the intensity. You can simply ask them to rate whether they experienced the emotion "a little," "a medium amount," "very," or "completely." If even that is difficult, drawing a scale can help:

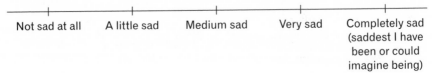

THERAPIST: How did you feel when your friend said, "Sorry, I don't have time now"?

PATIENT: Sad.

THERAPIST: How sad did you feel, 0 to 100%?

PATIENT: I'm not sure. I'm not too good with numbers.

THERAPIST: Do you think you felt a little sad? A medium amount sad? Very sad? Or completely sad?

PATIENT: What were the choices again?

THERAPIST: Here, let me draw a scale. Your sadness—would you say (*pointing to the scale*) that you were a just a little, a medium amount, very sad, or completely sad?

PATIENT: Oh, very sad.

THERAPIST: Okay, we've got our scale now. Let's see how useful it is. Were you sad any other times this week?

PATIENT: Yeah, last night when I locked myself out of my room.

THERAPIST: Use your new scale as a guide. About how sad did you feel?

PATIENT: Well, between a medium amount and very sad.

THERAPIST: Good. Now, do you think you could use this scale as a guide whenever you're trying to figure out how sad you are?

PATIENT: Yes, I can do that.

USING EMOTIONAL INTENSITY TO GUIDE THERAPY

Patients may not realize which situations they should bring up for discussion. You can ask them to rate the degree of distress they are still experiencing to decide whether discussion of a given situation is likely to help. In the next transcript, I quickly realize that Sally and I will probably not accomplish much by focusing on an initial situation that she has described:

THERAPIST: So a problem you want to talk about has to do with your roommate?

PATIENT: Yeah.

THERAPIST: Did something come up this week?

PATIENT: Well, I felt bad when she went out with her boyfriend instead of me.

THERAPIST: How bad did you feel, 0 to 100%?

PATIENT: I don't know. Maybe 25%?

THERAPIST: And now?

PATIENT: (*Thinks.*) Less.

THERAPIST: Sounds like this wasn't a terribly upsetting situation. Was there another time this week when you got pretty upset with her?

In summary, you aim to obtain a clear picture of situations that are distressing to patients. You help them clearly differentiate their thoughts from their emotions. You empathize with their emotions throughout this process and help them evaluate the dysfunctional thinking that has influenced their mood.

Chapter 11

EVALUATING
AUTOMATIC THOUGHTS

Patients have hundreds or thousands of thoughts a day, some dysfunctional, some not. You will have time to evaluate only few, at most, in a given session. This chapter describes how to:

- Select key automatic thoughts.
- Use Socratic questioning to evaluate automatic thoughts.
- Assess the outcome of the evaluation process.
- Conceptualize when evaluation is ineffective.
- Use alternate methods of questioning and responding to automatic thoughts.
- Respond when automatic thoughts are true.
- Teach patients to evaluate their automatic thoughts.

SELECTING KEY AUTOMATIC THOUGHTS

You have identified an automatic thought. Patients may have made a spontaneous utterance during a session (e.g., "I just don't think anything can help me"); related an automatic thought, often from the past week; or reported an automatic thought they predict will arise in the future. Next you need to conceptualize whether this is an important thought on which to focus; that is, is it currently distressing or dysfunctional or likely to recur? If it was an automatic thought from the past week, you might ask:

> "In what situation did you have this thought? How much did you believe it at the time? How much do you believe it now?"
>
> "How did it make you feel emotionally? How intense was the emotion then? How intense is the emotion now?"
>
> "What did you do?"

You will also ask yourself whether the patient is likely to have this kind of thought again and be distressed by it. You will vary these questions slightly if the patient spontaneously uttered the thought and/or if the thought is related to a future situation. You also should find out whether additional thoughts were more central or distressing:

> "What else went through your mind [in this situation]? Did you have any other thoughts or images?"
>
> "Which thought/image was most upsetting?"

In the transcript below, I determine that Sally's automatic thought was important:

THERAPIST: [summarizing] So you were in class on Thursday, and you didn't know the answers to questions that your professor threw out to the class, and you felt really sad because you thought, "I'll never make it here." How much did you believe that thought, and how sad did you feel?

PATIENT: I believed it a lot, and I felt really sad.

THERAPIST: How much do you believe it now, and how sad do you feel now?

PATIENT: I still think I won't make it.

THERAPIST: And is the thought still distressing?

PATIENT: Very.

This turned out to be an important automatic thought for us to evaluate. In another case, though, Sally and I judged that a different automatic thought was probably not worth discussing. Sally was describing a problem she had had in the library, and I asked her a few questions to evaluate whether this was an important situation to discuss.

THERAPIST: [summarizing] So you were in the library and you couldn't find the book you needed, and you thought, "They are so inefficient. The system is so bad," and you felt frustrated. How frustrated did you feel?

PATIENT: Oh, like 90%.

THERAPIST: Are you still that frustrated?

PATIENT: No, I got over it.

THERAPIST: What did you do when you were frustrated?

PATIENT: I went back to my room and worked on my chemistry problems instead. I ended up borrowing the book from Lisa. I have to give it back to her by Monday, though.

THERAPIST: So you solved the problem. Do you think the library could be a problem in the future? Might you get frustrated and leave, but not do something productive? Or not get the book you need another way?

PATIENT: I think I'm all right. I know what to expect. If I hadn't gotten the book from Lisa, I would have gone back to the library later and asked for help.

THERAPIST: That's good … Sounds like you've got a plan in case anything else comes up. Should we move on to something else?

Here I judge that the automatic thought, while upsetting at the time, did not warrant further discussion because (1) Sally was no longer distressed by it, (2) she had acted in a functional way, (3) the situation was resolved, and (4) she had a good solution if the same problem recurred.

Why do patients bring up problems and automatic thoughts that are not important? Most of the time, it is because they are simply not socialized enough to treatment. But they can learn the skill of figuring out what is most important to talk about.

Even if a patient reports an important automatic thought, you might decide not to focus on it, especially if:

- You judge that doing so might impair the therapeutic relationship (e.g., you perceive that the patient is feeling invalidated).
- The patient's level of distress is too high to evaluate his thinking.
- There's insufficient time in the session to help the patient respond effectively to the thought.

- You assess that it is more important to work on another element of the cognitive model (e.g., you might focus instead on solving the problematic situation, teaching the patient emotional regulation techniques, discussing more adaptive behavioral responses, or addressing the patient's physiological response).
- You assess that it is more important to elicit and work on a dysfunctional belief underlying the automatic thought.
- You assess that it is more important to discuss a different problem.

QUESTIONING TO EVALUATE AN AUTOMATIC THOUGHT

Having elicited an automatic thought, determined that it is important and distressing, and identified its accompanying reactions (emotional, physiological, and behavioral), you may collaboratively decide with the patient to evaluate it. *You would rarely directly challenge the automatic thought*, however, for three reasons.

1. You usually do not know in advance the degree to which any given automatic thought is distorted (e.g., Sally's thought that no one wanted to have dinner with her could have been valid).
2. A direct challenge can lead patients to feel invalidated (e.g., Sally might think, "[My therapist] is telling me I'm wrong").
3. Challenging a cognition violates a fundamental principal of cognitive behavior therapy, that of collaborative empiricism: You and the patient together examine the automatic thought, test its validity and/or utility, and develop a more adaptive response.

It is also important to keep in mind that automatic thoughts are rarely completely erroneous. Usually, they contain at least a grain of truth (which is important that you acknowledge).

Figure 11.1 contains a list of Socratic questions to help patients evaluate their thinking. (Actually, "Socratic" is a misnomer some of the time; the Socratic questioning method, derived from the philosopher Socrates, involves a dialectical discussion.) Patients need a structured method to evaluate their thinking; otherwise, their responses to automatic thoughts can be superficial and unconvincing and will fail to improve their mood or functioning. The evaluation should be even-handed. You do not want patients, for example, to ignore evidence that supports an automatic thought, devise an alternative explanation that is not likely, or adopt an unrealistically positive view of what might happen.

It is important to relate to patients that not all of the questions in Figure 11.1 are suitable for every automatic thought. Moreover, using all of the questions, even if they logically apply, may be too cumbersome and time consuming. Patients may not evaluate their thoughts at all if they consider the process too burdensome. Usually you will introduce just one or a few questions at a time.

You may use questioning from the very first session to evaluate a specific automatic thought. In a subsequent session, you will begin to explain the process more explicitly, so patients can learn to evaluate their thinking between sessions:

THERAPIST: (*Summarizes past portion of the session; writes automatic thoughts on paper for both to see*) So when you met your friend Karen on the way to the class, you had the thought, "She doesn't really care what happens to me," and that thought made you feel sad?

PATIENT: Yeah.

THERAPIST: And how much did you believe that thought at the time?

PATIENT: Oh, pretty much. About 90%.

THERAPIST: And how sad did you feel?

PATIENT: Maybe 80%.

THERAPIST: Do you remember what we said last week? Sometimes automatic thoughts are true, sometimes they turn out not to be true, and sometimes they have a grain of truth. Can we look at this thought about Karen now, and see how accurate it seems?

PATIENT: Okay.

You can use any set of questions to help patients evaluate their thinking, but Figure 11.1 can be helpful as it guides you and the patient to:

- Examine the validity of the automatic thought.
- Explore the possibility of other interpretations or viewpoints.
- Decatastrophize the problematic situation.
- Recognize the impact of believing the automatic thought.
- Gain distance from the thought.
- Take steps to solve the problem.

1. What is the evidence that supports this idea?
    What is the evidence against this idea?

2. Is there an alternative explanation or viewpoint?

3. What is the *worst* that could happen (if I'm not already thinking the worst)?
    If it happened, how could I cope?
    What is the best that could happen?
    What is the most realistic outcome?

4. What is the effect of my believing the automatic thought?
    What could be the effect of changing my thinking?

5. What would I tell _____ [a specific friend or family member]
    if he or she were in the same situation?

6. What should I do?

FIGURE 11.1. Questioning automatic thoughts.

Each of the questions is described below.

The "Evidence" Questions

Because automatic thoughts usually contain a grain of truth, patients usually do have some evidence that supports their accuracy (which you will seek first), but they often fail to recognize evidence to the contrary (which you will seek second):

THERAPIST: What's the evidence that Karen doesn't care what happens to you?

PATIENT: Well, when we passed on Locust Walk, she seemed like she was real rushed. She just quickly said, "Hi, Sally, see you later," and kept going fast. She hardly even looked at me.

THERAPIST: Anything else?

PATIENT: Well, sometimes she's pretty busy and doesn't have much time for me.

THERAPIST: Anything else?

PATIENT: (*Thinks.*) No. I guess not.

THERAPIST: Okay, now is there any evidence on the other side, that maybe she *does* care about what happens to you?

PATIENT: (*answering in general terms*) Well, she is pretty nice. We've been friends since school started.

THERAPIST: [helping Sally think more specifically] What kinds of things does she do or say that might show she likes you?

PATIENT: Ummm ... she usually asks if I want to go get something to eat with her. Sometimes we stay up pretty late just talking about things.

THERAPIST: Okay. So, on the one hand, on this occasion yesterday, she rushed by you, not saying much. And there have been other times, too, when she's been pretty busy. But on the other hand, she asks you to eat with her, and you stay up late talking sometimes. Right?

PATIENT: Yeah.

Here I gently probed to *uncover evidence* regarding the validity of Sally's thought. Having elicited evidence on both sides, I summarized what Sally said.

The "Alternative Explanation" Questions

Below, I help Sally *devise a reasonable alternative explanation* for what has happened.

THERAPIST: Good. Now, let's look at the situation again. Could there be an alternative explanation for what happened, other than she doesn't care about what happens to you?

PATIENT: I don't know.

THERAPIST: Why else might she have rushed by quickly?

PATIENT: I'm not sure. She might have had a class. She might have been late for something.

The "Decatastrophizing" Questions

Many patients predict a worst-case scenario. If a patient's automatic thought does not contain a catastrophe, it is often useful to ask the patients about their worst fear. In both cases, you should follow up by asking patients what they can do if the worst does happen.

THERAPIST: Okay. Now, what would be the *worst* that could happen in this situation?

PATIENT: That she would truly not like me, I guess. That I couldn't count on her for support.

THERAPIST: How could you cope with that?

PATIENT: Well, I wouldn't be happy about it. I guess I'd have to stop counting on her friendship.

THERAPIST: [asking leading questions to help her develop a robust response] Do you have other friends you could count on?

PATIENT: Yes.

THERAPIST: So you'd be okay?

PATIENT: Yes, I would.

Patients' worst fears are often unrealistic. Your objective is to help them think of more realistic outcomes, but many patients have difficulty doing so. You might help them extend their thinking by first asking for the best outcome.

THERAPIST: Now the worst may be unlikely to happen. What's the *best* that could happen?

PATIENT: That she'll realize she cut me off. That she'll apologize.

THERAPIST: And what's the *most realistic outcome*?

PATIENT: That she really was busy and we'll continue to be friends.

In the previous section, I help Sally see that even if the worst happened, she would cope. She also realizes that her worst fears are unlikely to come true.

> **Q:** What if ... patients' worst fears are that they will die?
>
> **A:** You obviously would not ask the "How would you cope?" question. Instead you might ask for the best and most realistic outcomes. You may also decide to explore what the worst part of dying would be: fears of the process of dying, fears of what they imagine an afterlife might be like for them, or fears of what would happen to loved ones after the patient's death.

The "Impact of the Automatic Thought" Questions

Below, I help Sally *assess the consequences of responding and not responding* to her distorted thinking.

THERAPIST: And what is the *effect of your thinking* that she doesn't like you?

PATIENT: It makes me sad. I think it kind of makes me withdraw from her.

THERAPIST: And what could be the *effect of changing your thinking?*
PATIENT: I'd feel better.

The "Distancing" Questions

Patients often benefit from getting some distance from their thoughts by imagining what they would tell a close friend or family member in a similar situation.

THERAPIST: Sally, let's say your friend Allison had a friend who sometimes was rushed, but seemed caring at other times. If Allison had the thought, "My friend doesn't care about me," what would you tell her?
PATIENT: I guess I'd tell her not to put too much importance on the times she seemed rushed, especially if her friend was nice about it.
THERAPIST: Does that apply to you?
PATIENT: Yes, I guess it does.

The "Problem-Solving" Questions

The answer to this question may be cognitive and/or behavioral in nature. The cognitive part would entail having patients remember their responses to the questions. In Sally's case, we came up with a behavioral plan:

THERAPIST: And what do you think you should *do* about this situation?
PATIENT: Uh ... I'm not sure what you mean.
THERAPIST: Well, have you withdrawn any since this happened yesterday?
PATIENT: Yeah, I think so. I didn't say much when I saw her this morning.
THERAPIST: So this morning you were still acting as if that original thought were true. How could you act differently?
PATIENT: I could talk to her more, be friendlier myself.

If I were unsure of Sally's social skills or motivation to carry through with this plan of being friendlier to Karen, I might have spent a few minutes asking Sally such questions as "When might you see her again?"; "Would it be worth it, do you think, to seek her out yourself?"; "What could you say to her when you do see her?"; "Anything you think could get in the way of your saying that?" (If needed, I might have modeled what she could say to Karen, and/or engaged Sally in a role play.)

ASSESSING THE OUTCOME
OF THE EVALUATION PROCESS

In the last part of this discussion, I assess how much Sally now believes the original automatic thought and how she feels emotionally, so I can decide what to do next in the session.

THERAPIST: Good. Now, how much do you believe this thought: "Karen doesn't really care what happens to me"?

PATIENT: Not very much. Maybe 20%.

THERAPIST: Okay. And how sad do you feel?

PATIENT: Not much either.

THERAPIST: Good. It sounds like this exercise was useful. Let's go back and see what we did that helped.

You and the patient will not use all the questions in Figure 11.1 for every automatic thought you evaluate. Sometimes none of the questions seems useful, and you might take another tack altogether (see pages 178–186).

CONCEPTUALIZING WHY THE EVALUATION
OF AN AUTOMATIC THOUGHT WAS INEFFECTIVE

If the patient still believes the automatic thought to a significant degree and does not feel better emotionally, you need to conceptualize why this initial attempt at cognitive restructuring has not been sufficiently effective. Common reasons to consider include the following:

1. There are other, more central automatic thoughts and/or images left unidentified or unevaluated.
2. The evaluation of the automatic thought is implausible, superficial, or inadequate.
3. The patient has not sufficiently expressed the evidence that he or she believes supports the automatic thought.
4. The automatic thought itself is also a core belief.
5. The patient understands intellectually that the automatic thought is distorted, but does not believe it on an emotional level.

In the first situation, *the patient has not verbalized the most central automatic thought or image.* John, for example, reports the thought, "If I try out [for the community basketball team], I probably won't make it." Evaluating this thought does not significantly affect his dysphoria because he has other important (but unrecognized) thoughts: "What if they think I'm a lousy player?" "What if I make stupid mistakes?" He also has an image of the coach and other players watching him with mocking, scornful faces.

In a second situation, *the patient responds to an automatic thought superficially.* John thinks, "I won't finish all my work. I have too much to do." Instead of carefully evaluating the thought, John merely responds, "No, I'll probably get it done." This response is insufficient, and his anxiety does not decrease.

In a third situation, *the therapist does not thoroughly probe for, and therefore the patient does not fully express the evidence that his or her automatic thought is true,* resulting in an ineffective adaptive response, as seen here:

THERAPIST: Okay, John, what evidence do you have that your sister doesn't want to bother with you?

PATIENT: Well, she hardly ever calls me. I always call her.

THERAPIST: Okay, anything on the other side? That she does care about you, that she does want a good relationship with you?

Had John's therapist queried him further, he would have uncovered other evidence that John has to support his automatic thought: that his sister spent more time with her girlfriends during vacations than with John, that she sounded impatient on the phone when he called, and that she had not sent him a birthday card. Having elicited this additional data, the therapist could have helped John weigh the evidence more effectively and investigated alternative explanations for his sister's behavior.

In a fourth situation, *the patient identifies an automatic thought that is also a core belief.* John often thinks, "I'm incompetent." He believes this idea so strongly that a single evaluation does not alter his perception or the associated affect. His therapist needs to use many techniques over time to alter this belief (see Chapter 14).

In a fifth situation, *the patient indicates that he believes an adaptive response "intellectually," in his mind, but not "emotionally," in his heart, soul, or gut.* He discounts the adaptive response. In this case, the therapist and patient need to explore an unarticulated belief that lies *behind* the automatic thought:

THERAPIST: How much do you believe that it's not your fault if you get laid off?

PATIENT: Well, I can see it intellectually.

THERAPIST: But?

PATIENT: Even though I know the economy is bad, I still think I should be able to hold on to my job.

THERAPIST: Okay, let's assume for a moment that you do get laid off. What would be the worst part about that, or what would that mean?

Here, John's therapist discovers that he does not really believe the adaptive response and uncovers an assumption: *If I lose my job, it means I'm incompetent.*

To summarize, having evaluated an automatic thought, you ask patients to rate how much they believe the adaptive response and how they feel emotionally. If their belief is low and they are still distressed, you conceptualize why examining the thought did not alleviate their distress and plan a strategy for what to do next.

USING ALTERNATE METHODS TO HELP PATIENTS EXAMINE THEIR THINKING

In lieu of or in addition to using the questions in Figure 11.1, you can do the following:

> • Vary your questions.
> • Identify the cognitive distortion.
> • Use self-disclosure.

These strategies are described below.

Using Alternative Questions

The following transcript is just one illustration of how to vary your questions when you predict that standard questions will be ineffective.

THERAPIST: What went through your mind [when you asked your mom if it was all right with her to shorten your time together, and she sounded hurt and angry]?

PATIENT: That I should have known it was a bad time to call. I shouldn't have called.

THERAPIST: What's the evidence that you shouldn't have called?

PATIENT: Well, my mother is usually rushed in the morning. If I had waited until after she got home from work, she might have been in a better frame of mind.

THERAPIST: Had that occurred to you?

PATIENT: Well, yeah, but I wanted to let my friend know right away whether I could visit, so she could make plans.

THERAPIST: So you actually had a reason for calling when you did, and it sounds as if you knew it might be risky, but you really wanted to let your friend know as soon as you could?

PATIENT: Yeah.

THERAPIST: Is it reasonable to be so hard on yourself for taking the risk?

PATIENT: No ...

THERAPIST: You don't sound convinced. How bad is it anyway, in the scheme of things, for your mom to feel hurt that you want to spend one week of your summer vacation with your friend?

I followed up these questions with others: How hurt did your mother feel? How long did the hurt last at that level? How does she probably feel now? Is it possible for you to spare your mother hurt all the time? Can you possibly do what is good for you and not hurt your mother at all, given that she wants to spend as much time with you as she can? Is it desirable to have a goal of *never* hurting someone else's feelings? What would you have to give up yourself?

The previous transcript demonstrates how to use nonstandard questions to help patients adopt a more functional perspective. Although I started out questioning the *validity* of the thought, I shifted the emphasis to the *implicit underlying belief* (which we had previously discussed in other contexts): "It's bad to hurt other people's feelings." At the end, I asked the patient an open-ended question ("How do you see the situation now?") to see whether she needed more help in responding to her thoughts. Note that many questions I asked were a variation of Question 2 in Figure 11.1: "Is there an alternative explanation [for why you called when you did and for why your mother was hurt, other than that you were bad and at fault]?"

Identifying Cognitive Distortions

Patients tend to make consistent errors in their thinking. Often there is a systematic negative bias in the cognitive processing of patients who suffer from a psychiatric disorder (Beck, 1976). The most common errors are presented in Figure 11.2 (see also Burns, 1980). It often helps to label distortions and to teach patients to do the same. You might make mental notes of a patient's common distortions and point out a specific distortion when you spot a pattern:

THERAPIST: Sally, this idea that you either get an "A" and you're a success, or you don't and you're a failure—that's what we call all-or-nothing thinking. Does it seem familiar? I remember you also thought that either you understood everything in a chapter, or you were stupid. Do you think it could be helpful to watch out for this kind of thinking?

You can also provide patients with a list of distortions, such as the one in Figure 11.2, if you judge that they will not be overwhelmed by it. At another session, I gave Sally the list, and together we identified her typical automatic thoughts and the distortions they represented. For example:

Catastrophizing: "I'll flunk out of school."

All-or-nothing thinking: "If I can't read the entire chapter, it's not worth reading any of it."

Mind reading: "My roommate doesn't want to be bothered with me."

Emotional reasoning: "I feel so incompetent."

Sally kept this list handy and often referred to it when she was evaluating her automatic thoughts. Doing so helped her gain additional distance from her thinking and allowed her to believe more strongly that perhaps an automatic thought was not true, or not completely true.

Using Self-Disclosure

At times, you might use judicious self-disclosure instead of or in addition to Socratic questioning or other methods, to demonstrate how you were able to change similar automatic thoughts that you had, as illustrated below:

THERAPIST: You know, Sally, sometimes I have thoughts like yours: "I have to make everyone happy." But then I remind myself that I have a responsibility to take care of myself, and that the world probably won't end if someone is disappointed. (*pause*) Do you think that applies to you, too?

Although some automatic thoughts are true, many are either untrue or have just a grain of truth. Typical mistakes in thinking include:

1. **All-or-nothing thinking** (also called black-and-white, polarized, or dichotomous thinking): You view a situation in only two categories instead of on a continuum.
   Example: "If I'm not a total success, I'm a failure."

2. **Catastrophizing** (also called fortune-telling): You predict the future negatively without considering other, more likely outcomes.
   Example: "I'll be so upset, I won't be able to function at all."

3. **Disqualifying or discounting the positive**: You unreasonably tell yourself that positive experiences, deeds, or qualities do not count.
   Example: "I did that project well, but that doesn't mean I'm competent; I just got lucky."

4. **Emotional reasoning**: You think something must be true because you "feel" (actually believe) it so strongly, ignoring or discounting evidence to the contrary.
   Example: "I know I do a lot of things okay at work, but I still feel like I'm a failure."

5. **Labeling**: You put a fixed, global label on yourself or others without considering that the evidence might more reasonably lead to a less disastrous conclusion.
   Example: "I'm a loser. He's no good."

6. **Magnification/minimization**: When you evaluate yourself, another person, or a situation, you unreasonably magnify the negative and/or minimize the positive.
   Example: "Getting a mediocre evaluation proves how inadequate I am. Getting high marks doesn't mean I'm smart."

7. **Mental filter** (also called selective abstraction): You pay undue attention to one negative detail instead of seeing the whole picture.
   Example: "Because I got one low rating on my evaluation [which also contained several high ratings] it means I'm doing a lousy job."

8. **Mind reading**: You believe you know what others are thinking, failing to consider other, more likely possibilities.
   Example: "He thinks that I don't know the first thing about this project."

(cont.)

FIGURE 11.2. Thinking errors. Adapted with permission from Aaron T. Beck.

9. **Overgeneralization**: You make a sweeping negative conclusion that goes far beyond the current situation.
   Example: "[Because I felt uncomfortable at the meeting] I don't have what it takes to make friends."

10. **Personalization**: You believe others are behaving negatively because of you, without considering more plausible explanations for their behavior.
   Example: "The repairman was curt to me because I did something wrong."

11. **"Should" and "must" statements** (also called imperatives): You have a precise, fixed idea of how you or others should behave, and you overestimate how bad it is that these expectations are not met.
   Example: "It's terrible that I made a mistake. I should always do my best."

12. **Tunnel vision**: You only see the negative aspects of a situation.
   Example: "My son's teacher can't do anything right. He's critical and insensitive and lousy at teaching."

FIGURE 11.2. *(cont.)*

WHEN AUTOMATIC THOUGHTS ARE TRUE

Sometimes automatic thoughts turn out to be true, and you may choose to do one or more of the following:

- Focus on problem solving.
- Investigate whether the patient has drawn an invalid or dysfunctional conclusion.
- Work on acceptance.

These strategies are described below.

Focus on Problem Solving

Not all problems can be solved, but if a patient's perception of a situation appears to be valid, you might investigate whether the problem can be solved, at least to some degree. In the transcript below, Sally and I have evaluated her automatic thought, "I'm going to run out of money," and the evidence seems clear that this is a valid perception.

THERAPIST: So even if you're careful, it looks as if you won't be able to come up with rent toward the end of the school year ... Have you already tried to do something about this?

PATIENT: No, not really. I don't want to ask my parents for more. They're pretty strapped as it is.

THERAPIST: But you might be able to use them as a last resort?

PATIENT: Maybe ...

THERAPIST: Have you thought of anything else?

PATIENT: No, I don't think there's anything else I can do.

THERAPIST: Have you talked to the dean of students?

PATIENT: I hadn't thought of that.

THERAPIST: Quite possibly he could help. I imagine there are other students who are also struggling financially. He might suggest another student loan, or a payment plan, or maybe there's some emergency fund you could tap into.

PATIENT: I hope so.

THERAPIST: Well, do you want to start with the dean? If that doesn't work out, we can brainstorm other ideas: getting a job, moving in with someone else, borrowing from another relative ... There might be lots of things that you could do that you haven't thought of because you've been so depressed.

Investigate Invalid Conclusions

While an automatic thought might be true, the *meaning* may be invalid or at least not completely valid (as illustrated below), and you can examine the underlying belief or conclusion.

THERAPIST: So it looks as if you really did hurt your friend's feelings.

PATIENT: Yeah, I feel so bad about it.

THERAPIST: What does it mean about you that you hurt her feelings? Or what are you afraid will happen?

PATIENT: I should never have said that to her. I'm a terrible friend ... I'm a terrible person! She'll never want to talk to me again!

THERAPIST: Okay, can we look at that first? What other evidence do you have that you're a terrible person? ... Is there evidence on the other side, that maybe you're not?

Work toward Acceptance

Some problems cannot be solved and may never be solved, and patients need help in accepting that outcome. They may continue to feel miserable if they have unrealistic expectations or hopes that an unresolvable problem will somehow, almost magically, improve. Meanwhile, they need assistance in learning to focus on their core values, emphasize the more rewarding parts of their lives, and enrich their experience in new ways. A number of strategies designed to enhance acceptance can be found in Hayes and colleagues (2004).

TEACHING PATIENTS TO EVALUATE THEIR THINKING

At some point, you may give a copy of the questions in Figure 11.1 to the patient. You could do so immediately following the part of a session in which you have verbally asked these questions. Or you would wait until a later time if your questioning was not very effective, if you don't have enough time to review Figure 11.1 with the patient, or if you think the patient would be overwhelmed. Many patients do better if you teach them just one or two questions, writing them on a separate piece of paper. You can give the full list to other patients and just mark the questions as you review them.

Learning to evaluate automatic thoughts is a skill. Some patients grasp it right away; others need much repeated, guided practice in a graded fashion. For example, one patient might be helped with a variation of the "evidence" question: "How do I know this thought is true?" Another patient who often catastrophizes might do better with a variation of the "decatastrophizing" question: "If the worst happens, how would I cope? What are the best and most realistic outcomes?" Still another patient might find it most useful to answer the "distancing" question: "If [my sister-in-law] were in this situation and had this thought, what would I tell her?"

When patients seem ready to learn this skill, select an automatic thought for which most of the questions in Figure 11.1 are likely to apply. Following an examination of one of Sally's automatic thoughts, I point out the process to her:

THERAPIST: If you're like most people, you may find that using these questions at home is sometimes harder than it looks. In fact, there will be lots of times when we really need to work together to help you examine a thought. But give it a try, and if you have trouble we can talk about it next week. Okay?

Predicting that patients may have some difficulty can help allay self-criticism or defeatism if the assignment doesn't go smoothly. Had I suspected, despite my admonition, that Sally would judge herself harshly for not being able to fulfill the homework assignment perfectly, I would have pursued the subject more thoroughly:

THERAPIST: Sally, if you do have trouble evaluating your thoughts this week, how are you likely to feel?

PATIENT: Frustrated, I guess.

THERAPIST: What's likely to go through your mind?

PATIENT: I don't know. I'll probably just quit.

THERAPIST: Can you imagine looking at the sheet of paper and not being able to figure out what to do?

PATIENT: Yeah.

THERAPIST: What's going through your mind as you look at the paper?

PATIENT: "I should be able to do this. I'm so stupid."

THERAPIST: Good! Do you think it would help to have a written reminder that it's just a skill you'll get better at as you learn more and more here with me?

PATIENT: Yes. (*Writes it in her therapy notes.*)

THERAPIST: Do you think this response will help enough? Or do you think we should put off this assignment until we have more time to practice together?

PATIENT: No. I think I can try it.

THERAPIST: Okay, now if you do get frustrated and have automatic thoughts, be sure to jot them down. Okay?

Here I make the assignment into a no-lose proposition: Either Sally does it successfully, or she has some difficulty that I can help her with at the next session. If frustrated, she either reads her therapy notes (and probably feels better), or keeps track of her thoughts so she can learn to respond to them in the next session.

TAKING A SHORTCUT: NOT USING THE QUESTIONS AT ALL

Finally, when patients have progressed in therapy and can automatically evaluate their thoughts, you may sometimes just ask them to *devise an adaptive response.*

PATIENT: [When I get ready to ask my roommate to keep the kitchen neater] I'll probably think I should just clean it better myself.

THERAPIST: Can you think of a more helpful way to view this?

PATIENT: Yeah. That it's better for me to stand up for myself. That I'm doing something reasonable. I'm not being mean or asking her to do more than her share. That she'll probably take it okay, like she did the last time I asked her to clean up.

THERAPIST: Good. What do you think will happen to your anxiety if you say that to yourself?

PATIENT: It'll go down.

Here's another example:

THERAPIST: Anything you can think of that might get in the way of your starting the chemistry assignment?

PATIENT: I might think there's too much to do and get overwhelmed.

THERAPIST: Okay, if you do have the thought, "There's too much to do," what can you tell yourself?

PATIENT: That I don't have to do it all in one night, that I don't have to understand it perfectly this first time through.

THERAPIST: Good. Will that be enough, do you think, to go ahead and start the assignment?

Evaluating automatic thoughts is a specific skill, one at which both therapists and patients improve with repeated practice. The next chapter describes how to help patients respond to their automatic thoughts.

Chapter 12

RESPONDING TO
AUTOMATIC THOUGHTS

The previous chapter demonstrated how to help patients evaluate important automatic thoughts and determine the effectiveness of their evaluation in session. This chapter describes how to facilitate patients' evaluation of and response to automatic thoughts *between sessions*. Patients experience two kinds of automatic thoughts outside of session: ones they have already identified and evaluated in session, and novel cognitions. For the former group, you will ensure that patients have recorded robust responses in writing (on paper or an index card, in a therapy notebook, or on a smartphone) or in an audio format (on an audiotape or CD, in a recorded message on their phone, etc.).

To respond to novel automatic thoughts between sessions, you will teach patients to use the list of questions in Figure 11.1 (either mentally or in writing), or to use a worksheet such as the Thought Record in Figure 12.1 or an easier version, the "Testing Your Thoughts" Worksheet in Figure 12.2. But there are other ways to respond to automatic thoughts. Patients can engage in problem solving, use distraction or relaxation techniques, or label and accept their thoughts and emotions without evaluation.

REVIEWING THERAPY NOTES

Having evaluated an automatic thought with patients (usually through Socratic questioning), you will ask them to summarize. For example, you might pose one of the following questions:

"Can you summarize what we've just been talking about?"

"What do you think would be important for you to remember this week?"

"If the situation comes up again, what do you wish you could tell yourself?"

When patients express a cogent summary, you can ask them if they would like to record it, so they can better remember the response when similar automatic thoughts arise in the future. In the following transcript, Sally and I have just evaluated her thought "I can't do it," using many of the questions in Figure 11.1 (page 172). I ask her to summarize.

THERAPIST: Okay, Sally, so if you open your chemistry text this week and again have the thought "I can't do it," what do you want to remind yourself?

PATIENT: That it's probably not true. That I can probably do at least some of it, because I have in the past, and I can get help if I don't understand all of it. I guess doing part of the reading is better than not doing any at all.

THERAPIST: That's good. Should we record that?

Q: What if ... patients' responses are superficial, confused, or too wordy?

A: You might say, "Well, I think that's close, but I wonder if it would be more helpful to remember it this way ..." If their answers are reasonable but incomplete, you might ask, "Do you also want to remind yourself that...?" If they agree, you or they can record your suggestions.

It is desirable to have patients read their therapy notes each morning and pull them out, as needed, during the day. Patients tend to integrate responses into their thinking when they have rehearsed them repeatedly. Reading notes only when encountering difficult situations is usually less effective than reading them regularly *in preparation for* difficult situations. Below are some of Sally's therapy notes. They contain:

- Responses to dysfunctional thinking,
- Behavioral assignments, or
- A combination of responses and behavioral assignments.

When I think "I'll never get all my work done," remind myself:

I just need to focus on what I need to do right now.

I don't have to do everything perfectly.

I can ask for help. It's not a sign of weakness.

When I think "I'd rather stay in bed," tell myself that I always

feel a little better when I get something done and worse when

I do nothing.

It might feel as if no one cares about me, but that's not true.

My family, Allison, and Joe do. It's harder to feel their caring,

but that's because I'm depressed. The best thing to do is to stay

in touch with them, so go call or text them.

When I want to ask the professor for help

1. Remind myself it's no big deal. The worst that'll happen is he'll act gruff.

2. Remember, this is an experiment. Even if it doesn't work this time,
   it's good practice for me.

3. If he is gruff, it probably has nothing to do with me. He may be busy or
   irritated by something else.

4. Even if he won't help me, so what? It's his failure as a professor, not mine
   as a student. It means he isn't doing his job properly. I can ask
   the department for a tutor, or ask someone else in the class to help.

5. So I should go knock on his door. At worst, it'll be good practice.

Strategies for when I'm anxious

1. Do a Thought Record.

2. Read coping cards.

3. Call [friend].

4. Go for a walk or run.

5. Tolerate the anxiety. It's an unpleasant feeling but it's not life
   threatening, and it will decrease once I turn my attention to
   something else.

On a practical note, you should keep copies of your patients' therapy notes, photocopying them or using carbonless paper. You will probably find that you refer back to these therapy notes often, especially when reviewing patients' homework or reinforcing ideas you had discussed with patients in prior sessions. Also, a certain number of patients lose their notes and benefit greatly from a photocopy of your copy.

Audio-Recorded Therapy Notes

Ensuring that patients have written therapy notes is ideal. They can carry around a notebook or index cards to read as needed, or they can read their therapy notes on their smartphone. But some patients cannot or do not like to read. Or they find listening to notes to be more effective. In any case, you can turn on an audio recorder or have patients push the record button on their phone when you and they develop responses to automatic thoughts; or you can note what the responses are and turn on the recorder for the last few minutes of a session, recording all responses at once. Recording and then having patients listen to an entire therapy session is usually not as useful. They are likely to listen to the recording only once during the week, instead of repeatedly listening to the most important points of the session.

Motivating patients to read therapy notes is similar to facilitating their doing any kind of homework (see Chapter 17). Initially, it is useful to have patients read their therapy notes at the end of a session and have them note that it takes less than a minute. When patients cannot read therapy notes, they may be able to listen to an audiotaped summary or find someone in their environment who can read the notes to them.

EVALUATING AND RESPONDING TO NOVEL AUTOMATIC THOUGHTS BETWEEN SESSIONS

The previous chapter provided a list of Socratic questions patients can ask themselves to evaluate their thinking. Before suggesting that they use these questions at home when they feel upset, you will make sure that:

> - They understand that evaluating their thinking can help them feel better.
> - They believe they will be able to use the questions effectively at home.
> - They understand that not all questions apply to all automatic thoughts.
> - You have shortened the list for patients who find the entire list daunting or overwhelming.

You also guide them as to when and how to use the questions, as I did with Sally:

THERAPIST: Sally, it would be too burdensome for you to use these questions for *every* automatic thought you have this week. That's one reason that you have therapy notes to read every morning and as needed during the day. But when you notice your mood getting worse and you catch your automatic thoughts, think to yourself, "Do I have therapy notes that cover this?" Okay?

PATIENT: Yes.

THERAPIST: If you do, you have a choice. Use these questions or pull out your notes.

PATIENT: Okay.

THERAPIST: If you don't have notes, then you definitely will want to pull out the list at least some of the time. Now, ideally, you'd not only ask yourself the questions, but you'd also *write down* your answers, if you can. How does that sound?

PATIENT: Fine.

Thought Records

The Thought Record (TR), also known in an earlier version as the Daily Record of Dysfunctional Thoughts (Beck et al., 1979), is a worksheet that prompts patients to evaluate their automatic thoughts when they feel distressed (see Figure 12.1). It elicits more information than just responding to the questions in Figure 11.1. It is not necessary for patients to use the TR if these questions are helpful, but many patients find the worksheet organizes their thinking and responses better. (The TR is not particularly useful, however, for patients who are low functioning, dislike writing, are unmotivated, or not well enough equipped intellectually to benefit from it.) You might first use the list of questions in Figure 11.1 (page 172) with patients, then show them how to write the answers and other information on a Thought Record.

In the following section, Sally and I have used the list of Socratic questions to evaluate her thought "Bob won't want to go with me," and she feels better.

THERAPIST: Good. Now I'd like to show you a worksheet that I think will help you at home, if that's okay. It's called a Thought Record—and it's just an organized way of writing down what we just did. Okay? (*Pulls out Figure 12.1.*)

PATIENT: Sure.

THERAPIST: Here it is. Now, before I start, I have to tell you a couple of things. First, spelling, handwriting, and grammar don't count. Second, this is a useful tool, and it may take some practice for you to get really good at it. So expect to make some mistakes along the way. These mistakes will actually be useful—we'll see what was confusing, so you can do it better the next time. Okay?

PATIENT: Okay.

THERAPIST: Here's how you'll know when you should pull it out (*pointing to the top of the sheet*). Do you see here at the top? It says, "Directions: When you notice your mood getting worse, ask yourself, 'What's going through my mind right now?' and as soon as possible jot down the thought or mental image in the Automatic Thought column."

PATIENT: Okay.

THERAPIST: Now, let's look at the columns. The directions are at the top of each. The first column is easy. When did you have that thought about Bob?

PATIENT: Friday afternoon, after class.

THERAPIST: Okay. You can write that in the first column.

PATIENT: (*Does so.*)

THERAPIST: Now, you'll see the second column prompts you to write down the situation. So you could put, "Thinking about asking Bob if he wants to have coffee." (*Pauses while Sally writes.*) Now, the third column is for your automatic thoughts and how much you believe them. Here's where you write down the actual words or pictures that went through your mind. In this case, you had the thought, "He won't want to go with me." How much did you believe the thought at that time?

PATIENT: A lot, maybe 90%.

THERAPIST: Good. You could write "90%" next to your thought, or "a lot." And in the fourth column, you write your emotion and how intense it was. In this case, how sad did you feel?

PATIENT: Pretty sad—75%.

THERAPIST: Okay, write that down. (*Waits for Sally to finish writing.*) Next, look at the fifth column. It tells you to identify the cognitive distortion. Can you look at your list and tell me if you think your automatic thought falls into one of those categories?

PATIENT: I think it's fortune telling or mind reading.

THERAPIST: Good. Actually, it's both. Next, column five tells you to use the questions at the bottom. Do you want to write down the answers we just went over?

PATIENT: Okay. (*Does so.*)

THERAPIST: Now, the last column tells us how helpful this was. How much do you now believe the automatic thought?

PATIENT: Less. Maybe 50%.

THERAPIST: And how sad are you feeling?

PATIENT: Less. About 50%, I guess.

THERAPIST: So you can write that down.

PATIENT: (*Does so.*)

THERAPIST: I want you to remember what I told you before. Don't expect all your negative emotion to go away. But if doing a Thought Record helps a little, even 10%, it was worth doing.

PATIENT: Okay.

THERAPIST: So what do you think of the Thought Record? Do you want to try it this week at home?

PATIENT: Yes, I will.

For some patients, it is better to introduce the Thought Record in two stages. In one session, you might teach patients to fill in the first four columns. If they successfully do so for homework, you can then teach them to use the final two columns.

Directions: When you notice your mood getting worse, ask yourself, "What's going through my mind right now?" and as soon as possible jot down the thought or mental image in the Automatic Thought(s) column.

Date/Time	Situation	Automatic Thought(s)	Emotion(s)	Adaptive Response	Outcome
	1. What actual event or stream of thoughts, or daydreams or recollection led to the unpleasant emotion? 2. What (if any) distressing physical sensations did you have?	1. What thought(s) and/or image(s) went through your mind? 2. How much did you believe each one at the time?	1. What emotion(s) (sad/anxious/angry/ etc.) did you feel at the time? 2. How intense (0–100%) was the emotion?	1. (optional) What cognitive distortion did you make? 2. Use questions at bottom to compose a response to the automatic thought(s). 3. How much do you believe each response?	1. How much do you now believe each automatic thought? 2. What emotion(s) do you feel now? How intense (0–100%) is the emotion? 3. What will you do (or did you do)?
Friday 3/8 3 P.M.	Thinking about asking Bob if he wants to have coffee.	He won't want to go with me. (90%)	Sad (75%)	(Fortune telling and mind reading) I don't really know if he wants to or not. (90%) He is friendly to me in class. (90%) The worst that'll happen is he'll say no and I'll feel bad for a while, but I could go talk to Allison about it. (90%) The best is he'll say yes. (100%) The most realistic is he may say he's busy but still act friendly. (80%) If I keep on assuming he doesn't want to go with me, I won't ask him at all. (100%) I should just go up and ask him. (50%) What's the big deal, anyway? (75%)	1. AT (50%) 2. Sad (50%) 3. I'll ask him.

Questions to help compose an alternative response: (1) What is the evidence that the automatic thought is true? Not true? (2) Is there an alternative explanation? (3) What's the worst that could happen? How could I cope? What's the best that could happen? What's the most realistic outcome? (4) What's the effect of my believing the automatic thought? What could be the effect of my changing my thinking? (5) What should I do about it? (6) If _____ [friend's name] was in the situation and had this thought, what would I tell him/her?

FIGURE 12.1. Thought Record. From *Cognitive behavior therapy worksheet packet.* Copyright 2011 by Judith S. Beck. Bala Cynwyd, PA: Beck Institute for Cognitive Behavior Therapy.

"Testing Your Thoughts" Worksheet

When you predict that the Thought Record could be too confusing or elaborate for patients, you can consider using a simplified version, the "Testing Your Thoughts" Worksheet (Figure 12.2). It contains similar questions, is worded at a lower readability level, and its more structured format is easier to complete.

What is the situation? *Joanne yelled at me.*

What am I thinking or imagining? *She'll never call me again.*

What makes me think the thought is true? *She seemed pretty mad.*

What makes me think the thought is not true or not completely true? *She's gotten mad at me before, but she seems to get over it.*

What's another way to look at this? *She's got a real temper, but she doesn't stay mad.*

What's the worst that could happen? What could I do then? *I'd lose my best friend. I would have to concentrate on my other friends.*

What's the best that could happen? *She'll call back right away and apologize.*

What will probably happen? *She'll act kind of cold for a few days, but then I'll call her.*

What will happen if I keep telling myself the same thought? *I'll keep being really upset.*

What could happen if I changed my thinking? *I could feel better, maybe call her sooner.*

What would I tell my friend [think of a specific person] *Emily* if this happened to him or her? *Don't worry, just wait 2 days and call.*

FIGURE 12.2. "Testing Your Thoughts" Worksheet. From *Cognitive behavior therapy worksheet packet.* Copyright 2011 by Judith S. Beck. Bala Cynwyd, PA: Beck Institute for Cognitive Behavior Therapy.

When a Worksheet Is Not Sufficiently Helpful

As with any technique in cognitive behavior therapy, it is important not to overemphasize the importance of worksheets. Most patients, at some point, find that completing a particular worksheet did not provide much relief. If you emphasize its *general* usefulness and "stuck points" as an opportunity for learning, you help patients avoid automatic thoughts critical of themselves, the therapy, the worksheet, or you.

As described in the previous chapter, evaluation of an automatic thought (with or without a worksheet) may be less than optimal if patients fail to respond to their most upsetting thought or image, if their automatic thought is a core belief or activated an underlying belief, if their evaluation and response are superficial, or if they discount their response.

RESPONDING TO AUTOMATIC THOUGHTS IN OTHER WAYS

Sometimes you will use other methods to respond to automatic thoughts. For example, when patients have anxious, obsessive thoughts, you may teach them the "AWARE" technique (Beck & Emery, 1985) in which patients practice:

> **A:** Accepting their anxiety.
> **W:** Watching their anxiety without judgment.
> **A:** Acting with their anxiety, as if they aren't anxious.
> **R:** Repeating the first three steps.
> **E:** Expecting the best.

When patients' emotions are too high to effectively use their executive function to evaluate their thoughts, you might use distraction or relaxation techniques, described in Chapter 15.

Chapter 13

IDENTIFYING AND MODIFYING
INTERMEDIATE BELIEFS

Previous chapters described the identification and modification of automatic thoughts, the actual words or images that go through a patient's mind in a given situation and lead to distress. This chapter and the next describe the deeper, often unarticulated ideas or understandings that patients have about themselves, others, and their personal worlds, that give rise to specific automatic thoughts. These ideas often are not expressed before therapy but can easily be elicited from the patient, or inferred and then tested.

As described in Chapter 3, these beliefs may be classified in two categories: intermediate beliefs (composed of rules, attitudes, and assumptions) and core beliefs (rigid, global ideas about oneself, others, or the world). Intermediate beliefs, while not as easily modifiable as automatic thoughts, are still more malleable than core beliefs.

This chapter is divided into two parts. In the first part, *cognitive conceptualization* (initially introduced in Chapter 3) is described, and the process of developing a Cognitive Conceptualization Diagram is illustrated. Conceptualization is emphasized throughout this volume to help the therapist plan therapy, become adept at choosing appropriate interventions, and overcome stuck points when standard interventions fail. *Eliciting and modifying intermediate beliefs* are the focus of the second part of this chapter. These techniques also apply to the next chapter, which presents additional specialized techniques for eliciting and modifying core beliefs.

COGNITIVE CONCEPTUALIZATION

Generally, you will guide patients to work on automatic thoughts before directly modifying their beliefs. From the beginning, though, you start formulating a conceptualization, which logically connects automatic thoughts to the deeper-level beliefs. If you fail to see this larger picture, you will be less likely to direct therapy in an effective, efficient way.

You can start filling out a Cognitive Conceptualization Diagram (Figures 13.1 and 13.2) after the first session with a patient, if you have collected data in the form of the cognitive model (the bottom part of the diagram); that is, you have data about the patient's typical automatic thoughts, emotions, behavior, and/or beliefs. This diagram depicts, among other things, the relationship between core beliefs, intermediate beliefs, and current automatic thoughts. It provides a cognitive map of the patient's psychopathology and helps organize the multitude of data that the patient presents. The diagram in Figure 13.1 illustrates the basic questions you will ask yourself to complete the diagram.

When filling in data after the initial session, you should regard your first efforts as tentative; you have not yet collected enough data to determine the extent to which the automatic thoughts patients have expressed are very typical for them. The completed diagram will mislead you if you choose situations in which the themes of patients' automatic thoughts are not part of an overall pattern. After three or four sessions, you should be able to complete the bottom half with more confidence, as patterns should have emerged.

You share your partial conceptualization with patients verbally (and sometimes on a blank piece of paper) at every session as you summarize their experience in the form of the cognitive model. Generally you will not share the worksheet, however, as many patients would find it confusing (or occasionally demeaning if they interpret the diagram as your attempt to "fit" them into boxes).

Initially, you may have data to complete only a portion of the diagram. You either leave the other boxes blank, or fill in items you have inferred with a question mark to indicate their tentative status. You will check out missing or inferred items with the patient at future sessions. At some point you will share both the top and bottom parts of the conceptualization, when your goal for a session is to help patients understand the broader picture of their difficulties. At that time, you will review the conceptualization verbally, share a simplified version on a blank sheet of paper, or (for patients whom you judge will benefit) present a blank conceptualization diagram and fill it out together. Whenever you present your interpretations, you will do so tentatively and label them as hypotheses, asking patients whether they "ring true." Correct hypotheses generally resonate with the patient.

Patient's name: _____ Date: _____

Diagnosis: Axis I _____ Axis II _____

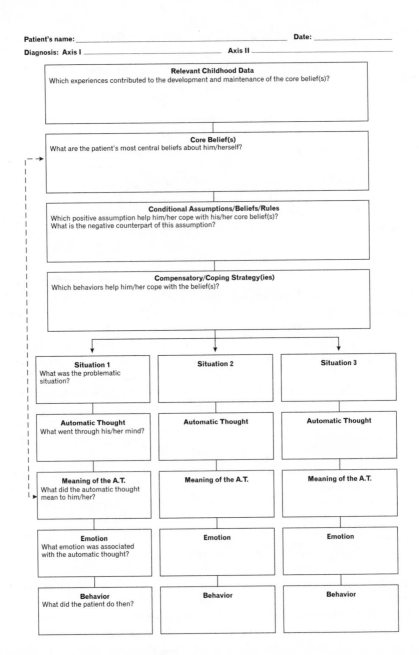

FIGURE 13.1. Cognitive Conceptualization Diagram. Adapted from *Cognitive behavior therapy worksheet packet.* Copyright 2011 by Judith S. Beck. Bala Cynwyd, PA: Beck Institute for Cognitive Behavior Therapy.

Reprinted by permission in *Cognitive Behavior Therapy: Basics and Beyond, Second Edition,* by Judith S. Beck (Guilford Press, 2011). Permission to photocopy this material is granted to purchasers of this book for personal use only (see copyright page for details). Purchasers may download a larger version of this material from *www.guilford.com/p/beck4.*

Usually it is best to start with the bottom half of the conceptualization diagram. You jot down three *typical* situations in which the
patient became upset. Then, for each situation, fill in the key automatic
thought, its meaning, and the patient's subsequent emotion and relevant behavior (if any). If you have not directly asked patients for the
meaning of their automatic thoughts, you either hypothesize (with a
written question mark) or, better still, do the downward arrow technique (pages 206–208) at the next session to uncover the meaning for
each thought.

The meaning of the automatic thought for each situation should
be logically connected with the Core Belief box near the top of the
diagram. For example, Sally's diagram (Figure 13.2) clearly shows how
her automatic thoughts, and the meaning of those thoughts are related
to her core belief of incompetence.

To complete the top box of the diagram, ask yourself (and the
patient): How did the core belief originate and become maintained?
What life events (especially those in childhood) did the patient experience that might be related to the development and maintenance of the
belief? Typical relevant childhood data include such significant events
as continual or periodic strife among parents or other family members;
parental divorce; negative interactions with parents, siblings, teachers,
peers, or others in which the child felt blamed, criticized, or otherwise
devalued; serious illness; death of significant others; physical or sexual
abuse; and other adverse life conditions, such as moving frequently,
experiencing trauma, growing up in poverty, or facing chronic discrim-
ination, to name a few.

The relevant childhood data may, however, be more subtle: for
example, children's perceptions (which may or may not have been
valid) that they did not measure up in important ways to their siblings;
that they were different from or demeaned by peers; that they did not
meet expectations of parents, teachers, or others; or that their parents
favored a sibling over them.

Next ask yourself, "How did the patient cope with this painful core
belief? Which intermediate beliefs (i.e., underlying assumptions, rules,
and attitudes) has the patient developed?"

Sally's beliefs are depicted hierarchically in Figure 13.3. As Sally
has many intermediate beliefs that could be classified as attitudes or
rules, it is particularly useful to list the key *assumptions* in the box below
the core belief. (See page 211 on how you can help a patient re-express
an attitude or rule as an assumption.) Sally, for example, developed
an assumption that helped her cope with the painful idea of incompetence: "If I work very hard, then I can do okay." Like most patients,
she also had the flip side of the same assumption: "If I don't work hard,
then I'll fail." Most Axis I patients tend to operate according to the first

Patient's name: _Sally_   Date: _2/22_
Diagnosis: Axis I _Major depressive episode_   Axis II _None_

Relevant Childhood Data
Which experiences contributed to the development and maintenance of the core belief(s)?
Compared self with older brother and peers
Critical mother

Core Belief(s)
What are the patient's most central beliefs about him/herself?
I'm incompetent.

Conditional Assumptions/Beliefs/Rules
Which positive assumption help him/her cope with his/her core belief(s)?
What is the negative counterpart of this assumption?
(positive) If I work very hard, I can do okay.
(negative) If I don't do great, then I've failed.

Compensatory/Coping Strategy(ies)
Which behaviors help him/her cope with the belief(s)?

Develop high standards   Look for shortcomings and correct
Work very hard   Avoid seeking help
Overprepare

Situation 1	**Situation 2**	**Situation 3**
What was the problematic situation?	Thinking about course requirements	Reflecting on difficulty of textbook
Talking to freshmen about advanced placement credits		
Automatic Thought	**Automatic Thought**	**Automatic Thought**
What went through his/her mind?	I won't be able to do it (research paper).	I won't make it through the course.
They're all smarter than me.		
Meaning of the A.T.	**Meaning of the A.T.**	**Meaning of the A.T.**
What did the automatic thought mean to him/her?	I'm incompetent.	I'm incompetent.
I'm incompetent.		
Emotion	**Emotion**	**Emotion**
What emotion was associated with the automatic thought?	Sad	Sad
Sad		
Behavior	**Behavior**	**Behavior**
What did the patient do then?	Cried	Closed the book; stopped studying
Kept quiet.		

FIGURE 13.2. Sally's Cognitive Conceptualization Diagram. Adapted from *Cognitive behavior therapy worksheet packet*. Copyright 2011 by Judith S. Beck. Bala Cynwyd, PA: Beck Institute for Cognitive Behavior Therapy.

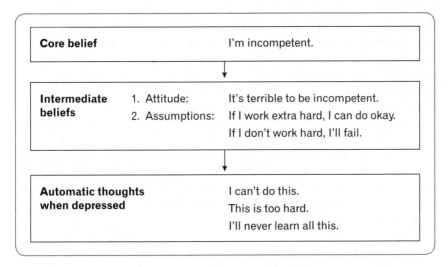

FIGURE 13.3. Sally's hierarchy of beliefs and automatic thoughts.

assumption, the one phrased in a more positive way, until they become psychologically distressed, at which time the negative assumption surfaces. Note that the designation "positive" does not necessarily mean the belief is adaptive.

To complete the next box, "coping strategies," you ask yourself, "Which behavioral strategies did the patient develop to cope with the painful core belief?" Note that the patient's broad assumptions often link the coping strategies to the core belief:

> "If I [engage in the coping strategy], then [my core belief may not come true; I'll be okay]. However, if I [do *not* engage in my coping strategy], then [my core belief is likely to come true]."

Sally's strategies were to develop high standards for herself, work very hard, overprepare for exams and presentations, remain vigilant for her shortcomings, and avoid seeking help (especially in situations in which asking for assistance could, in her mind, expose her incompetence). She believes that engaging in these behaviors will protect her from failure and the exposure of her incompetence (and that not doing them *could* lead to failure and exposure of incompetence).

Another patient might have developed strategies that are the opposite of Sally's behaviors: avoiding hard work, developing few goals, underpreparing, and asking for excessive help. Why did Sally develop a particular set of coping strategies while a second patient developed the opposite set? Perhaps nature endowed them with different cognitive and behavioral styles; in interaction with the environment they developed different intermediate beliefs that reinforced their particular behavioral strategies. The second patient, perhaps because of his childhood experiences, had the same core belief of incompetence, but coped with it by developing a different set of beliefs: "If I set low goals for myself I'll be okay, but if I set high goals I'll fail." "If I rely on others I'll be okay, but if I rely on myself I'll fail."

Note that most coping strategies are *normal* behaviors that everyone engages in at times. The difficulty of patients in distress lies in the *overuse* of these strategies at the expense of more functional strategies. Figure 13.4 lists a few examples of strategies that patients develop to cope with painful core beliefs.

To summarize, the Cognitive Conceptualization Diagram is based on data patients present, their actual words. You should regard your hypotheses as tentative until confirmed by the patient. You will continually reevaluate and refine the diagram as you collect additional data, and your conceptualization is not complete until the patient terminates treatment. While you might not show the actual diagram to patients, you will verbally (and often on paper) conceptualize their experience from the first session on, to help them make sense of their current reactions to situations. At some point, you will present the larger picture to patients so they can understand:

Avoid negative emotion	Display high emotion (e.g., to attract attention)
Try to be perfect	Purposely appear incompetent or helpless
Be overly responsible	Avoid responsibility
Avoid intimacy	Seek inappropriate intimacy
Seek recognition	Avoid attention
Avoid confrontation	Provoke others
Try to control situations	Abdicate control to others
Act childlike	Act in an authoritarian manner
Try to please others	Distance self from others or try to please only oneself

FIGURE 13.4. Typical coping strategies.

> - How their earlier experiences contributed to the development of core beliefs about themselves, their worlds, and others.
> - How they developed certain assumptions or rules for living to help them cope with their painful core beliefs.
> - How these assumptions led to the development of particular coping strategies or patterns of behavior that may (or may not) have been adaptive at the time but are no longer adaptive in many situations.

Some patients are intellectually and emotionally ready to see the larger picture early on in therapy; you should wait to present it to others (especially those with whom you do not have a sound therapeutic relationship, or who do not really believe in the cognitive model). As mentioned previously, whenever you present your conceptualization, ask the patient for confirmation, disconfirmation, or modification of each part.

Identifying Intermediate and Core Beliefs

You will identify intermediate beliefs by:

> 1. Recognizing when a belief is expressed as an automatic thought.
> 2. Providing the first part of an assumption.
> 3. Directly eliciting a rule or attitude.
> 4. Using the downward arrow technique.
> 5. Examining the patient's automatic thoughts and looking for common themes.
> 6. Asking the patient directly.
> 7. Reviewing a belief questionnaire completed by the patient.

These strategies are illustrated below.

1. First, a patient may actually articulate a belief as an automatic thought, especially when depressed.

THERAPIST: What went through your mind when you got the quiz back?

PATIENT: I should have done better. I can't do anything right. I'm so incompetent. [core belief]

2. Second, you may be able to elicit a full assumption by providing the first half of it.

THERAPIST: So you had the thought "I'll have to stay up all night working."

PATIENT: Yes.

THERAPIST: And if you don't work as hard as you possibly can on a paper or a project...?

PATIENT: Then I haven't done my best. I've failed.

THERAPIST: Does this sound familiar, based on what we've talked about before in therapy? Is this generally how you view your efforts, that if you don't work as hard as you can, then you've failed?

PATIENT: Yes, I think so.

THERAPIST: Can you give me some more examples so we can see how widespread this belief is?

Q: What if ... patients have difficulty providing the second part of the assumption?

A: Rephrase the question.

> THERAPIST: Let me ask you about it this way: If you don't work as hard as you possibly can on a paper or project, what bad thing could happen? Or what bad thing would it mean?

3. Third, you can identify a rule or an attitude by direct elicitation.

THERAPIST: So it's pretty important to you to do really well in your volunteer tutoring job?

PATIENT: Oh, yes.

THERAPIST: Do you remember our talking about this kind of thing before, having to do very well? Do you have a rule about that?

PATIENT: Oh ... I hadn't really thought of it ... I guess I have to do whatever I do really well.

4. More often, you will use a fourth technique to identify intermediate (and core) beliefs: the *downward arrow technique* (Burns, 1980).

First, you identify a key automatic thought that you suspect may stem directly from a dysfunctional belief. Then you ask the patient for the *meaning* of this cognition, assuming the automatic thought is true. Continue to do so until you have uncovered one or more important beliefs. Asking what a thought means *to* the patient often elicits an intermediate belief; asking what it means *about* the patient usually uncovers the core belief.

THERAPIST: Okay, to summarize, you were studying late last night, you were looking over your class notes, you had the thought, "These notes make no sense," and you felt sad.

PATIENT: Yes.

THERAPIST: Okay, now we haven't yet looked at the evidence to see if you're right. But I'd like to see if we can figure out *why* that thought made you feel so sad. To do that, we have to assume for a moment that you *are* right, your notes don't make sense. What would that mean to you?

PATIENT: I didn't do a very good job in class.

THERAPIST: Okay, if it's true that you didn't do a very good job in class, what would that mean?

PATIENT: I'm a lousy student. [The assumption is, "If I don't do a good job in school, it means I'm a lousy student."]

THERAPIST: Okay, if you're a lousy student, what does *that* mean about you?

PATIENT: [core belief] I'm not good enough. [I am incompetent.]

Sometimes you can get stuck in the course of a downward arrow technique when the patient answers with a "feeling" response, such as "That would be terrible," or "I'd be so anxious." As in the example below, you will gently empathize, and then try to get back on track. To minimize the possibility that the patient will react negatively to your probing, you will provide a rationale for your repeated questioning and vary your inquiry through questions such as the following:

> "If that's true, so what?"
> "What's so bad about ..."
> "What's the worst part about ..."
> "What does that mean *about you*?"

The transcript below demonstrates the provision of a brief rationale and the variation of questions in the downward arrow technique.

THERAPIST: It's important for us to understand what part of this is most upsetting to you. What would it mean if your roommate and friends *did* get better grades than you?

PATIENT: Oh, I couldn't stand it.

THERAPIST: So you'd be pretty upset, but what would be the worst part about it?

PATIENT: They'd probably look down on me.

THERAPIST: And if they did look down on you, what would be so bad about that?

PATIENT: I'd hate that.

THERAPIST: Sure, you'd be distressed if that happened. But so what if they looked down on you?

PATIENT: I don't know. That would be pretty bad.

THERAPIST: Would it mean something *about you,* if they looked down on you?

PATIENT: That I'm inferior, not as good as they are. [The assumption is "If people look down on me, it means I'm inferior." The core belief is "I'm inferior."]

How do you know when to stop the downward arrow technique? Generally you have uncovered the important intermediate beliefs and/ or core belief when the patient shows a negative shift in affect, and/or begins to state the belief in the same or similar words.

THERAPIST: And what would it mean if you are inferior and not as good as they are?

PATIENT: Just that, I'm inferior.

5. A fifth way to identify beliefs is to look for common themes in a patient's automatic thoughts across situations. You can ask insightful patients whether they can identify a recurrent theme or you can make a hypothesis about a belief and ask the patient to reflect on its validity:

THERAPIST: Sally, in a number of situations you seem to think, "I can't do it," or "It's too hard," or "I won't be able to get it done." I wonder whether you believe that you are somehow incompetent or inadequate?

PATIENT: Yes, I think I do. I do think I'm incompetent.

6. A sixth way to identify beliefs is to ask the patient directly. Some patients are able to articulate their beliefs fairly easily.

THERAPIST: Sally, what is your belief about asking for help?

PATIENT: Oh, asking for help is a sign of weakness.

7. Finally, a patient may be asked to complete a belief questionnaire, such as the Dysfunctional Attitude Scale (Weissman & Beck, 1978) or the Personality Belief Questionnaire (A. T. Beck & Beck, 1991). Careful review of items that are strongly endorsed can highlight problematic beliefs. The use of such questionnaires is a useful adjunct to the techniques described above.

To summarize, you can identify both intermediate and core beliefs in a number of ways. You can look for the expression of a belief in an automatic thought; provide the conditional clause ("If …) of an assumption and ask the patient to complete it; directly elicit a rule; use the downward arrow technique; recognize a common theme among automatic thoughts; ask patients what they think their belief is; or you can review the patient's belief questionnaire.

Deciding Whether to Modify a Belief

Having identified a belief, you need to determine whether the intermediate belief is central or more peripheral. Generally, to conduct therapy as efficiently as possible, you focus on the most important intermediate beliefs (Safran, Vallis, Segal, & Shaw, 1986). It is not worth the time or effort to work on dysfunctional beliefs that are tangential, or that patients believe only slightly.

THERAPIST: It sounds as if you believe if people don't accept you, then you're inferior.

PATIENT: I guess.

THERAPIST: How much do you believe that?

PATIENT: Not that much, maybe 20%.

THERAPIST: It doesn't sound as if we have to work on that belief, then. How about if we get back to the problem we were discussing before?

Having identified an important intermediate belief, you decide whether you will make the belief explicit to the patient and, if so, whether you will merely identify the belief as one to be worked on in the future, or whether you will work on it at the present time. Ask yourself:

"What is the belief?"

"How strongly does the patient believe it?"

"If strongly, how broadly and how strongly does it affect the patient's life?"

"If broadly and strongly, should I work on it now? Is it likely the patient will be able to evaluate it with sufficient objectivity at this point? Do we have enough time in the session today to begin working on it?"

You will begin belief modification as soon as possible. When patients no longer endorse their beliefs or do not believe them as strongly, they will be able to interpret their experiences in a more realistic, functional way. But some beliefs are very deeply held, and it is advisable to teach patients to evaluate their more superficial cognitions (automatic thoughts) first, so they can learn that just because they think or believe something doesn't necessarily mean it is true. Belief modification is relatively easy with some patients and much more difficult with others. Modifying intermediate beliefs is generally accomplished before modifying core beliefs, as the latter may be quite rigid.

Educating Patients about Beliefs

Having identified an important belief and checked that the patient believes it strongly, you may decide to educate the patient about the nature of beliefs in general, using a specific belief as an example. You might stress that there is a range of potential beliefs that the patient could adopt, and that beliefs are learned, not innate, and can be revised.

THERAPIST: Okay, we've identified some of your beliefs: "It's terrible to do a mediocre job"; "I have to do everything great"; "If I do less than my best, I'm a failure." Where do you think you learned these ideas?

PATIENT: Growing up, I guess.

THERAPIST: Does everyone have these same beliefs?

PATIENT: (*Thinks.*) No. Some people don't seem to care.

THERAPIST: Can you think of someone specifically who seems to have different beliefs?

PATIENT: Well, my cousin Emily, for one.

THERAPIST: What belief does she have?

PATIENT: I think she thinks it's okay to be mediocre. She's more interested in having a good time.

THERAPIST: So she learned different beliefs?

PATIENT: I guess so.

THERAPIST: Well, the bad news is that you currently have a set of beliefs that aren't bringing you much satisfaction, right? The good news is that since you *learned* this current set of beliefs, you can unlearn them and learn others—maybe not as extreme as Emily's, but somewhere in between hers and yours. How does that sound?

Changing Rules and Attitudes into Assumption Form

It is often easier for patients to see the distortion in and test an intermediate belief that is in the form of an assumption, rather than an intermediate belief that is in the form of a rule or an attitude. Having identified a rule or an attitude, you use the downward arrow technique to ascertain its meaning.

THERAPIST: So you believe pretty strongly that you should do things yourself [rule], and that it's terrible to ask for help [attitude]. What does it *mean* to you to ask for help, for example with your schoolwork, instead of doing it yourself?

PATIENT: It means I'm incompetent.

THERAPIST: How much do you believe this idea right now, "If I ask for help, I'm incompetent?"

Logical evaluation of this conditional assumption through questioning or other methods often creates greater cognitive dissonance than does evaluation of the rule or attitude. It is easier for Sally to recognize the distortion and/or dysfunctionality in the assumption "If I ask for help, it means I'm incompetent" than in her rule "I shouldn't ask for help."

Examining Advantages and Disadvantages of Beliefs

Often it is useful for patients to examine the advantages and disadvantages of continuing to hold a given belief. You then strive to minimize or undermine the advantages and emphasize and reinforce the disadvantages. (A similar process was previously described in the section on evaluating the utility of automatic thoughts on pages 174–175.)

THERAPIST: What are the *advantages* of believing if you don't do your best, then you're a failure?

PATIENT: Well, it might make me work harder.

THERAPIST: It'd be interesting to see whether you actually *need* such an extreme belief to keep you working hard. We'll get back to that idea later. Any other advantages?

PATIENT: … No, not that I can think of.

THERAPIST: What are the *disadvantages* of believing you're a failure if you don't do your best?

PATIENT: Well, I feel miserable when I don't do well on an exam … I get really nervous before presentations … I don't have as much time to do other things I like because I'm so busy studying …

THERAPIST: And does it cut some enjoyment out of studying and learning itself?

PATIENT: Oh, definitely.

THERAPIST: Okay, so on one hand, it may or may not actually be true that this belief is the only thing that makes you work hard. On the other hand, this belief about having to live up to your potential makes you feel miserable when you don't do great, makes you more nervous than you have to be before presentations, cuts into your enjoyment of your work, and stops you from doing other things you like. Is that right?

PATIENT: Yes.

THERAPIST: Is this an idea, then, that you'd like to change?

Formulating a New Belief

In order to decide which strategies to use to modify a given belief, you clearly formulate to yourself a more adaptive belief. Ask yourself, "What belief would be more functional for the patient?"

For example, Figure 13.5 lists Sally's current beliefs and the new beliefs I have in mind. Although constructing a new belief is a *collaborative* process, you nevertheless mentally formulate a range of more reasonable beliefs so you can appropriately choose strategies to change the old belief.

Sally's old beliefs	More functional beliefs
1. If I don't do as well as others, I'm a failure.	If I don't do as well as others, I'm not a failure, just human.
2. If I ask for help, it's a sign of weakness.	If I ask for help when I need it, I'm showing good problem-solving abilities (which is a sign of strength).
3. If I fail at work/school, I'm a failure as a person.	If I fail at work/school, it's not a reflection of my whole self. (My whole self includes how I am as a friend, daughter, sister, relative, citizen, and community member, and my qualities of kindness, sensitivity to others, helpfulness, etc.) Also, failure is not a permanent condition.
4. I should be able to excel at everything I try.	I shouldn't be able to excel at something unless I am gifted in that area (and am willing and able to devote considerable time and effort toward it at the expense of other things).
5. I should always work hard and do my best.	I should put in a reasonable amount of effort much of the time.
6. If I don't live up to my potential, I have failed.	If I do less than my best, I have succeeded perhaps 70%, 80%, or 90%; not 0%.
7. If I don't work hard all the time, I'll fail.	If I don't work hard all the time, I'll probably do reasonably well and have a more balanced life.

FIGURE 13.5. Formulation of more functional beliefs.

To summarize, before you try to modify a patient's belief, you confirm that it is a central, strongly held belief, and you formulate in your own mind a more functional, less rigid belief that is thematically *related* to the dysfunctional one, but which you believe is more realistic and adaptive for the patient. You do not impose this belief on the patient, but rather you guide the patient in a collaborative manner, using Socratic questioning, to construct an alternative belief. You may also educate the patient about the nature of beliefs (e.g., that they are ideas, not necessarily truths; that they have been learned and so can be unlearned; that they can be evaluated and modified) and/or help the patient assess the advantages and disadvantages of continuing to hold the belief.

MODIFYING BELIEFS

A number of strategies are useful in modifying both intermediate and core beliefs. (Additional techniques for modifying core beliefs are presented in more detail in the next chapter.) Some beliefs may change easily, but many take concerted effort over a period of time. You continue to ask patients how much they currently believe a given belief (0–100%), at both an "intellectual" and at a "gut" or "emotional" level, to gauge whether further work is needed.

It is usually neither possible nor necessarily desirable to reduce degrees of belief to 0%. Knowing when to stop working on a belief is therefore a judgment call. Generally, beliefs have been sufficiently attenuated when patients endorse them less than 30% and when they are likely to continue modifying their dysfunctional behavior despite still holding on to a remnant of the belief.

It is advisable for patients to keep track, in their therapy notes, of the beliefs they have examined. A useful format includes the dysfunctional belief; the new, more functional belief; and the strength of each belief, expressed in a percentage, as in the following example:

> *Old belief*: "If I don't achieve highly, I'm a failure." (50%)
>
> *New belief*: "I'm only an overall failure if I actually fail at almost everything." (80%)

A typical homework assignment is to read and rerate daily how strongly the patient endorses both beliefs.

Techniques to modify beliefs are listed below. Some are the same as those used to modify automatic thoughts.

> 1. Socratic questioning.
> 2. Behavioral experiments.
> 3. Cognitive continuum.
> 4. Intellectual–emotional role plays.
> 5. Using others as a reference point.
> 6. Acting "as if."
> 7. Self-disclosure.

Socratic Questioning to Modify Beliefs

As illustrated in the next transcript, I use the same kinds of questions to examine Sally's belief that I used in evaluating her automatic thoughts. Even when I identify a general belief, I help her evaluate it in the context of specific situations. This specificity helps make the evaluation more concrete and meaningful, and less abstract and intellectual.

THERAPIST: [summarizing what they learned from the just-completed downward arrow technique] Okay, so you believe about 90% that if you ask for help, it means you're incompetent. Is that right?

PATIENT: Yes.

THERAPIST: Could there be another way of viewing asking for help?

PATIENT: I'm not sure.

THERAPIST: Take therapy, for example. Are you incompetent because you came for help here?

PATIENT: A little, maybe.

THERAPIST: Hmmm. That's interesting, because I usually view it in the opposite way. Is it possible it's actually a sign of *strength* and *competence* that you came to therapy? Because what would have happened if you hadn't?

PATIENT: I might still be pulling the covers over my head.

THERAPIST: Are you suggesting that asking for appropriate help when you have an illness like depression is a more competent thing to do than remaining depressed?

PATIENT: Yeah ... I guess so.

THERAPIST: Well, you tell me. Let's say we have two depressed college students. One seeks treatment and the other doesn't, but continues to have depressive symptoms. Which do you consider more competent?

PATIENT: Well, the one who goes for help.

THERAPIST: Now how about another situation you've mentioned—your volunteer job. Again, we have two college students. This is their first tutoring experience. They're not sure what to do because they've never done it before. One seeks help; the other doesn't, but continues to struggle. Who's the more competent?

PATIENT: (*hesitantly*) The one who goes for help?

THERAPIST: Are you sure?

PATIENT: (*Thinks for a moment.*) Yeah. It's not a sign of competence to just struggle if you could get help and do better.

THERAPIST: How much do you believe that?

PATIENT: Pretty much—80%.

THERAPIST: And how do these two situations—therapy and help in tutoring—apply to you?

PATIENT: I guess they do.

THERAPIST: Let's have you write something down about this ... Let's call the first idea "old belief"—now what did you say?

PATIENT: If I ask for help, I'm incompetent.

THERAPIST: How much do you believe it now?

PATIENT: Less. Maybe 40%.

THERAPIST: Okay, write "40%" next to it.

PATIENT: (*Does so.*)

THERAPIST: Now, write "new belief." How would you put that?

PATIENT: If I ask for help, I'm not incompetent?

THERAPIST: You don't sound convinced. Would it be better if you phrased it, "If I ask for help when it's reasonable, it's a sign of competence"?

PATIENT: Yes. (*Writes that.*)

THERAPIST: How much do you believe the new belief now?

PATIENT: A lot ... (*Reads and ponders the new belief.*) Maybe 70 to 80%. (*Writes that down.*)

THERAPIST: Okay, Sally, we'll be coming back to these beliefs again. How about for homework this week you do two things? One is to read these beliefs every day and rate how much you believe them— actually write down the percentage next to the beliefs themselves.

PATIENT: Okay.

THERAPIST: [providing a rationale] Writing down how much you believe them will make you really think about them. That's why I didn't say just read them.

PATIENT: Okay. (*Writes down the assignment.*)

THERAPIST: Second, could you be on the lookout for other situations this week where you *could* reasonably ask for help? That is, let's imagine that you believe the new belief 100%, that asking for reasonable help *is* a sign of competence. When during this coming week might you ask for help? Jot down those situations.

PATIENT: Okay.

In the previous segment, I use Socratic questioning in the context of specific situations to help Sally evaluate an intermediate belief. I judge that the standard questions of examining the evidence and evaluating outcomes will be less effective than leading Sally to develop an alternative viewpoint. My questions are much more persuasive and less even-handed than when I help her evaluate more malleable cognitions at the automatic thought level. We devise a follow-up homework assignment that is designed to have Sally continue to reflect daily on both the dysfunctional assumption and the new belief.

Behavioral Experiments to Test Beliefs

As with automatic thoughts, you can help patients devise behavioral tests to evaluate the validity of a belief. Behavioral experiments, when properly designed and carried out, can modify a patient's beliefs more powerfully than verbal techniques in the office.

THERAPIST: Okay, Sally, we've identified another belief: "If I ask for help, others will belittle me," and you believe that 60%. Of course, *I* haven't actually belittled you, have I?

PATIENT: No, of course not. But that's your job, to help people.

THERAPIST: True, but it would be useful to find out if other people, in general, are more like me or not. How could you find out?

PATIENT: Ask other people for help, I guess.

THERAPIST: Okay, whom could you ask and for what kind of help?

PATIENT: Ummm. I'm not sure.

THERAPIST: Could you ask your roommate?

PATIENT: Yeah, actually I already do. And I guess I could ask my resident adviser for help with something.

THERAPIST: Good. How about your academic adviser?

PATIENT: Uh-huh. I could also ask my brother. No. I won't ask my roommate or my brother. I know they wouldn't belittle me.

THERAPIST: Oh, so you know already there are some exceptions?

PATIENT: Yes. But I guess I could go to my adviser or my teaching assistants.

THERAPIST: What could you ask for help with?

PATIENT: Well, the teaching assistants ... I could ask questions about the papers I have due or about the readings. The resident adviser, I don't know. My academic adviser ... I would feel a little funny going to her. I don't really even know what I want to major in.

THERAPIST: That would be an interesting experiment—going for help in deciding a major to the person whose job it is to help students make those kinds of decisions.

PATIENT: True ...

THERAPIST: So you might kill two birds with one stone—testing the belief that you'll be belittled *and* getting some guidance for a real-life problem you have.

PATIENT: I guess I could.

THERAPIST: Good. So would you like to test the belief, "If I ask others for help, they'll belittle me"? How would you like to do that this week?

In the previous segment, I suggested a behavioral experiment to test a belief. Had I sensed that Sally felt hesitant, I would have asked her how likely she was to do the experiment and what practical problems or thoughts might get in her way. I might also have her do covert rehearsal (see pages 303–305) to increase the likelihood of her following through. In addition, if I judged that there was the possibility of others' belittling Sally, I might have discussed in advance what such belittling would mean to her and how she could cope if the belittling did occur. Also, I might have asked Sally for a description of belittling to ensure that she would not inaccurately perceive others' behavior as belittling when they did not intend it to be.

For an extensive description and discussion of behavioral experiments, see Bennett-Levy and colleagues (2004).

Cognitive Continuum to Modify Beliefs

This technique is useful to modify both automatic thoughts and beliefs that reflect polarized thinking (i.e., when the patient sees something in all-or-nothing terms). Sally, for example, believed that if she was not a superior student, she was a failure. Building a cognitive continuum for the concept in question facilitates the patient's recognition of the middle ground, as the following transcript illustrates:

THERAPIST: Okay, you believe pretty strongly that if you're not a superior student, you're a failure. Let's see what that looks like graphically. (*Draws a number line.*)

THERAPIST: Now, where does the superior student go?

PATIENT: Up here. I guess 90–100%.

THERAPIST: Okay. And, you're a failure. Where are you?

PATIENT: At 0%, I guess.

Initial Graph of Success

```
┌─────────────────────────────────────────┬──────────┬─────┐
0%                                         90%        100%
Sally                                      Superior
                                           student
```

THERAPIST: Now, is there anyone else who more realistically belongs at 0% than you?

PATIENT: Ummm ... Maybe this guy, Jack, who's in my economics class. I know he's doing worse than I am.

THERAPIST: Okay. We'll put Jack at 0%. But I wonder if there is anyone who's doing even worse than Jack?

PATIENT: Probably.

THERAPIST: Is it conceivable that there is someone who is failing almost every test, every paper?

PATIENT: Yeah.

THERAPIST: Okay, now if we put that person at 0%, a real failure, where does that put Jack? Where does that put you?

PATIENT: Probably Jack's at 30%. And I'm at 50%.

THERAPIST: Now, how about a person who is actually failing *everything*, and he isn't even showing up at any classes or doing any of the reading or turning in any papers?

PATIENT: I guess *he* would be at 0%.

THERAPIST: Where does that put the student who is at least trying but not passing much?

PATIENT: I guess he would be at 10%.

THERAPIST: Where does that put you and Jack?

PATIENT: Jack goes to about 50%; I guess I'm at 75%.

Revised Success Graph

```
┌─────────┬──────────┬─────┬──────┬──────┬─────┐
0%        10%        50%   75%    90%    100%
Student   Student    Jack  Sally  Superior students
who does  who tries,
nothing   but gets
          failing
          grades
```

THERAPIST: How about for homework if you see whether even 75% is accurate? Even if it is for this school, perhaps for schools and students in general, you would rank higher. In any case, how accurate is it to call someone a failure who is at the 75% mark?

PATIENT: Not very.

THERAPIST: Maybe the *worst* thing you can say is that he or she is 75% successful.

PATIENT: Yeah. (*Brightens visibly.*)

THERAPIST: Okay, to get back to your original idea, how much do you believe now that if you are not a superior student, you're a failure?

PATIENT: Not as much. Maybe 25%.

THERAPIST: Good!

The cognitive continuum technique is often useful when the patient is displaying dichotomous thinking. As with most techniques, you may directly teach the patient how to employ the technique herself so she can use it when it is applicable:

THERAPIST: Sally, let's review what we did here. We identified an all-or-nothing error in your thinking. Then we drew a number line to see whether there were really only two categories—success and failure—or whether it's more accurate to consider *degrees* of success. Can you think of anything else that you see in only two categories and that distresses you?

Intellectual–Emotional Role Play

This technique, also called point–counterpoint (Young, 1999), is usually employed after you have tried other techniques such as those described in this chapter. It is particularly useful when patients say that *intellectually* they can see that a belief is dysfunctional, but that *emotionally* or in their gut it still "feels" true. You first provide a rationale for asking patients to play the "emotional" part of their mind that strongly endorses the dysfunctional belief, while you play the "intellectual" part. In the second segment you switch roles. Note in both segments you and patients both speak as the patient; that is, you both use the word "I."

THERAPIST: It sounds from what you're saying that you still believe to some extent that you're incompetent because you didn't do as well in school last semester as you would have liked.

PATIENT: Yeah.

THERAPIST: I'd like to get a better sense of what evidence you still have that supports your belief.

PATIENT: Okay.

THERAPIST: Can we do a role play? I'll play the "intellectual" part of your mind that intellectually knows that just because you didn't get all A's doesn't mean you are incompetent through and through. I'd like you to play the "emotional" part of your mind, that voice from your gut that still really believes you *are* incompetent. I want you to argue against me as hard as you can, so I can really see what's maintaining the belief. Okay?

PATIENT: Yeah.

THERAPIST: Okay, you start. Say "I'm incompetent because I didn't get all A's."

PATIENT: I'm incompetent because I didn't get all A's.

THERAPIST: No, I'm not. I have a *belief* that I'm incompetent, but I am reasonably competent most of the time.

PATIENT: No, I'm not. If I were truly competent, I *would* have gotten all A's last semester.

THERAPIST: That's not true. Competence doesn't equal total academic perfection. If that were true, only 1% of the students in the world would be competent, and everyone else would be incompetent.

PATIENT: Well, I got a C in chemistry. That *proves* I'm incompetent.

THERAPIST: That's not right, either. If I had flunked the course *perhaps* it might be reasonable to say I wasn't competent in chemistry, but it doesn't make me incompetent in *everything*. Besides, maybe I really am competent in chemistry, but I flunked for other reasons; for example, I was depressed and couldn't concentrate on my studying.

PATIENT: But a truly competent person wouldn't become depressed in the first place.

THERAPIST: Actually, even truly competent people get depressed. There isn't a connection there. And when truly competent people get depressed, their concentration and motivation definitely suffer and they don't perform as well as usual. But that doesn't mean they are incompetent through and through.

PATIENT: I guess that's true. They're just depressed.

THERAPIST: You're right, but you're out of role. Any more evidence that you're completely incompetent?

PATIENT: (*Thinks for a moment.*) No, I guess not.

THERAPIST: Well, how about if we trade roles now, and this time you be the "intellectual" part who disputes my "emotional" part? And I'll use your same arguments.

PATIENT: Okay.

THERAPIST: I'll start. "I'm incompetent because I don't get all A's."

Switching roles provides patients with an opportunity to speak with the intellectual voice that you have just modeled. You use the same emotional reasoning and the same words that the patients used. Using their own words and not introducing new material help patients to respond more precisely to their specific concerns.

If patients are unable to formulate a response while in the intellectual role, you can either switch roles temporarily or come out of role to discuss the stuck point. As with any belief modification technique, you will evaluate both its effectiveness and the degree to which patients need further work on the belief. You do so by asking patients to rate how much they believe the belief after the intervention.

Many patients find the intellectual–emotional role play useful. A few, however, feel uncomfortable doing it. As with any intervention, the decision to use it should be collaborative. Because it is a slightly argumentative technique, take special note of patients' nonverbal reactions during the role play. Also take care to ensure that patients do not feel criticized or denigrated by the elevation of the intellectual part of their mind over the emotional part.

Using Other People as a Reference Point in Belief Modification

When patients consider *other* people's beliefs, they often obtain psychological distance from their own dysfunctional beliefs. They begin to see an inconsistency between what they believe is true or right for themselves and what they more objectively believe is true about other people. Following are four examples of using other people as a reference point to gain distance.

Example 1

THERAPIST: Sally, you mentioned last week that you think your cousin Emily has a different belief about having to do everything great.

PATIENT: Yeah.

THERAPIST: Could you put what you think her belief is into words?

PATIENT: She thinks she doesn't have to do great. She's an okay person, no matter what.

THERAPIST: Do you believe she's right? That she doesn't have to do great to be an okay person?

PATIENT: Oh, yes.

THERAPIST: Do you see her as incompetent, through and through?

PATIENT: Oh, no. She might not get good grades, but she's competent in lots of other ways.

THERAPIST: I wonder if Emily's belief could apply to you: "If I don't do great, I'm still an okay, competent person."

PATIENT: Hmmm.

THERAPIST: Is there something different about Emily that makes her okay and competent no matter how well or poorly she does, but not you?

PATIENT: (*Thinks for a moment.*) No. I don't think so. I guess I hadn't really thought of it that way.

THERAPIST: How much do you believe right now, "If I don't do great, I'm incompetent"?

PATIENT: Less, maybe 60%.

THERAPIST: And how much do you believe this new belief, "If I don't do great, I'm still an okay, competent person"?

PATIENT: More than before. Maybe 70%.

THERAPIST: Good. How about if we have you write down the new belief and start making a list of the evidence that supports this new belief.

At this point, you might introduce the Core Belief Worksheet, described in Chapter 14, which can be used for both core beliefs and intermediate beliefs.

Example 2

Another way to help patients modify an intermediate or core belief is to have them identify someone else who plainly seems to have the same dysfunctional belief. Sometimes patients can see the distortion in someone else's thinking and apply this insight to themselves. This technique is analogous to the Thought Record question: "If [friend's name] was in this situation and had this thought, what would I tell [him/her]?"

THERAPIST: Is there someone else you know who has your same belief, "If I don't work hard, I'll fail"?

PATIENT: I'm sure my friend Rebecca, from high school, believes that. She's always studying, night and day.

THERAPIST: How accurate do you think that belief is for her?

PATIENT: Oh, not at all. She's very bright. She probably couldn't fail if she tried.

THERAPIST: Is it possible that she might consider anything less than an A a failure, too?

PATIENT: Yes, I know she does.

THERAPIST: And do you agree with her, that if she gets a B, then she's failed?

PATIENT: No, of course not.

THERAPIST: How would you view it?

PATIENT: She got a B. An okay grade, not the best, but not a *failure*.

THERAPIST: What belief would you like her to have?

PATIENT: It's good to work hard and try for A's, but it's not the end of the world if you don't get them. And it doesn't mean you've failed.

THERAPIST: How does all this apply to you?

PATIENT: Hmmm. I guess it's the same.

THERAPIST: Could you spell out what's the same?

PATIENT: That if I don't get all A's, I haven't failed. I still think I should work hard, though.

THERAPIST: Sure. It's reasonable to want to work hard and do well. The unreasonable part is to believe you've failed if you haven't done perfectly. Do you agree with that?

Example 3

You could also do a role play with patients in which you instruct them to convince another person that the belief they both share is invalid for the other person.

THERAPIST: Sally, you say you think your roommate also believes that she shouldn't go to a professor for help because he might think she's unprepared or not smart enough?

PATIENT: Yes.

THERAPIST: Do you agree with her?

PATIENT: No. She's probably wrong. But even if he is critical, it doesn't mean he's right.

THERAPIST: Could we try to role-play this? I'll be your roommate; you give me advice. Don't let me get away with any distorted thinking.

PATIENT: Okay.

THERAPIST: I'll start. Sally, I don't understand this stuff. What should I do?

PATIENT: Go to the professor.

THERAPIST: Oh, I couldn't do that. He'll think I'm dumb. He'll think I'm wasting his time.

PATIENT: Hey, it's his job to help students.

THERAPIST: But he probably doesn't like students bothering him.

PATIENT: Tough, that's what he's getting paid for. Anyway, good professors like to help students. If he's impatient, that says something about him, not about you.

THERAPIST: But even if he doesn't mind helping, he'll find out how confused I am.

PATIENT: That's okay. He won't expect you to know everything. That's why you're coming to him.

THERAPIST: What if he thinks I'm dumb?

PATIENT: First of all, you wouldn't be here if you were dumb. Second, if he does expect you to know everything, he's just wrong. If you did know everything, you wouldn't be taking his course.

THERAPIST: I still think I shouldn't go.

PATIENT: No, you should. Don't let his snobby attitude make you feel like you're imposing or you're dumb. You're not.

THERAPIST: Okay. I'm convinced. Out of role, how does what you told your roommate apply to you?

Example 4

Finally, many patients can get distance from a belief by using their own children (or children they know) as a reference point, or by imagining that they have children.

THERAPIST: Sally, so you believe 80% that if you don't do as well as everyone else, then you've failed?

PATIENT: Yeah.

THERAPIST: I wonder, can you imagine that you have a daughter? She's 10 years old and in fifth grade, and she comes home one day very, very upset because her friends got A's on a test and she got a C. Would you want her to believe that she's a failure?

PATIENT: No, of course not.

THERAPIST: Why not? ... What would you like her to believe? (*Sally responds.*) Now how does what you've just said apply to you?

Acting "As If"

Changes in belief often lead to corresponding changes in behavior. And changes in behavior, in turn, often lead to corresponding changes in belief. If a belief is fairly weak, the patient may be able to change a target behavior easily and quickly, without much cognitive intervention. Many beliefs do require some modification before the patient is willing to change behaviorally. However, frequently only *some* belief modification, not complete belief change, is needed. And once patients begin to change their behavior, the belief itself becomes somewhat more attenuated (which makes it easier to continue the new behavior, which further attenuates the belief, and so on, in a positive upward spiral).

THERAPIST: Okay, Sally, how much do you believe *now* that it's a sign of weakness to ask for help?

PATIENT: Not as much. Maybe 50%.

THERAPIST: That's a good drop. Would it be to your benefit to act as if you don't believe it at all?

PATIENT: I'm not sure what you mean.

THERAPIST: If you didn't believe it was a sign of weakness, in fact, if you believed it was *good* to ask for help, what might you do this week?

PATIENT: Well, we've been talking about my going to see the teaching assistant. I guess if I really believed it was *good* to ask for help, I would go.

THERAPIST: Anything else?

PATIENT: I might try to find a tutor for Economics ... I might ask to borrow notes from the guy down the hall ...

THERAPIST: Hey, that's good. And what positive things could happen if you did some of these things?

PATIENT: (*Laughs.*) I could get the help that I need.

THERAPIST: Do you think you're ready this week to act as if you believe it's a good thing to ask for help?

PATIENT: Maybe.

THERAPIST: Okay, in a minute, we'll find out what thoughts might get in the way, but first, how about if you jot down those ideas you had. And do you want to write down this technique to get you going? Act *as if* you believe the new belief, even if you don't totally.

This acting "as if" technique is equally applicable to core beliefs as are the preceding intermediate belief modification techniques.

Using Self-Disclosure to Modify Beliefs

Using appropriate and judicious self-disclosure can help some patients view their problems or beliefs in a different way. The self-disclosure, of course, should be genuine and relevant:

THERAPIST: You know, Sally, when I was in college, I had some trouble going to professors for help because I thought I'd be showing my ignorance too. And to tell you the truth, the few times I did end up doing it anyway, I had mixed results. Sometimes the professors were really nice and helpful. But a couple of times, they were pretty brusque, just told me to reread a chapter or something. The point is, just because I didn't understand something didn't mean I was incompetent. And the professors who were brusque—well, I think that said a lot more about them than about me. (*pause*) What do you think?

In summary, you help patients to *identify* intermediate beliefs by recognizing when a belief has been expressed as an automatic thought, by providing part of an assumption, by directly eliciting a rule or an attitude, by using the downward arrow technique, by looking for common themes among the patient's automatic thoughts, and/or by reviewing a belief questionnaire completed by the patient. You next determine how *important* the belief is by ascertaining how strongly the patient believes it, and how broadly and strongly it affects her functioning. Then you decide whether to begin the task of *modifying* it in the current session or wait for future sessions. When beginning belief modification work, you *educate* the patient about the nature of beliefs, *change rules and attitudes into assumption form,* and explore the *advantages and disadvantages* of a given belief. You mentally *formulate a new, more functional belief* and guide the patient toward its adoption through many *belief modification techniques,* including Socratic questioning, behavioral experiments, cognitive continua, intellectual–emotional role plays, using others as a reference point, acting "as if," and self-disclosure. Some of these techniques are more persuasive than standard Socratic questioning of automatic thoughts, because the beliefs are much more rigidly held. These same techniques can also be used to modify core beliefs.

Chapter 14

IDENTIFYING AND MODIFYING
CORE BELIEFS

Core beliefs, as described in Chapter 3, are one's most central ideas about the self. Some authors refer to these beliefs as schemas. Beck (1964) differentiates the two by suggesting that schemas are cognitive structures within the mind, the specific content of which are core beliefs. Furthermore, he theorizes that negative core beliefs essentially fall into two broad categories: those associated with helplessness and those associated with unlovability (Beck, 1999). A third category, associated with worthlessness, has also been described (J. S. Beck, 2005). Some patients have core beliefs that fall in one category; others have core beliefs in two or all three categories.

People develop these beliefs from an early age, as children, with their genetic predisposition toward certain personality traits, interact with significant others, and encounter a series of situations. For much of their lives, most people maintain relatively positive and realistic core beliefs (e.g., "I am substantially in control"; "I can do most things competently"; "I am a functional human being"; "I am likable"; "I am worthwhile"). Negative core beliefs may surface only during times of psychological distress. (Some patients with personality disorders, however, may have almost continuously activated negative core beliefs.) Often, unlike automatic thoughts, core beliefs that patients "know" to be true about themselves are not fully articulated until you peel back the layers by continuing to ask for the meaning of their thoughts.

It is important to note that patients may also have negative core beliefs about other people and their worlds: "Other people are untrustworthy"; "Other people will hurt me"; "The world is a rotten place"; "The world is dangerous." Fixed, overgeneralized ideas such as these often need to be evaluated and modified, in addition to core beliefs about the self.

Before Sally became depressed, she recognized when she was acting competently and interpreted signs of possible incompetence as situation specific; for example, when she got a lower grade than expected on a paper in high school, she took it as an instance of inadequacy, but she did not interpret this situation as meaning she was an overall incompetent person.

As Sally was becoming depressed, her positive schema became deactivated and her negative schema containing the cognition "I am incompetent" became almost fully activated. As illustrated on page 34, Sally began to overemphasize and overgeneralize negative data, contained in negative rectangles, continually reinforcing her belief that she was incompetent. At the same time, Sally was failing to recognize a significant amount of positive data related to her schema (such as resuming her usual activities even though the depression made it very difficult to do so); these positive triangles "bounced off" the schema and did not get incorporated. Sally also discounted much positive information through her "Yes, but . . ." interpretations of her experiences ("Yes, I did well on the quiz, but it was easy."; "Yes, I helped the kid I was tutoring, but I got lucky because I really didn't know what I was doing."). These positive triangles were, in essence, changed into negative rectangles.

Sally was not volitionally processing information in this dysfunctional way. This kind of information processing is automatic and a symptom of depression. I recognized that it would be important to work directly on modifying her negative core belief, not only to alleviate her current depression, but also to prevent or reduce the severity of future episodes.

For example, one day when Sally was depressed, she received a B– on an exam. She immediately understood this data as signifying that she was an incompetent person. When she received an A on a paper the next day, her mind automatically discounted this positive evidence that was contrary to her negative core belief. She believed the good grade was not an indication of competence; in fact, she believed that she was incompetent and that she had merely "fooled" the professor. She also failed to recognize other positive data; for example, that she got to every class on time. (Note that had she gotten to class late or skipped class, she would have interpreted those experiences in a negative light, as confirming her negative core belief.)

You will begin to work directly on belief modification as early in treatment as possible. Once patients change their beliefs, they are less likely to process data in a maladaptive way. In specific situations, they have different (more adaptive and realistic) automatic thoughts and improved reactions. You may not succeed with early belief modification, though, if patients:

- Have core beliefs that are quite rigid and overgeneralized.
- Do not yet believe that cognitions are ideas and not necessarily truths.
- Experience very high levels of affect when beliefs are elicited or questioned.
- Do not have a strong enough alliance with you (they may not trust you sufficiently; they may not perceive you as understanding who they really are; they may feel invalidated by the process of belief evaluation).

In these cases, you will teach patients the tools of identifying, evaluating, and adaptively responding to automatic thoughts and intermediate beliefs before using the same tools for core beliefs.

You may unwittingly try to evaluate a core belief early in treatment because it has been expressed as an automatic thought. Such evaluation may have little effect. In another case, you may intentionally test the modifiability of a core belief even before you have done much work at the automatic thought and intermediate belief level.

The degree of difficulty in identifying and modifying core beliefs varies from patient to patient. In general, patients who are in significant emotional distress are more easily able than others to express their core beliefs (because the beliefs are activated in session). And, in general, it is far easier to modify the negative core beliefs of Axis I patients whose counterbalancing positive core beliefs have been activated throughout much of their lives. Negative core beliefs of patients with personality disorders are usually much more difficult to modify (J. S. Beck, 2005; Beck et al., 2004; Young, 1999) because they typically have fewer positive core beliefs, their positive core beliefs are weaker, and they have developed a multitude of strongly held negative core beliefs that interconnect and support each other like a network.

In identifying and modifying core beliefs, you do the following during the course of treatment (each step is described later in this chapter):

1. Mentally hypothesize from which category of core belief ("helplessness" or "unlovability" or "worthlessness") specific automatic thoughts appear to have arisen (see Figure 14.1).
2. Specify the core belief (to yourself) using the same techniques you use to identify patients' intermediate beliefs.
3. Present your hypothesis about the core belief to patients, asking for confirmation or disconfirmation; refine your hypothesis about the core belief as patients provide additional data about current and childhood situations and their reactions to them.
4. Educate patients about core beliefs in general and about their specific core beliefs; guide patients in monitoring the operation of the core belief in the present.
5. Help patients specify and strengthen a new, more adaptive core belief.
6. Begin to evaluate and modify the negative core belief with patients; examine the childhood origin of the core belief (if applicable), its maintenance through the years, and its contribution to patients' present difficulties; continue to monitor the activation of the core belief in the present; use both "intellectual" and "emotional" or experiential methods to decrease the strength of the old core belief and to increase the strength of the new core belief.

CATEGORIZING CORE BELIEFS

As mentioned previously, patients' core beliefs may be categorized in the helplessness realm, the unlovability realm, and/or the worthlessness realm. Whenever patients present data (problems, automatic thoughts, emotions, behavior, history), you "listen" for the category of core belief that seems to have been activated. For example, when Sally expresses thoughts about her work being too hard, about her inability to concentrate, and about her fears of failing, I hypothesize that a core belief in the helpless category was operating. Sally occasionally mentions automatic thoughts that her friends might not want to spend time with her because she is depressed. When I do the downward arrow technique, asking what that means about her, she shrugs and says, with little emotion: "I just won't have anyone to hang out with." Sally does not seem to have a significant core belief of unlovability.

Another patient consistently expresses thoughts of others not caring about him and fears that he is too different from others to sustain a relationship. This patient has a core belief in the category of unlovability. A third patient is frustrated by her inability to get others to listen to her. Although her distress occurs only in interpersonal situations, she does not believe that she is unlovable. Her core belief of helplessness is what gets activated. Finally, a fourth patient feels like a worthless human being, not because he cannot achieve (a helpless belief), and not related to his relationships (which might possibly be an unlovable belief). He believes that morally, he is a bad person (a worthless belief).

The top of Figure 14.1 lists typical core beliefs in the helpless category. Themes include being ineffective:

- In getting things done ("I'm inadequate"; "I'm incompetent"; "I can't do anything right").
- In protecting oneself ("I'm vulnerable, weak, powerless, trapped").
- In achievement ("I'm a failure, I don't measure up, I'm a loser").

The middle of Figure 14.1 lists typical core beliefs in the unlovable category. Themes include being unlikable, undesirable, unappealing, or defective (not in achievement or morality, but being defective in character so as to preclude gaining the sustained love and caring of others). The bottom of Figure 14.1 lists worthless core beliefs. When patients have beliefs in this category, they are not unduly concerned with their efffectiveness or lovability. They just believe that they are bad, unworthy, or even dangerous to other people.

Sometimes it is clear in which category a given core belief belongs, especially when patients actually use words such as "I am helpless," or "I am unlovable." At other times, you may not know initially which category of core belief has been activated. For example, depressed patients may say, "I'm not good enough." You need to ascertain the meaning of the cognition to determine whether they believe they are not good enough to achieve or to gain respect (helpless category), or if they are not good enough for others to love them (unlovable category).

To summarize, you begin mentally to formulate a hypothesis about patients' core beliefs whenever they provide data in the form of their automatic thoughts (and associated meanings) and reactions (emotions and behaviors). You first make a gross distinction (to yourself) among cognitions that seem to fall in the helpless, unlovable, or worthless categories.

Helpless core beliefs

"I am incompetent."
"I am ineffective."
"I can't do anything right."
"I am helpless."
"I am powerless."
"I am weak."
"I am vulnerable."
"I am a victim."

"I am needy."
"I am trapped."
"I am out of control."
"I am a failure."
"I am defective" [i.e., I do not measure up to others].
"I am not good enough" [in terms of achievement].
"I am a loser."

Unlovable core beliefs

"I am unlovable."
"I am unlikeable."
"I am undesirable."
"I am unattractive."
"I am unwanted."
"I am uncared for."

"I am different."
"I am bad [so others will not love me]."
"I am defective [so others will not love me]."
"I am not good enough [to be loved by others]."
"I am bound to be rejected."
"I am bound to be abandoned."
"I am bound to be alone."

Worthless core beliefs

"I am worthless."
"I am unacceptable."
"I am bad."
"I am a waste."

"I am immoral."
"I am dangerous."
"I am toxic."
"I am evil."
"I don't deserve to live."

FIGURE 14.1. Categories of core beliefs. Adapted from *Cognitive therapy for challenging problems: What to do when the basics don't work.* Copyright 2005 by Judith S. Beck. New York: Guilford Press.

IDENTIFYING CORE BELIEFS

You use the same techniques to identify patients' specific core beliefs that you used when identifying their intermediate beliefs (see Chapter 13). In addition to the *downward arrow* technique, you look for *central themes in patients' automatic thoughts,* watch for *core beliefs expressed as automatic thoughts,* and *directly elicit* the core belief.

You will often identify a core belief early in therapy to conceptualize patients and plan treatment. You may gather data about and even try to help patients evaluate their core beliefs early on. In some cases, such early evaluation is ineffective but helps you test the strength, breadth, and modifiability of the core belief.

THERAPIST: What went through your mind when you couldn't finish the statistics assignment?

PATIENT: I can't do anything right. I'll never be able to make it here.

THERAPIST: [downward arrow technique] And if that's true, that you can't do anything right and you can't make it here, what does that mean?

PATIENT: [core belief] I'm hopeless. I'm so incompetent.

THERAPIST: How much do you believe you're incompetent?

PATIENT: Oh, 100%.

THERAPIST: And how incompetent are you: a little, a lot?

PATIENT: Completely. I'm completely incompetent.

THERAPIST: In every way?

PATIENT: Just about.

THERAPIST: Any evidence that you're not incompetent?

PATIENT: No ... No, I don't think so.

THERAPIST: Did you say you're doing okay in your other courses?

PATIENT: Yes, but not as well as I should be.

THERAPIST: Does the fact that you're doing okay in them contradict this idea that you're incompetent?

PATIENT: No, if I were really competent, I'd be doing much better.

THERAPIST: How about other areas of your life—managing your apartment, managing your finances, taking care of yourself ...?

PATIENT: I'm doing pretty badly at them, too.

THERAPIST: So this idea that you're incompetent extends to other things, too?

PATIENT: Just about everything.

THERAPIST: Okay, I can see how strongly you believe this idea. Can we go back to the situation in which you couldn't finish the statistics assignment and you had the thoughts: "I can't do anything right. I'll never be able to make it here."

In this example, I use the downward arrow technique to identify an idea I conceptualize as a core belief. I gently test its strength, breadth, and modifiability, and decide not to pursue further evaluation at this time. However, I label it as an "idea" (implying it is not necessarily a truth) and mark it as a future topic.

PRESENTING CORE BELIEFS

When you believe that you have collected sufficient data to hypothesize about the core belief, and when you believe patients will be sufficiently receptive, you tentatively pose your conceptualization to them, as I did below.

THERAPIST: Sally, we've talked about a number of different problems in the past few weeks—your schoolwork, decisions about how to spend the summer, your volunteer job. Whenever we examine your thoughts, and ask you what they mean about you, you consistently say they mean that you're incompetent ... Is that right?

PATIENT: Yes. I still think I'm incompetent.

Or you might review with patients a number of related automatic thoughts they had in a variety of situations and then ask them to draw a conclusion as to an underlying pattern ("Sally, do you see a common theme in these automatic thoughts?").

With certain patients you can use a hand-drawn diagram, a simplified version of the Cognitive Conceptualization Diagram (page 200), early in treatment. Either with or without the diagram, you might briefly explore childhood precursors.

THERAPIST: Do you remember feeling incompetent like this at other times in your life, too? As a child?

PATIENT: Yeah, sometimes. I remember never being able to do things my brother could.

THERAPIST: Can you give me some examples?

You will use historical data later, when you hypothesize to patients how they came to believe a core belief, and explain how the core belief could be untrue or mostly untrue even though they currently believe it so strongly.

EDUCATING PATIENTS ABOUT CORE BELIEFS
AND MONITORING THEIR OPERATION

It is important for patients to understand the following about a core belief:

- That it is an idea, not necessarily a truth.
- That they can believe it quite strongly, even "feel" it to be true, and yet it might be mostly or entirely untrue.
- That, as an idea, it can be tested.
- That it may be rooted in childhood events, and may or may not have been true at the time they first came to believe it.
- That it continues to be maintained through the operation of their schemas, in which they readily recognize data that support the core belief while ignoring or discounting data to the contrary.
- That you and they, working together, can use a variety of strategies over time to change this idea so that they can view themselves in a more realistic way.

In the transcript that follows, I educate Sally about her core belief. (She had previously confirmed the conceptualization I had presented.)

THERAPIST: Sally, does this [automatic thought that she will not be able to write her economics paper] sound familiar? Do you think your idea that you're incompetent could be getting in the way?

PATIENT: Yeah. I do feel incompetent.

THERAPIST: Well, Sally, one of two things has been going on. The problem is either you really *are* incompetent, and we'll have to do some work together to make you more competent ... or the problem is that you *believe* you are incompetent; and sometimes, you believe it so strongly that you actually *act* in an incompetent way, like not going to the library to start researching your paper. (*pause*) What do you think?

PATIENT: I don't know.

THERAPIST: Why don't we write these two possibilities on paper? This is what I'd like to start doing in therapy, if it is okay with you, seeing which possibility seems more true—that you really *are* incompetent, or that you *believe* you're incompetent.

Later I explain core beliefs to Sally, in small parts, making sure she understands as I proceed.

THERAPIST: This idea, "I'm incompetent," is what we call a core belief. Let me tell you a little bit about core beliefs so you'll understand why they're more difficult to evaluate and respond to. Okay?

PATIENT: Yes.

THERAPIST: First of all, a core belief is an idea that you may not believe very strongly when you're not depressed. On the other hand, we'd expect you to believe it almost completely when you *are* depressed, even if there's evidence to the contrary. (*pause*) Follow me so far?

PATIENT: Yes.

THERAPIST: When you get depressed, this idea becomes activated. When it's activated, you'll easily notice any evidence that seems to support it, and you'll tend to ignore any evidence that contradicts it. It's as if there is a screen around your head. Anything that fits in with the idea that you are incompetent sails straight through the screen and into your head. Any information that contradicts the idea won't fit through the screen, and so either you don't notice it, or you change it in some way so it *will* fit through the screen. Do you think you might be screening information like this?

PATIENT: I'm not sure.

THERAPIST: Well, let's see. Looking back at the past few weeks, what evidence is there that you *might* be competent?

PATIENT: Ummm ... I got an A on my statistics exam.

THERAPIST: Good! And did that evidence go right through the screen? Did you tell yourself, "I got an A. That means I'm smart or competent or a good student," or anything like that?

PATIENT: No. I said, "Well, the exam was easy. I learned some of that stuff last year."

THERAPIST: Oh, so it looks like the screen *was* operating. Do you see how you discounted information that contradicted your core belief, "I am incompetent"?

PATIENT: Hmmm.

THERAPIST: Can you think of any other examples from this week? Situations where a reasonable person might think something you did showed you were competent, even if you didn't?

PATIENT: (*Thinks for a moment.*) Well, I helped my roommate figure out how to solve a problem with her father. But that doesn't count; anyone could have done what I did.

THERAPIST: Good example. Again, it sounds as if you didn't recognize information that doesn't fit in with your idea: "I'm incompetent."

I'm going to let you think about how true the idea is that *anyone* could have done what you did. Maybe this is another instance of not giving yourself credit, when another person might have thought it was evidence that you are *not* incompetent.

PATIENT: Well, my roommate did think I helped her a lot.

THERAPIST: Okay, just to summarize: "I'm incompetent" seems to be a core belief that goes back a long time with you, and which you believe much more strongly when you're depressed. Can you summarize how it seems to work?

PATIENT: Well, you're saying that when I'm depressed, I screen in information that agrees with it and I screen out information that doesn't agree with it.

THERAPIST: Right. How about for homework this week if you try to notice each day how the screen is operating—jot down information that seems to support the idea that you're incompetent. And here's the harder part. Really hunt for and jot down any information that another person might think contradicts it. Okay?

In the next session, I explain why Sally believes her core belief so strongly and how it could still be untrue.

THERAPIST: Okay, you did a good job this week noticing how you tend to let in only the negative information that seems to support your idea that you're incompetent. As we predicted, it was much harder to recognize positive information that contradicts your idea.

PATIENT: Yeah. I didn't do it very well.

THERAPIST: Are you feeling incompetent now?

PATIENT: (*Laughs.*) Yes. I guess so.

THERAPIST: Is the screen operating right now? Did you put more emphasis on the part of the homework you didn't do as well, and forget about the part you did do well?

PATIENT: I guess I did.

THERAPIST: What do you think is the effect of having a screen like this?

PATIENT: Makes me not notice the good things.

THERAPIST: Right. And, day after day, what happens to this idea, "I'm incompetent"?

PATIENT: Gets stronger, I guess.

THERAPIST: Right. To the point where it "feels" true, even if it's not.

PATIENT: Hmmm.

THERAPIST: Do you see now how the idea that you're incompetent *could* be false, even though it feels so true?

PATIENT: Well, I can kind of see it intellectually, but I still do *feel* incompetent.

THERAPIST: That's pretty common. In the next few weeks, we'll keep evaluating this idea. And then we'll work together on helping the more reasonable, intellectual part of your mind talk to the more emotional side. Okay?

PATIENT: Yeah.

Alternatively, I could have drawn the schema diagram from page 34 and elicited the same examples of positive and negative data, and asked Sally whether she thought the diagram accurately illustrated how she was processing information. I would then ask her, "Sally, if it's true that you've been overemphasizing the negative data and ignoring or discounting the positive data, can you see how your idea that you're incompetent could grow stronger with each passing hour and each passing day and week and month—but it might not be true, or not completely true?"

Bibliotherapy can reinforce important core belief work. *Prisoners of Belief* (McKay & Fanning, 1991) and *Reinventing Your Life* (Young & Klosko, 1994) are helpful in this phase of treatment.

DEVELOPING A NEW CORE BELIEF

Many depressed patients had a different core belief, a more positive, reality-based, and functional idea about themselves, before the onset of their Axis I disorder. They may easily identify this belief.

THERAPIST: Before you got depressed, say a year ago, how did you see yourself? Did you think you were unlikable?

PATIENT: No; I mean, not everyone liked me, but I basically thought I was a good person. People liked me.

THERAPIST: So was your belief "I'm likable"?

PATIENT: Yeah, it was.

When patients cannot express their former idea, you mentally devise a new, more realistic, and functional belief and guide patients toward it. A relatively positive belief is generally easier for patients to adopt than a belief that is at an extreme.

For example:

Old core belief	New core belief
"I'm (completely) unlovable."	"I'm generally a likable person"
"I'm bad."	"I'm okay."
"I'm powerless."	"I have control over many things."
"I'm defective."	"I'm normal, with both strengths and weaknesses."

THERAPIST: Sally, we've been talking about this core belief, "I'm incompetent." What do you intellectually think a more accurate belief might be?

PATIENT: I am competent?

THERAPIST: That's good. Or we could work on a new belief that might be easier for you to adopt, say, "I'm competent in most ways, but I'm only human, too." Which sounds better?

PATIENT: The second.

Having identified a negative core belief and devised a positive belief, you will simultaneously work on weakening the first and strengthening the latter.

STRENGTHENING NEW CORE BELIEFS

You will primarily strengthen new core beliefs in two ways. One, from the beginning of treatment, as described on pages 26–27, you deliberately elicit positive data from patients through questioning, and you also point out positive data to them—especially when the data contradict the old, negative core belief but support a new, more reality-based belief. Two, when specifically working on strengthening their new core beliefs, you ask patients to examine their experiences in a new way that facilitates their ability to recognize positive data themselves.

I accomplished the tasks of eliciting and pointing out positive data in several ways with Sally. For example:

- At the evaluation, I asked Sally what her strengths were.
- Later, whenever applicable, I asked her whether certain data indicated other strengths. ("So you did all these things: you made a list of all your assignments for this week and figured out when you would do them and what resources you would need. Is being organized a strength of yours?")
- During the first part of the session, I asked Sally about her positive experiences ("What positive things happened since I saw

you last?"). Finishing a paper, doing reasonably well on an exam, being assertive with her roommate, figuring out which classes to sign up for, starting a self-defense class, to name a few examples, all provided data that I emphasized at the time and later that supported her new core belief.

- I suggested that Sally keep a credit list (page 275).
- I continually asked Sally for (positive) evidence that her cognitions were not true, or not completely true.
- I asked for her attribution when she displayed positive behaviors ("What does it say about you that *you* were the one to initiate the recycling project?").
- I provided her with feedback about her accomplishments and positive qualities ("It sounds like you did a great job organizing the get-together for the dorm").

The second strategy involves helping patients adopt a different view of their experiences. They do so by asking themselves what they are doing or what is happening that could lend support to the new core belief. ("Sally, can you keep track this coming week of anything that shows that you are competent?") If patients have difficulty with this assignment, you can modify it. ("Sally, could you pretend I'm following you around this week? Notice the times when you think *I* would say, 'That shows you're competent,' or could you notice what your roommate does that shows you *she's* competent—and then see whether you're doing the same thing?")

Most patients need a visual or audio cue to remind themselves to look for positive data throughout the day, for example, they can wear a rubber band around their wrist, post sticky notes, have pop-up reminders on their computers or smartphones, or set the alarm on their cell phone to ring periodically. Encourage them to record the data in some way, instead of just making mental notes that they are likely to forget. A Core Belief Worksheet (Figure 14.3) can help them organize their note taking.

Finally, it is important to track with patients how strongly they believe their new core belief over time, both at an intellectual level and an emotional level. You will elicit instances in which their degree of belief was relatively higher and reinforce their interpretation, and you will help them reframe the meaning of experiences in which their belief was relatively lower.

MODIFYING NEGATIVE CORE BELIEFS

To help patients change their negative core beliefs, you will use many techniques described in the previous chapter, as well as others that are

Already described	Additional techniques
Socratic questioning techniques	Core Belief Worksheet
Examining advantages and disadvantages	Extreme contrasts
Intellectual–emotional role plays	Stories and metaphors
Acting "as if"	Historical tests
Behavioral experiments	Restructuring early memories
Cognitive continuum	Coping cards
Self-disclosure	

FIGURE 14.2. Techniques to modify core beliefs.

described below (see Figure 14.2). Core beliefs usually change at the intellectual level first, especially when you have been employing intellectual-level techniques. Patients may need emotional-level techniques to change their core beliefs at the emotional level.

THE CORE BELIEF WORKSHEET

Having identified the old core belief and developed a new one, you may introduce the Core Belief Worksheet (CBW; see Figure 14.3), or draw a modified chart.

Patients fill out the CBW in session and for homework as they monitor the operation of their beliefs and reframe evidence that seemed to support the old belief.

THERAPIST: Sally, let me show you a Core Belief Worksheet, which is just an organized way of working on your beliefs. I'd like us to keep this sheet in front of us during our sessions to see whether the topic we're discussing is relevant to competency.

PATIENT: Okay.

THERAPIST: Learning to fill out this sheet takes time and practice, just as it took you a while to get good at the Thought Record. Okay?

PATIENT: Yes.

THERAPIST: All right. Is it okay if we start with the right side, evidence that you're incompetent?

PATIENT: Sure.

Evidence supporting new core belief *I'm competent but human*	Evidence supporting old core belief *I'm incompetent* with reframe
Did well on literature paper. Asked a question in statistics. Understood this worksheet. Made decisions about next year. Arranged to switch phones, bank accounts, insurance, etc. Got together all the references I need for econ paper. Understood most of Chapter 6 in statistics book. Explained statistics concept to guy down the hall.	Didn't understand econ concept in class *BUT* I hadn't read about it and I'll probably understand it later. At worst it's *an* incompetency but maybe it's actually her fault for not explaining it well enough. Didn't go to the teaching assistant for help *BUT* that doesn't mean I'm incompetent. I was nervous about going because I think I should be able to figure out these things myself and I thought he'd think I was unprepared. Got a B on my literature paper, *BUT* it's an okay grade. If I were really incompetent, I wouldn't even be here.

FIGURE 14.3. Sally's Core Belief Worksheet. From *Cognitive behavior therapy worksheet packet.* Copyright 2011 by Judith S. Beck. Bala Cynwyd, PA: Beck Institute for Cognitive Behavior Therapy.

THERAPIST: Okay, think over what you did *today*. What evidence do you have that you're incompetent?

PATIENT: Well, I didn't understand something my economics professor presented in class today.

THERAPIST: Okay, write that down on the right side, then put a big "BUT" next to it. Now, let's think if there could be another explanation for why you might not have understood the concept *other* than that you're incompetent.

PATIENT: Well, it was the first time she talked about it. And it wasn't in the readings.

THERAPIST: Good. Now might you be able to understand it after she has reviewed it, or you've read something about it, or asked someone else to explain it better?

PATIENT: Probably.

THERAPIST: Okay. Now next to the "BUT" you'll write what we call the "reframe"—another, more helpful way of looking at the evidence. What could you say here?

244 COGNITIVE BEHAVIOR THERAPY: BASICS AND BEYOND

PATIENT: I guess I could say, "But I hadn't read about it, and I'll probably understand it later."

THERAPIST: Okay, write that down ... Now let's see if we can make the reframe even stronger. Would you agree that not understanding a concept at worst means a person has *an* incompetency, not that she's completely incompetent as a person?

PATIENT: Yes, that's true.

THERAPIST: Is it possible that *many* competent people don't necessarily grasp concepts at the first presentation?

PATIENT: True.

THERAPIST: I wonder, is it possible that it was actually an incompetency of the *professor*, because if she had explained it more clearly, you might have understood it?

PATIENT: That's possible.

THERAPIST: Why don't you take a minute and see if there is anything else you want to add in writing?... Okay, let's try the left side now. What evidence do you have from *today* that you *are* competent at many things? I'll warn you, this can be hard if your screen is operating.

PATIENT: Well, I worked on my literature paper.

THERAPIST: Good. Write that down. What else?

PATIENT: I asked a question in my statistics course.

THERAPIST: You did! Good. What else?

PATIENT: (*No response.*)

THERAPIST: How about the fact that you seem to grasp how to do this worksheet?

PATIENT: I guess so.

THERAPIST: Okay, how about for homework if you try to add to this sheet every day? Can you see that to start, doing the first part of the right side will be easiest, but the second part and the left side will probably be harder?

PATIENT: Yeah.

THERAPIST: So do what you can. It may be that we'll have to work together to do the reframes and look for positive evidence. I'll give you a clue, though. If you have trouble with these two parts, pretend someone else, your roommate, for example, has done exactly what you've done, and see how you'd view her actions. Okay?

PATIENT: Sure.

THERAPIST: Can you think of anything that might get in the way of your doing this assignment this week?

PATIENT: No, I'll try it.

THERAPIST: Good.

Had Sally displayed difficulty in identifying positive data during the session, I might have postponed this homework assignment, trying different techniques in session first to help her successfully elicit items for the left side. For example, I might use a contrasting technique:

THERAPIST: How about the fact that you battled your way through the student health system so you would get seen right away? Doesn't that belong on the left side?

PATIENT: I don't know. I was just so mad; it was easy.

THERAPIST: Wait a minute. If you *hadn't* asserted yourself, wouldn't you have put that on the right side as a sign of incompetence?

PATIENT: Probably.

THERAPIST: So think of it this way: Anything that you would criticize yourself for or put on the right side if you *didn't* do it probably belongs on the left.

Other ways of having patients recognize positive data that belong on the left side of the worksheet include asking patients:

1. To think of data that they would say were positive evidence for *another* person: "Sally, can you think of someone else who you consider is competent in most ways? Who would that be? What have *you* done today that you would say shows that [this person] is competent if *she* or *he* had done it?"

2. To name another person who would say the data indicate positive evidence about the patient: "Sally, who's someone you think knows you pretty well, whose judgment you trust? What would [this person] say you had done today that's evidence you're competent?" or "Sally, what have you done today that *I* probably think indicates you're competent?"

3. To reflect on whether they would discount specific positive evidence if they compared what they did to a hypothetical *negative* model: "Sally, you don't believe that finishing that brief paper is a sign of competence. But would a *truly* incompetent person have

been able to write it? Would a truly incompetent person even have made it to where you are now?"

4. To rate the strength of their beliefs at the intellectual and emotional levels at the beginning of each session, before setting the agenda. Then you can ask, "When you believed *least* strongly that you were incompetent or most strongly that you were competent, what was going on? Is this something we should put on the agenda?" Discussing these (more positive) situations provides an opportunity to gather or reinforce evidence for the left side.

You may also take the opportunity throughout the session to question patients about the applicability of the CBW to the topic at hand.

THERAPIST: Sally, can you summarize what we've just been talking about?

PATIENT: Well, I was pretty down because I didn't get the summer job I wanted, and where anyone would probably be disappointed, I got pretty depressed because I was thinking it meant that I was incompetent.

THERAPIST: Good. Can you see how this is relevant to the Core Belief Worksheet?

PATIENT: Yes. It's the same idea.

THERAPIST: How can you write it down on the worksheet?

PATIENT: I guess it goes on the *right side* ... I didn't get the research assistant job ... but that doesn't mean I'm completely incompetent. A lot of people applied for it, some with lots more experience than me.

Using Extreme Contrasts to Modify Core Beliefs

At times, it is helpful for patients to compare themselves with someone, either real or imagined, who is at a negative extreme of the quality related to their core belief. You suggest that patients imagine someone within their frame of reference. (This technique is similar to the cognitive continuum described in Chapter 13.)

THERAPIST: I wonder, do you know anyone at your school who truly *is* incompetent or at least *behaves* very incompetently?

PATIENT: Ummm ... There is one guy in my dorm who never, I think, goes to classes or does work. He just seems to party all the time. I think he's failing.

THERAPIST: Okay, so compared to him, how incompetent are you?

PATIENT: (*Pauses.*) Not very.

THERAPIST: If you truly were an incompetent person, through and through, what would you be doing differently?

PATIENT: ... I guess I'd drop out of college, sit around all day ... not support myself ... not do anything worthwhile ... not have any friends ...

THERAPIST: How close are you to that now?

PATIENT: Not at all, I guess.

THERAPIST: So how accurate would you say it is to label yourself as truly incompetent?

PATIENT: I guess it's really not accurate.

Using Stories, Movies, and Metaphors

You can help patients develop a different idea about themselves by encouraging them to reflect on their view of characters or people who share the same negative core belief. When patients experience vivid examples of the invalidity of others' very strongly held core beliefs, they begin to understand how they, too, could have a very strong core belief that is not accurate.

One patient was sure that she was bad because as a child, and later as an adult, her mother had been physically and emotionally abusive to her, often telling the patient how bad she was. It was helpful for this patient to reflect on the story of Cinderella, in which a wicked step-mother treats a child quite badly without the child's being at fault.

Historical Tests of the Core Belief

When patients' core beliefs stem from early experiences, it is often useful to have them examine how their belief originated and was maintained through the years (Young, 1999). You elicit and help patients reframe evidence that seemed to support the core belief from an early age, and also to uncover evidence that contradicted it. (You can use the CBW to collect data.) Usually, this process is initiated after patients have been monitoring the operation of their core belief in the *present* and have started the process of modifying it. First you provide a rationale:

THERAPIST: Sally, I'd like to see where this idea that you're incompetent started.

PATIENT: Okay.

THERAPIST: Let's pull out the Core Belief Worksheet. Do you remember anything when you were quite young that made you believe at the time that you were incompetent? Say, before elementary school?

PATIENT: I remember preschool. I remember doing something with puzzles and the teacher yelling at me. I was crying ...

THERAPIST: Were you slow to finish it?

PATIENT: Yes, something like that.

THERAPIST: And you felt pretty incompetent?

PATIENT: Uh-huh.

THERAPIST: Okay, write that down on the right-hand side. We'll fill in the reframes later. What else?

PATIENT: I remember this time my family went to the state park. Everyone else could ride their bikes around, but I couldn't keep up, and I got left really far behind.

Either in session or for homework, patients continue this first step: recording memories that may have contributed to the establishment or maintenance of the core belief. They may reflect on preschool, elementary school, high school, college, their 20s, and succeeding decades. The second step of the historical review involves searching for and recording evidence that supports the new, positive belief for each period. Having evoked more positive memories, patients are ready for the third step: reframing each piece of negative evidence. Finally, in the fourth step, patients summarize each period. For example:

> High School Years—I did a lot of things competently, from sports to being responsible for a lot of things at home to doing well at school. It's true that I didn't get all A's, and I wasn't good at everything, and I felt incompetent at times, but basically I was competent.

Restructuring Early Memories

For many Axis I patients, the "intellectual" techniques that have already been presented are sufficient to modify a core belief, as long as they are employed in the presence of emotion (i.e., that the core belief has been activated and the patient is experiencing negative affect). For others, special "emotional" or experiential techniques, in which patients' affect is aroused, are also indicated. One such technique involves role-playing, reenacting an event to help patients reinterpret an earlier, traumatic experience. In the transcript that follows, I help a patient restructure the meaning of an earlier event related to a current distressing situation.

THERAPIST: Annie, you look pretty down today.

PATIENT: Yes. (*crying*) ... My boss called me into his office this afternoon. He said I made a couple of typos in an e-mail I sent out for him, and that I have to be more careful and proofread my e-mails better.

THERAPIST: What went through your mind when he said that?

PATIENT: I'm a terrible secretary. I can't do anything right.

THERAPIST: How are you feeling?

PATIENT: [expressing her emotion] Sad. Real sad. [expressing her core belief] And, you know, incompetent.

THERAPIST: In proofreading some e-mails or overall?

PATIENT: Overall, I'm completely incompetent.

THERAPIST: [heightening her affect to facilitate memory retrieval] Do you feel this sadness and incompetency somewhere in your body?

PATIENT: Behind my eyes. And my shoulders feel heavy.

Instead of focusing on this current situation, I elicit a past experience with the same theme. First we talk about it on the intellectual level.

THERAPIST: When is the first time you remember feeling this way, as a kid?

PATIENT: (*pause*) When I was 6. I was in first grade. I remember I brought home my report card, and I was a little scared because I hadn't done very well. My dad was okay about it, but my mom got pretty mad.

THERAPIST: What did she say?

PATIENT: She yelled, "Annie, what am I going to do with you? Just look at this report card!"

THERAPIST: What did you say?

PATIENT: I don't think I said anything. My mom kept saying, "Don't you know what will happen if you don't get good grades? Your brother always does well. Why can't you? I'm so ashamed of you. What are you going to amount to?"

THERAPIST: [empathizing] You must have felt pretty bad.

PATIENT: I did.

THERAPIST: Do you think this was a reasonable way for her to act?

PATIENT: (*Thinks.*) No ... I guess not.

THERAPIST: Well, is this something you'd say to your own kids some day?

PATIENT: No. I'd never say that.

THERAPIST: What would *you* say if you had a 6-year-old daughter who brought home a report card like that?

PATIENT: Ummm ... I guess I'd say what my father did, "That's okay. Don't feel bad. I didn't do great in school either, and it didn't matter one bit."

THERAPIST: That's good. Do you have any idea why your mother didn't say that?

PATIENT: I'm not sure.

THERAPIST: I wonder, from what you've told me before, if it could be because she thought other people might look down on *her* if her kids didn't do well.

PATIENT: That's probably right. She was always bragging about my brother to her friends. I think she was always trying to keep up with the Joneses.

Next I change the focus of our discussion so the patient can engage in experiential learning:

THERAPIST: Okay, how about if we do a role play. I'll play you at age 6; you play your mom. Try to see things from her point of view as much as you can. I'll start ... Mom, here's my report card.

PATIENT: Annie, I'm ashamed of you. Look at these grades. What am I going to do with you?

THERAPIST: Mom, I'm only 6. My grades aren't great like Robert's, but they're okay.

PATIENT: Don't you know what will happen if you don't get good grades? You'll never amount to anything.

THERAPIST: That's silly, Mom. I'm only 6.

PATIENT: But next year, you will be 7, and after that 8 ...

THERAPIST: Mom, I didn't do that bad. Why are you making such a big deal? You're making me feel like I'm completely incompetent. Is that what you mean to do?

PATIENT: No, of course not. I don't want you to think that. It's not true. I just want you to do better.

Next I help the patient draw a different conclusion about the experience:

THERAPIST: Okay, out of role. What do you think?

PATIENT: I wasn't really incompetent. I did okay. Mom probably was hard on me because *she* didn't want to be criticized.

THERAPIST: How much do you believe that?

PATIENT: I think I do believe it.

THERAPIST: How about if we do the role play again, but this time we'll switch parts. Let's see how well the 6-year-old Annie can talk back to her mother.

Following this second role play, I ask Annie what she learned, and how this learning applies to the situation that upset her this week (getting criticized by her boss).

Another technique uses imagery to restructure early memories in the presence of affect (J. S. Beck, 2005; Edwards, 1989; Layden, Newman, Freeman, & Morse, 1993; Smucker & Dancu, 1999; Young, Klosko, & Weishaar, 2006). This Gestalt type technique has been adapted specifically to change core beliefs and is more often used with patients with personality disorders than with Axis I patients. In the following case example, I help a patient reexperience an early distressing event that seems to have contributed to the origin or maintenance of a key core belief. I do the following:

1. Identify a specific situation that is currently quite distressing to the patient and seems linked to an important core belief.
2. Heighten the patient's affect by focusing on automatic thoughts, emotions, and somatic sensations linked with this situation.
3. Help the patient identify and reexperience a relevant early experience.
4. Talk to the "younger" part of the patient to identify automatic thoughts, emotions, and beliefs.
5. Help the patient develop a different understanding of the experience through guided imagery, Socratic questioning, dialogue, and/or role play.

In the following transcript, Annie reports an upsetting experience from the previous day in which she felt criticized by women in her church group with whom she was working on a fundraising project.

THERAPIST: Can you imagine this scene again, as if it's happening right now? You're all sitting around the table ... (*I have Annie vividly picture and describe the distressing incident in the present tense.*)

PATIENT: Peggy is saying, "Annie, you've got to go back to the stores and find out who the managers or owners are and talk to *them* about contributing—the clerks don't have the authority." And I'm feeling so down, so sad. [I'm thinking] "I'm letting everyone down. I'm not good enough. I can't do anything right."

THERAPIST: Are you feeling the sadness right now?

PATIENT: (*Nods.*)

THERAPIST: [questioning her about her physiological response to heighten her affective response] Where in your body do you feel it?

PATIENT: Behind my eyes.

THERAPIST: Anywhere else? Where else is the sadness?

PATIENT: In my chest ... and my stomach. There's a heaviness.

THERAPIST: Okay, can you focus on the heaviness? Can you really feel it now, in your stomach, in your chest? And behind your eyes?

PATIENT: (*Nods.*)

THERAPIST: Okay, just focus on your eyes, your stomach, your chest ... (*Waits about 10 seconds.*) Annie, when do you remember feeling this heaviness before, when you were a kid? When's the *first* time you remember feeling like this?

In the next section, I have Annie relate a distressing, significant memory with the same theme as the current upsetting experience. Annie describes (in the past tense) how critical her mother was when Annie stayed up late to do a homework assignment in second grade and how incompetent she felt. I then ask Annie to relate this experience again, this time telling it to me as her younger self, as if experience is happening right now. I interview the "child" part of Annie, continually reinforcing the emotional immediacy of the experience by having the patient use the present tense throughout.

THERAPIST: Seven-year-old Annie, where are you?

PATIENT: I'm home. In the kitchen. I'm doing my homework.

THERAPIST: Is it hard?

PATIENT: Yes. I don't know what to do.

THERAPIST: [asking questions to deepen the experience, affect, and cognitions] Can you see your mom come into the kitchen? How does she look?

PATIENT: She looks mad. Really mad.

THERAPIST: How can you tell?

PATIENT: (*Eyes begin to tear.*) Her face is scrunched up. It's all red.

THERAPIST: What is she saying to you?

PATIENT: "Annie, go to bed."

THERAPIST: Keep going.

PATIENT: "Mom, I can't. I have to finish this."

THERAPIST: What is Mom saying?

PATIENT: "Get to bed! What's the matter with you? This stuff is easy. Are you stupid?" (*Sobs.*)

THERAPIST: (*gently*) Seven-year-old Annie, how are you feeling?

PATIENT: Sad. (*Cries a little.*)

THERAPIST: Real sad?

PATIENT: (*Nods.*)

THERAPIST: (*softly*) Seven-year-old Annie, what's going through your mind right now?

PATIENT: I *am* stupid. I can't do anything right.

THERAPIST: How much do you believe that? (*gesturing with her hands*) A little? A medium amount? A whole lot?

PATIENT: A whole lot.

THERAPIST: What else are you thinking?

PATIENT: I'll never be able to do stuff right.

Note that the intensification of Annie's affect verifies this as a core issue. In the next section, I help Annie reinterpret this experience.

THERAPIST: Seven-year-old Annie, I'd like to help you see this in a different way. Is it okay if we get your older self to come talk to you?

PATIENT: (*Nods.*)

THERAPIST: Okay, 7-year-old Annie, can you imagine that your mom walks out of the kitchen and your 45-year-old self walks in? Where would you like her to be?

PATIENT: Next to me, I guess.

THERAPIST: Real close?

PATIENT: (*Nods.*)

THERAPIST: Would you like her to put her arm around you?

PATIENT: (*Nods.*)

THERAPIST: Okay. Let's have older Annie talk to 7-year-old Annie. Have her ask 7-year-old Annie what's wrong.

PATIENT: What's wrong?

THERAPIST: What does 7-year-old Annie say?

PATIENT: I feel so stupid. I can't do anything right.

THERAPIST: What does your older self answer back?

PATIENT: No, you're not. This homework is too hard. It's not your fault. You're not stupid.

THERAPIST: What does 7-year-old Annie say?

PATIENT: But I should be able to do it.

THERAPIST: Have your older self keep talking to her.

PATIENT: No, that's not true. You shouldn't be able to do it. You've been absent. You were never taught this. Actually, it's your teacher's fault for giving you something too hard.

THERAPIST: Seven-year-old Annie, do you believe her?

PATIENT: A little.

THERAPIST: Seven-year old Annie, what do you want to ask your older self?

PATIENT: Why does everything have to be so hard? Why can't I do anything right?

THERAPIST: What does older Annie say?

PATIENT: You do lots of things right. Some things like math papers are easy, and getting dressed all by yourself and playing soccer ...

THERAPIST: Seven-year-old Annie, what are you thinking?

PATIENT: But I can't play soccer well. Robert is so much better.

THERAPIST: Older Annie, help her understand.

PATIENT: Listen, he *is* better at baseball than you. But he's *older.* When he was your age, he could only do what you can do now. You'll get better, just wait.

THERAPIST: Seven-year-old Annie, how are you feeling now?

When Annie reports that her younger self is feeling significantly less sad, I wrap up the exercise (e.g., "Is there anything else you want to ask your older self, 7-year-old Annie?"). I then ask Annie to write down the old belief that was activated in this memory and the new belief, and to rate how much she now believes each one at an intellectual level and at an emotional level.

Then we discuss the present distressing incident involving her friend Peggy and the church group, and help Annie draw a more reality-based, adaptive conclusion. By the end of the session, Annie believes only 20% that she is incompetent and 70% that she is competent. She believes an alternative explanation quite strongly: that her contribution may not live up to Peggy's expectations, but that does not mean that she is incompetent. This was her first experience with fundraising, and the more experienced members had not given her enough information. Even if someone else in the group could have done a better job, it does not mean that Annie is completely incompetent as a person.

In summary, core beliefs require consistent, systematic work. A number of techniques applicable to restructuring automatic thoughts and intermediate beliefs may be used along with more specialized techniques oriented specifically toward core beliefs. Additional strategies to modify core beliefs can be found in J. S. Beck (2005), Beck and colleagues (2004), and Young (1999). Typical core beliefs of patients with a variety of psychiatric disorders are described in Riso, du Toit, Stein, and Young (2007).

Chapter 15

ADDITIONAL COGNITIVE AND BEHAVIORAL TECHNIQUES

A number of cognitive and behavioral techniques have previously been introduced, among them Socratic questioning, behavioral experiments, intellectual–emotional role-playing, Core Belief Worksheets, imagery, and listing advantages and disadvantages of beliefs. This chapter describes other important techniques, many of which are both cognitive and behavioral in nature. As described more fully in Chapter 19, you will choose techniques according to your overall conceptualization and goals for a particular session. You will also create your own techniques as you become more proficient as a cognitive behavior therapist.

The techniques described in this chapter, as is the case for all cognitive behavior therapy techniques, aim to influence the patient's thinking, behavior, mood, and physiological arousal. They include problem solving, making decisions, refocusing, relaxation and mindfulness, coping cards, graded task assignments, exposure, role play, the "pie" technique, self-comparisons, and credit lists. Additional techniques are described in various sources (Beck et al., 1979; Beck & Emery, 1985; Leahy, 2003; McMullin, 1986).

PROBLEM SOLVING AND SKILLS TRAINING

Associated with or in addition to their psychological disorders, patients have real-life problems. At every session, you will encourage patients to put on the agenda problems that have come up during the week that still distress them and problems they anticipate in the coming weeks. You will encourage patients to devise solutions to their problems, asking them how they have solved similar problems in the past, or how they might advise a close friend or family member to solve the same kind of problem. You will then offer potential solutions, if needed. To spur your thinking, you might ask yourself how you have solved or would have solved a similar problem.

Some patients are deficient in problem-solving skills. They may benefit from direct instruction in problem solving, where they learn to specify a problem, devise solutions, select a solution, implement it, and evaluate its effectiveness (see, e.g., D'Zurilla & Nezu, 2006). And many patients also have skill deficits. They require skills training from you or from an outside source in such areas as effective parenting, job interviewing, budgeting, and relationship skills. Self-help books can be useful; for example, McKay, Davis, and Fanning (2009) offer a client guide to improving communication.

Other patients, however, already have good problem-solving and other skills. They may need help in testing dysfunctional beliefs that impede problem solving or using the skills they already possess. A problem-solving worksheet (J. S. Beck, 2011) helps patients specify a problem and identify and respond to interfering cognitions before discussing potential solutions.

Sally, for example, had difficulty concentrating when she was studying. She and I brainstormed solutions. She could start with the easiest assignment first, review relevant class notes before reading the textbook, write down questions when she was unsure of her understanding, and pause every few minutes to rehearse mentally what she had just read. We agreed she would try these strategies as experiments to see which, if any, facilitated her concentration and comprehension.

A few sessions later, Sally put her volunteer job on the agenda. She had started tutoring a child at a nearby elementary school. Although the child was cooperative, Sally felt unsure of what she was doing. Intellectually she knew how to solve the problem; she realized she should contact the agency that coordinated the volunteers and/or the child's teacher. Her belief that she should not ask for help, however, inhibited her. After evaluating her automatic thoughts and beliefs about this specific situation, Sally implemented the solution she herself had initially conceived.

I used self-disclosure to help Sally when she brought up the problem of procrastination. She was avoiding doing research for a paper she had to write. I told her that I often find the few moments or minutes just before starting a task I was avoiding the most unpleasant. Once I actually start doing the task, I invariably feel better. Sally recognized that she often had the same experience, and we set up a behavioral experiment to see what would happen later that afternoon when she went online to start her research.

Some problem solving may involve significant life changes. After careful evaluation of a situation, you might encourage battered spouses to seek refuge or take legal action. If you have patients who are chronically dissatisfied with their job, you might guide them in analyzing the advantages and disadvantages of staying in their current job versus looking for another job. Not all problems, of course, can be ameliorated. In such cases, however, patients may be able to change their *response* to problems by modifying their cognitions. They may need to accept the status quo and work on making other aspects of their lives more satisfying.

Some patients are chronic worriers about problems that are highly unlikely to occur. For these patients, you may need to help them differentiate between low-probability and higher-probability problems and between taking reasonable and unreasonable precautions. You also need to help them accept uncertainty, recognize and build personal and external resources, and increase their sense of self-efficacy, so they will have more confidence that if problems do arise, they will be able (by themselves or with the help of others) to handle them.

MAKING DECISIONS

Many patients, especially those who are depressed, have difficulty making decisions. When patients want your help in this area, you will ask them to list the advantages and disadvantages of each option and then help them devise a system for weighing each item and drawing a conclusion about which option seems best (see Figure 15.1).

THERAPIST: You mentioned that you wanted help in deciding whether to go to summer school or to get a job?

PATIENT: Yes.

THERAPIST: Okay. (*Pulls out a piece of paper.*) Let me show you how to weigh advantages and disadvantages. Have you ever done that?

PATIENT: No. At least not in writing. I've been going over some of the pros and cons in my head.

THERAPIST: Good. That'll help us get started. I think you'll find that writing them down will make the decision clearer. Which one do you want to start with—school or a job?

PATIENT: Getting a job, I guess.

Advantages of job	Disadvantages of job
1. Make money.	1. Have to find one.
2. Maybe learn skills.	2. Less free time.
3. Break from what I've been doing.	3. Might not like it.
4. Meet different people.	
5. Make me feel more productive.	
6. Good for resumé.	

Advantages of summer school	Disadvantages of summer school
1. Two friends are going.	1. Not making money and it costs money.
2. Could take one less course in the fall.	2. Doesn't increase my skills.
3. Lots of free time.	3. More of the same of what I've been doing.
4. It's a known quantity.	4. Doesn't make me feel as productive.
5. Could meet new people.	5. Doesn't help my resumé.
6. Easier to enroll than to find a job.	

FIGURE 15.1. Sally's advantages–disadvantages analysis.

THERAPIST: Okay. Write "Advantages of job" at the top left of this paper and "Disadvantages of job" on the top right, and "Advantages of summer school" and "Disadvantages of summer school" at the bottom.

PATIENT: (*Does so.*) Okay.

THERAPIST: What have you been thinking? Could you jot down some advantages and disadvantages of getting a job? (*Sally writes down the ideas she has had so far. I ask some questions to guide her.*) How about the fact that you'd be doing something different—taking a break from schoolwork—is that an advantage?

PATIENT: Yeah. (*Writes it down.*)

THERAPIST: Would a job cut into your vacation time?

PATIENT: No, I'd only take a job that would let me spend the last 2 weeks of August with my family.

Sally and I continue this process until she feels she has recorded both sides fairly and thoroughly. We repeat the process with the second option. Examining advantages and disadvantages of summer school reminds Sally of additional items to add to the "job" lists. Likewise, she also reviews the "job" items to see whether their counterparts are relevant to the "summer school" lists.

Next, I help Sally evaluate the items:

THERAPIST: Okay, this looks pretty complete. Now you need to weigh the items in some way. Do you want to circle the most important items—or rate the importance of each one on a 1–10 scale?

PATIENT: Circle the items, I guess.

THERAPIST: Okay, let's look at the "job" lists. Which items are most important to you? (*Sally circles items in each column in Figure 15.1.*) Just looking over what you've circled, what do you think?

PATIENT: I'd like to get a job, because if I had one, I'd make money and feel productive, and it would be good to get a break from school. But it feels like it would be really hard to get one.

THERAPIST: Should we spend a few minutes now talking about how you might go about looking for a job? Then we can come back to this list and see if you're still leaning that way.

At the end of the discussion, I increase the probability that Sally will use this technique again:

THERAPIST: Did you find this [process of listing and weighing advantages and disadvantages] useful? Can you think of any other decisions you might have to make where it would be good to do the same thing? How will you remember to do it this way?

REFOCUSING

As described in Chapter 11, it is often best for patients to evaluate their automatic thoughts on the spot and evaluate them or read relevant therapy notes. In some situations, however, this strategy is unfeasible or undesirable, and refocusing their attention is indicated. Refocusing is particularly useful when concentration is needed for the task at hand, such as completing a work assignment, carrying on a conversation, or driving. It is also useful when patients are having obsessive thoughts for which rational evaluation is ineffective. You will teach patients to label and accept their experience: "I'm just having automatic thoughts. I can accept the fact that I'm having them and that I'm feeling badly and refocus on what I was doing." Then patients should deliberately turn their attention to the report they are writing, to what their fellow conversationalists are saying, to the road ahead. You will rehearse the strategy with them, trying to elicit how they have refocused their attention in the past or how they believe they could in the future.

THERAPIST: Okay, so one alternative when you're feeling anxious in class is to answer back those thoughts. But sometimes you may be better off just changing your focus to what's going on in class. Have you done this before, made an effort to concentrate on the class?

PATIENT: Ah ... yeah, I guess so.

THERAPIST: How did you do that?

PATIENT: Well, it helps if I start taking lots of notes.

THERAPIST: Good. How about this week if you try *not* to let yourself just feel overwhelmed by your negative thoughts and anxiety and sadness, but instead either answer back your thoughts, or refocus and take lots of notes, or both.

PATIENT: Okay.

THERAPIST: How will you remember to do that?

At other times, patients may be too distressed to refocus their attention on a task, or may not have a specific task to which to attend. Distracting activities can be useful in these circumstances. While distraction is not the ultimate solution, it can be a helpful short-term technique. Again, elicit what has worked for the patient in the past and then offer other suggestions, if needed.

THERAPIST: So you got really worked up about the report you have to write?

PATIENT: Yes, I couldn't concentrate. I just got more and more anxious.

THERAPIST: What did you do?

PATIENT: I just started to pace around my room.

THERAPIST: Did that help?

PATIENT: Not really.

THERAPIST: Did you try to answer back your thoughts?

PATIENT: I read my therapy notes, but they didn't help. I didn't believe them, I guess.

THERAPIST: (*Jots down a note.*) Let's try to figure out why they weren't helpful in a few minutes, but first let me ask you, how long were you anxious?

PATIENT: A long time. I don't know, maybe a couple of hours. I kept going back to my desk to try to read, but I just couldn't.

THERAPIST: Did you try to distract yourself?

PATIENT: No. I finally decided not to try and I just went to dinner.

THERAPIST: Do you ever try to distract yourself? What have you done?

PATIENT: Usually, I turn on the TV.

THERAPIST: How well does that usually work?

PATIENT: Sometimes I can lose myself and feel better, sometimes not.

THERAPIST: Okay, if it doesn't work well, what else do you try?

PATIENT: Sometimes I pick up the newspaper or do a crossword puzzle, but that doesn't always work either.

THERAPIST: Any other ideas?

PATIENT: ... No, not really.

THERAPIST: Can I mention some things that other people find helpful? You might try some of these things as an experiment this week: take a walk or go running, call or e-mail a friend or someone in your family, clean your closet or desk, balance your checkbook, go to the grocery store, knock on a neighbor's door, play a video game, visit your favorite websites ... What do you think? Do you want to try any of these things this week?

PATIENT: Yes. I could do that.

THERAPIST: Sometimes people find that soothing activities are better: taking a long bath, listening to uplifting music, reading prayers. What do you think? Would you like to write down a few possibilities?

PATIENT: Yes.

THERAPIST: Once you're feeling less distressed, you may be able to answer your thoughts better, or just return to what you were doing. Now, ultimately, we don't want you to have to distract yourself. But it may help for now.

On the other hand, you may find that patients are distracting themselves too much. If they do not fear negative emotion, the following type of discussion can be useful.

THERAPIST: So, what you're saying is that you tend to try to push your thoughts out of your mind when you're feeling upset? Is that right?

PATIENT: Yes.

THERAPIST: And do these thoughts, for example, that you can't do something, vanish from your mind completely?

PATIENT: No, they usually come back.

THERAPIST: So you're not really pushing them completely out of mind, just to the back of your mind, where they wait for another opportunity to pop out and make you miserable?

PATIENT: I guess so.

THERAPIST: I wonder this week if you would be willing, at least some of the time, to stop distracting yourself and instead really work on these thoughts, evaluate them as you've been learning to do in session?

PATIENT: Okay.

THERAPIST: Even if it's impossible to do a Thought Record at the time, maybe you could do it as soon as you have a free moment.

Patients may use distraction to avoid the experience of negative emotion. It is imperative for them to fully understand that they do not need to distract themselves because while feeling upset can feel painful, it is not harmful. If patients consistently distract themselves, they cannot learn this important lesson, and you may need to set up behavioral experiments to test their fears about experiencing strong affect. It may be beneficial for you to teach them the AWARE technique on page 197 (Beck & Emery, 1985), in which they are instructed to accept the anxiety, watch it, act with the anxiety, repeat these steps, and expect the best.

MEASURING MOODS AND BEHAVIOR USING THE ACTIVITY CHART

For some patients, it is helpful to use the activity chart, not to schedule activities, but to monitor their moods while engaged in various activities, to look for patterns of occurrence. For example, a patient with an anxiety disorder might fill in the boxes listing activities and rating levels of anxiety 0–10 (or mild, moderate, severe). A patient who is chronically irritated or angry might do likewise with an anger scale. Using such a scale is particularly useful for patients who either do not seem to notice small to moderate shifts in affect, or patients who chronically over- or underestimate degrees of emotion.

Patients with a problematic behavior such as binge eating, smoking, overspending, gambling, substance use, or angry outbursts might record all their activities to investigate patterns of occurrence, or might just record the maladaptive behaviors themselves.

RELAXATION AND MINDFULNESS

Many patients benefit from learning relaxation techniques, described in detail elsewhere (Benson, 1975; Davis, Eshelman, & McKay, 2008; Jacobson, 1974). There are several kinds of relaxation exercises, including progressive muscle relaxation, imagery, and controlled breathing. Patients can obtain commercially produced relaxation tapes or you can follow a script and make a recording for them during the session. You should teach relaxation exercises in session, where you can deal with problems and assess efficacy. Be aware that some patients experience a paradoxical arousal effect from relaxation exercises; they actually become more tense and anxious (Barlow, 2002; Clark, 1989). As with all techniques, you will propose that patients try relaxation as an experiment; either it will help reduce anxiety or it will lead to anxious thoughts that can be evaluated.

Mindfulness techniques help patients nonjudgmentally observe and accept their internal experiences, without evaluating or trying to change them. A short summary of techniques, particularly for people with rumination, can be found in Leahy (2010). Mindfulness is currently being integrated with cognitive behavior therapy for a number of problems, including psychiatric disorders, medical conditions, and stress (Chiesa & Serretti, 2010a, 2010b). For extended discussions of mindfulness, see Hayes and colleagues (2004); McCown, Reibel, and Micozzi (2010); Williams, Teasdale, Segal, and Kabat-Zinn (2007); and Kabat-Zinn (1990).

GRADED TASK ASSIGNMENTS

To reach a goal, it is usually necessary to accomplish a number of steps along the way. Patients tend to become overwhelmed when they focus on how far they are from a goal, instead of focusing on their current step. A graphic depiction of the steps is often reassuring (see Figure 15.2).

THERAPIST: Sally, it sounds like you get nervous just thinking about voluntarily talking in class, though it's something you want to be able to do.

PATIENT: Yeah.

THERAPIST: I wonder how we could break it down into steps; for example, could you start by just asking a question *after* class, either to another student or to the professor?

PATIENT: Yeah. I guess I could do that.

THERAPIST: What could the next step be? (*Guides Sally in identifying the steps presented in Figure 15.2.*)

THERAPIST: Does it still seem scary to think about talking in class?

PATIENT: Yeah, some.

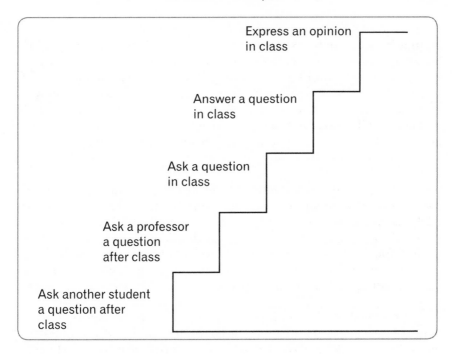

FIGURE 15.2. Breaking down goals into steps.

THERAPIST: (*Draws a staircase.*) Okay, here's what you have to remember. You're going to start down here, doing something that's just a little hard, and you'll get really comfortable on this step before trying the next step, and so on. And remember, before you try the final step, you'll have gotten really good at the step just below it. Okay?

PATIENT: Uh-huh.

THERAPIST: So every time you start thinking about the final goal, how about reminding yourself of this staircase and especially of the step you're now on, and how you're going to go up the staircase one step at a time. Do you think that'll help bring down the anxiety?

EXPOSURE

Depressed and anxious patients often engage in avoidance, a coping strategy. They may feel hopeless about engaging in certain activities ("It won't do any good to call my friends. They won't want to see me") or fearful ("If I [do this activity], something bad will happen"). The avoidance may be quite apparent (e.g., patients who spend a great deal of time in bed, avoiding self-care activities, household tasks, socializing, and errands.) Or the avoidance may be more subtle (e.g., socially anxious patients who avoid making eye contact, smiling at others, making small talk, and volunteering their opinions). These latter avoidances are *safety behaviors* (Salkovskis, 1996) that patients believe will ward off anxiety. While avoidance tends to bring immediate relief (and so is quite reinforcing), it perpetuates the problem. Patients do not get the opportunity to test their automatic thoughts and receive disconfirming data.

When patients are anxious and significantly avoidant, you will provide a strong rationale for exposing themselves to feared situations. Help them identify an activity that is associated with low to moderate discomfort and ask them to engage in this activity every day (or even several times a day, if feasible), until their anxiety has decreased significantly. Then identify a new situation that is just a little more difficult, and encourage frequent exposure until they can do it with relative ease, and so on.

You may discuss various coping techniques to use before, during, and after each task: Thought Records, coping cards, or relaxation exercises, for example. For particularly avoidant patients, covert rehearsal (pages 303–305) to identify either dysphoric automatic thoughts or excuses not to do an assignment is useful. In addition, you may find that patients are more likely to do daily work on a graded exposure hierarchy if you ask them to fill out a daily monitor, which can be simple, listing just the date, activity, and level of anxiety, or it can be more elaborate (see Figure 15.3).

In a more elaborate monitor, you can also ask patients to record and then *cross off* predictions that did not come true, a task that further reminds them of the inaccuracy of many of their thoughts. Detailed descriptions of the process used to develop agoraphobic hierarchies can be found in various sources (e.g., Goldstein & Stainback, 1987).

Date	Activity	Predicted level of anxiety 0–100	Actual level of anxiety 1–100	Predictions
4/4	Asking questions in class	80	50	I won't be able to do it. Nothing will come out of my mouth. I'll make a fool of myself.

FIGURE 15.3. Custom-made monitor.

Dobson and Dobson (2009) describe plans for effective exposure sessions, possible targets, and factors that decrease the effectiveness of exposure.

ROLE-PLAYING

Role-playing is a technique that can be used for a wide variety of purposes. Descriptions of role-playing can be found throughout this volume, including role-playing to uncover automatic thoughts, to develop an adaptive response, and to modify intermediate and core beliefs. Role-playing is also useful in learning and practicing social skills.

Some patients have weak social skills in general, or are proficient at one style of communication but lack skills to adapt their style when needed. Sally, for example, is reasonably good at normal social conversation and situations that call for a caring, empathic stance. She is far less skilled, however, in situations in which assertion is appropriate. She and I engaged in a number of role plays to practice assertiveness.

PATIENT: I don't even know how I'd begin to talk to my professor.

THERAPIST: Well, you want him to help you understand this concept better, right? What would you like to say?

PATIENT: ... I don't know.

THERAPIST: Well, how about if we do a role play. I'll be you; you play your professor. You can play him as being as unreasonable as you'd like.

PATIENT: Okay.

THERAPIST: I'll start: Uh, Professor X, could you explain this concept?

PATIENT: (*gruffly*) I did that already last week in class. Weren't you there?

THERAPIST: Actually, I was. But I don't understand it well enough yet.

PATIENT: Well, you should go read the chapter in your textbook.

THERAPIST: I've done that already. It didn't help enough either. That's why I'm here now.

PATIENT: Okay, what don't you understand about it?

THERAPIST: I tried to think of a specific question before I came, but I couldn't quite think of how to phrase it. Could you spend a couple of minutes just describing it, and then I can see if I can put it in my own words?

PATIENT: You know, I don't have much time now. Why don't you see someone else in the class?

THERAPIST: I'd rather get it straight from you. That's why I came now during office hours. But if you'd rather, I could come back on Thursday when you have office hours again.

PATIENT: This is a simple concept. You should really ask some other student.

THERAPIST: I'll try that first. If I need more help, I'll come back Thursday ... Okay, out of role. Let's review what I did and then we can switch roles.

Before teaching patients social skills, you should assess the level of skill they already possess. Many patients know precisely what to do and say, but have difficulty using this knowledge because of dysfunctional assumptions (e.g., "If I express an opinion, I'll get shot down"; "If I assert myself, the other person will be hurt/get mad/think I'm out of line"). One way of assessing skills is to have patients assume a positive outcome: "If you knew for sure the teaching assistant would be willing to talk to you, what would you say?" "If you really believed it was your right to get help, what would you say?" "If you knew the professor would back down and realize he was being unreasonable, what would you say?"

Another indication that the problem is associated with dysfunctional beliefs rather than with a skill deficit is the patient's use of these skills in another context. Patients may be quite appropriately assertive at work, for example, but not with friends. In this case, you might not need to use role-playing to teach assertiveness skills (although you could use role-playing to have the patients identify their automatic thoughts while they are being assertive, or to predict thoughts and feelings of the other person when roles are switched).

USING THE "PIE" TECHNIQUE

It is often helpful to patients to see their ideas in graphic form. A pie chart can be used in many ways, for instance, helping patients set goals or determining relative responsibility for a given outcome, both of which are illustrated below (see Figure 15.4).

Setting Goals

When patients have difficulty specifying their problems and the changes they would like to make in their lives, or when they lack insight into how

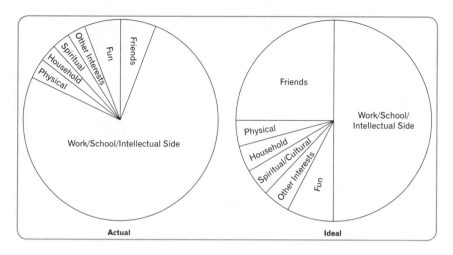

FIGURE 15.4. Use of pie charts in setting goals.

imbalanced their lives are, they may benefit from a graphic depiction of their ideal versus actual expenditure of time.

THERAPIST: It sounds as if you know your life isn't quite in balance, but you don't know what to change—is that right?

PATIENT: Yes, I guess so.

THERAPIST: How about we draw a pie diagram to help figure it out?

PATIENT: Okay.

THERAPIST: First, we'll create a diagram of your life now, then an ideal one. Think about how much time you are actually spending in these areas:

Work	Taking care of your physical self
Friends	Taking care of your household
Fun	Taking care of your spiritual/
Family	cultural/intellectual side
Other interests	

THERAPIST: Can you draw a pie and put in divisions to give me a *rough* idea of how you're spending your time now?

PATIENT: (*Does so.*)

THERAPIST: Okay, next, what would you change about it in an ideal world?

PATIENT: Well ... I guess I'd work less, probably try to have more fun ... spend more time with friends, exercise more, read more, things like that.

THERAPIST: Good. How would that look on this ideal pie?

PATIENT: (*Fills in "ideal" pie.*) [expressing an automatic thought] But I'm afraid if I spend less time working, I'll accomplish even less than I am now.

THERAPIST: Okay, let's write down that prediction. Now, you may be right, in which case you could always go back to the amount of work you're doing now. Or you may be wrong. It's possible if you work a little less and do more pleasurable things, your mood will improve. If your mood improves, is it possible that you might concentrate better and work more efficiently? What do you think?

PATIENT: I'm not sure.

THERAPIST: In any case, we can test your prediction and see what happens.

PATIENT: I know for a fact that I'm not working too efficiently right now.

THERAPIST: Then it may well be that once we get your life back in balance and you're getting positive inputs from doing things you like, that you'll be able to do better with less work.

Following a discussion such as this, you would work with patients to set specific goals to move their expenditure of time closer to their ideal.

Determining Responsibility

Another technique allows the patient to see graphically the possible causes for a given outcome (see Figure 15.5).

THERAPIST: Sally, how much do you believe you got a C on your exam because you're basically incompetent?

PATIENT: Oh, close to 100%.

THERAPIST: I wonder if there might be any other reasons?

PATIENT: ... Well, there were some things on it that we had never really covered in class.

THERAPIST: Okay, anything else?

PATIENT: I missed two classes, so I had to borrow notes, and Lisa's notes weren't that good.

THERAPIST: Anything else?

PATIENT: I don't know. I studied some things a lot that turned out not to be on the exam.

THERAPIST: Sounds like you weren't very lucky in that regard.

PATIENT: No, and I hardly studied other things that *were* on the exam. I guessed wrong.

THERAPIST: Any other reason to explain why you didn't do as well as you would have liked?

PATIENT: Hmmm. Can't think of any.

THERAPIST: Did everyone else do pretty well?

PATIENT: I don't know.

THERAPIST: Would you say it was a hard test?

PATIENT: Yeah, too hard.

THERAPIST: Would you say the professor had done a really good job of explaining the material?

PATIENT: No. I don't think he did a great job. I had to rely on the readings, mostly. A couple of times, I heard people saying that they hadn't been able to follow what he was talking about.

THERAPIST: I wonder if you also might have trouble concentrating because of your depression and anxiety?

PATIENT: Definitely.

THERAPIST: Okay, let's see how all this would look graphically. Here's a pie chart; let's have you divide up sections to explain why you got a C on the exam, including (1) the professor didn't teach that great; (2) the test was really hard; (3) you hadn't guessed right about which material to study; (4) you borrowed class notes that weren't great; (5) there was material on the exam that wasn't even covered in class; (6) your depression and anxiety interfered with your concentration; and (7) at heart, you're an incompetent person.

PATIENT: (*Fills in pie diagram* [Figure 15.5].)

THERAPIST: Looks like you divided up the sections pretty evenly. How much do you believe now that you got a C on the exam because you're an incompetent person?

PATIENT: Less. 50%, maybe.

THERAPIST: Good. That's quite a drop.

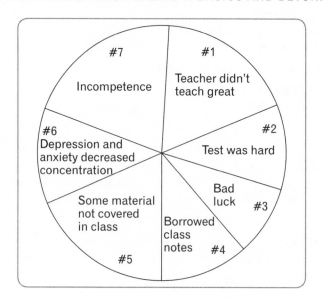

FIGURE 15.5. Pie chart for causality.

When investigating the contribution of alternative explanations, ask patients to estimate the dysfunctional attribution (in this case, "I'm incompetent") last so they will more fully consider all explanations.

SELF-COMPARISONS AND CREDIT LISTS

Patients with psychiatric disorders have a negative bias in information processing, especially when evaluating themselves. They tend to notice data that could be construed as negative and to ignore, discount, or even forget information that is positive. In addition, they often make dysfunctional comparisons: They compare themselves at present with how they were before the onset of their disorder, or with how they would like to be, or they compare themselves with others who do not have a psychiatric disorder. This negative attentional bias helps to maintain or increase their dysphoria.

Changing the Self-Comparison

In the following transcript, I help Sally see that her selective negative attention and comparisons are dysfunctional. I then teach her to make more functional comparisons (with herself at her worst point) and to keep a credit list.

THERAPIST: Sally, it sounds as if you're pretty down on yourself. Do you think there's anything you did this week that you deserve credit for?

PATIENT: Well, I did finish my lit paper.

THERAPIST: Anything else?

PATIENT: Ummm ... can't think of anything.

THERAPIST: I wonder whether you might not have noticed some things.

PATIENT: I don't know.

THERAPIST: For instance, how many classes did you go to?

PATIENT: All of them.

THERAPIST: In how many did you take notes?

PATIENT: All of them.

THERAPIST: Was that easy to do? Or did you have to push yourself to go and concentrate?

PATIENT: It was hard. But I should have been able to do it easily. No one else probably had to push.

THERAPIST: Oh ... Sounds as if you might be comparing yourself with other people again. Do you do that a lot?

PATIENT: Yeah, I guess so.

THERAPIST: Does that seem like a fair comparison to you? Would you be as hard on yourself, for example, if you had to push yourself to go to class and concentrate if you had pneumonia?

PATIENT: No, I'd have a legitimate reason to be tired.

THERAPIST: Exactly. I wonder if you have a legitimate reason to be tired now? Maybe you *do* deserve credit when you push yourself. Do you remember at the first session when we talked about the symptoms of depression: tiredness, low energy, trouble concentrating, distur-bances in sleep and appetite, and so on?

PATIENT: Uh-huh.

THERAPIST: So maybe you *do* deserve credit for pushing ahead, given that you are depressed?

PATIENT: I hadn't thought of it that way.

THERAPIST: Okay, let's go over two things now: what to do when you compare yourself with others, and how to keep track of what you deserve credit for. Okay, what happens to your mood when you compare yourself to others, for example, when you think, "No one else has to push to go to class and take notes?"

PATIENT: I feel pretty bad.

THERAPIST: And what would happen if you said to yourself, "Now wait a minute. That's not a reasonable comparison. Let me compare myself to *me* at my worst point, when I was in my room a lot and couldn't concentrate in class."

PATIENT: Well, I'd realize that I'm doing more now.

THERAPIST: And would your mood get worse?

PATIENT: No, probably better.

THERAPIST: Would you like to try this comparison for homework?

PATIENT: Uh-huh.

THERAPIST: Okay, let's have you write this down on your assignment sheet, "Catch myself when I compare myself to nondepressed people. Then remind myself this isn't reasonable, and compare myself to me at my worst point instead."

Patients may also have automatic thoughts in which they compare themselves at present to where they would like to be (e.g., "I should be able to read this chapter easily"), or to where they were before they became depressed (e.g., "This used to be so easy for me"). In this case, help them focus on how far they have progressed since their worst point, rather than on far they are from their best point or on how far they have to go.

When patients are at their lowest point, you will modify the approach:

THERAPIST: It sounds as if you feel pretty down when you compare yourself with other people, or with how you wish you were. I wonder if it might be helpful at these times to remind yourself that you have a goal list, and that together we're developing a plan to help you make changes. If you reminded yourself that you and I are a team working to get you to where you want to be, what could happen to your mood?

Credit Lists

Credit lists are simply daily lists (mental or written) of positive things the patient is doing or items she deserves credit for (see Figure 15.6). As with all assignments, I first explain the rationale:

THERAPIST: Sally, I'd like to describe a homework assignment that I think could help. You know, we've talked about how you have lots and lots of self-critical thoughts. And what happens to your mood every time you have a thought like, "I should be doing this better," or "I did a lousy job on that"?

(Things that I did that were positive or were a little hard but I did them anyway)

1. Tried to follow what was said in statistics class.
2. Finished paper and e-mailed it to [the professor].
3. Talked to Julie at lunch.
4. Called Jeremy to confirm chemistry assignment.
5. Went for a run instead of taking a nap.
6. Read Chapter 5 of econ book.

FIGURE 15.6. Sally's credit list.

PATIENT: I feel worse.

THERAPIST: Right. And what would happen, do you think, if you started noticing more *good* things you're doing?

PATIENT: I'd probably feel better.

THERAPIST: Okay, now would you say that it would be reasonable for *me* to give myself credit if I were tired from either pneumonia or depression, but I pushed ahead anyway and got out of bed and came to work and saw my patients and wrote e-mails and so on?

PATIENT: Sure.

THERAPIST: Even if I didn't do these things as well as usual?

PATIENT: Well, sure.

THERAPIST: Because I suppose I could have stayed in bed and pulled the covers over my head instead.

PATIENT: Right.

THERAPIST: Now, does that same thing apply to you? Do *you* deserve credit for pushing ahead?

PATIENT: I guess so.

THERAPIST: You know, it's probably hard for you to remember to give yourself credit outside of our session. That's why I'm suggesting you keep a written list of things you deserve credit for. What do you think?

PATIENT: I could try it.

THERAPIST: (*beginning the assignment in session*) Here, let's start it now, if that's okay with you. What do you want to call it—"credit list"? Something else?

PATIENT: Credit list is fine.

THERAPIST: Good. Now on this list you can either just write positive things you've done, or you can think to yourself, "What did I do today that was even a little hard, but I did it anyway?"

PATIENT: Okay. (*Writes down instructions.*)

THERAPIST: Let's start with today. What have you already done today?

PATIENT: (*Writes as she speaks.*) Let's see, I went to my statistics class ... it was kind of hard to follow, but I tried ... I finished my paper and e-mailed it to the professor ... I talked to my roommate's friend, who had lunch with us ...

THERAPIST: That's a good start. How do you feel about doing this every day?

PATIENT: Okay.

THERAPIST: I think that you'll remember things ten times better if you write them down immediately. But if you can't, you might at least try to write things down at lunch, dinner, and before bed. Think you can do that?

PATIENT: Yeah.

THERAPIST: Do you think you need to write down *why* you're doing this assignment?

PATIENT: No, I'll remember. It makes me focus on good things, and that makes me feel better.

Completing credit lists early in treatment also helps prepare patients for the later task of uncovering positive data for the Core Belief Worksheet (Chapter 11).

In summary, there are many cognitive and behavioral techniques; this volume describes some of the most common. Readers are encouraged to do additional reading to add to their repertoire.

Chapter 16

IMAGERY

M any patients experience automatic thoughts not only as unspoken words in their mind, but also in the form of mental pictures or images (Beck & Emery, 1985). Sally had the thought "[My classmate] will think I'm imposing on him if I ask [for a copy of his notes]." Upon questioning, I determined that when Sally experienced this thought, she simultaneously envisioned her classmate with an irritated look on his face. This image was an imaginal automatic thought.

This chapter demonstrates how to teach patients to identify their spontaneous images and how to intervene therapeutically with both spontaneous and induced images. Although many patients have visual images, few report them. Merely asking about images, even repeatedly, sometimes is not sufficient to elicit them. Images usually are quite brief and are often upsetting; many patients push them out of mind quite quickly. Failure to identify and respond to upsetting images may result in continued distress for the patient.

IDENTIFYING IMAGES

You will need to be alert to the possibility of patients' thoughts occurring in imaginal form, because few patients spontaneously report images and some have difficulty identifying them even when prompted. In the following transcript, I try to ascertain whether Sally has had a spontaneous image simultaneous with a verbal automatic thought.

THERAPIST: So you had the thought "I won't be able to handle a part-time job," and you felt sad?

PATIENT: Yes.

THERAPIST: I wonder, when you had that thought, did you get a picture in your head?

PATIENT: I'm not sure what you mean.

THERAPIST: Did "not handling" a job look like something?

PATIENT: I guess I pictured myself walking back to my dorm late at night, just feeling overwhelmed and kind of burdened.

THERAPIST: Anything else?

PATIENT: I was walking really slowly, just feeling exhausted, with a really heavy backpack.

THERAPIST: Okay. That picture, or imagining, is what we call an image.

At times, patients fail to grasp the concept when the therapist only uses the word "image." Synonyms include mental picture, daydream, fantasy, imagining, and memory. Had Sally failed to report an image, I might have tried using one of these different words. Or I might have chosen to help her create an image (if a therapeutic goal for that session was to help her recognize images). I could have induced a neutral or positive image ("Describe for me what the outside of your home looks like," or "Imagine you're walking into this building. What do you see?"). Or I might have tried to induce an image about a distressing situation, as below:

THERAPIST: Did you imagine what your professor might look like when you asked him for help? Did he look happy?

PATIENT: I don't think I pictured what he looked like.

THERAPIST: [helping Sally to think very specifically] Could you picture it now? Can you imagine going up to him? When would you approach him, anyway?

PATIENT: Oh, probably on Tuesday. That's when he has office hours.

THERAPIST: So he'd be in his office?

PATIENT: Yeah.

THERAPIST: What building is he in?

PATIENT: Bennett Hall.

THERAPIST: Okay, can you picture it now? It's Tuesday, you're coming up to Bennett Hall ... You're coming to his office ... Can you see it in your mind? Is the door open or closed?

PATIENT: Closed.

THERAPIST: Okay, can you see yourself knocking on the door? What does he say when he hears your knock?

PATIENT: He says, "Come in." (*Imitates professor's gruff voice.*)

THERAPIST: Okay, can you see yourself go in? What does his face look like?

PATIENT: He's scowling.

THERAPIST: And then what happens? (*Sally and I follow the image out to its most distressing point.*) Okay, this scene you've just visualized is what we call an "image." Do you think you might have had an image like this when you were considering going to see him this week?

PATIENT: Maybe ... I'm not sure.

THERAPIST: How about for homework if you look for images when you realize you're getting upset, along with looking for automatic thoughts?

PATIENT: Okay.

EDUCATING PATIENTS ABOUT IMAGERY

Some patients can identify images, but do not report them because their images are graphic and distressing. They may be reluctant to reexperience the distress or fear you will view them as disturbed. If you suspect either scenario, normalize the experience of images.

THERAPIST: Sally, I don't know whether you *are* having images. Most people do, but usually they're more aware of the emotion that accompanies the image than they are of the image itself. Sometimes images seem pretty strange, but actually it's common to have all kinds of images—sad, scary, even violent ones. The only problem is if *you* think you're strange for having the images. Can you recall any images you've had recently?

PATIENT: No, I don't think so.

THERAPIST: Well, we've agreed this week that you're going to be on the lookout for images when you notice your mood changing. If you *are* having distressing images, I'll teach you what you can do about them.

Normalizing and teaching patients about images helps reduce their anxiety and makes it more likely that they will be able to identify their images. In the previous transcript, I indicate that Sally will learn to respond to images, implying that she can gain control over her distress.

You must often be diligent in teaching patients to identify images until they "catch on." Most patients simply are unaware of images initially, and many therapists, after a few tries, abandon the attempt. If you get a visual image yourself as the patient is describing a situation, you can use the image as a cue to probe further for an image your patient may have experienced:

THERAPIST: Sally, as you were just describing how you're afraid your roommate will react, I got a picture of her in *my* head, even though I don't know her. Have you been imagining how she might look when you bring up the problem of noise with her?

RESPONDING TO SPONTANEOUS IMAGES

When patients do have distressing images, there are several strategies you can teach them. The first seven techniques help patients reduce their distress by viewing a situation in a different way; the last one offers temporary respite by having the patient focus on something else. It is important for you to advise patients that they will need to practice the techniques in and out of session to use them effectively.

Following Images to Completion

This technique is often the most helpful. It can help you and patients conceptualize their problem better, lead to cognitive restructuring of the image, and provide relief. You will encourage patients to continue visualizing a spontaneous image until one of two things occurs: Either patients imagine getting through a crisis and feeling better, or they imagine an ultimate catastrophe, such as death. (In the latter case, you can then explore the feared consequences and meaning of the ultimate catastrophe and intervene further.) The first transcript illustrates the first scenario; the patient imagines getting through a particular difficulty.

THERAPIST: Okay, Sally, can you get that image in mind again? Tell it to me aloud as you imagine it as vividly as you can.

PATIENT: I'm sitting in class. My professor is passing out the exam. I'm looking at it. My mind is going blank. I read the first question. Nothing is making sense. I see everyone else busy writing. I'm thinking, "I'm paralyzed. I'm going to fail."

THERAPIST: And you're feeling ...?

PATIENT: Really, really anxious.

THERAPIST: Anything else happen?

PATIENT: No.

THERAPIST: Okay. [providing psychoeducation] This is very typical. You've stopped the image at the very *worst* point, where you're feeling blank and paralyzed. Now I'd like you to imagine what happens next.

PATIENT: Hmmm. I'm not sure.

THERAPIST: Well, do you stay that way for the whole hour?

PATIENT: No, I guess not.

THERAPIST: Can you picture what happens next?... If you're looking around and seeing the other students, are you actually paralyzed?

PATIENT: No, I guess not.

THERAPIST: What do you see happening next?

PATIENT: I look at my exam again, but I can't focus.

THERAPIST: Then what happens?

PATIENT: I blink. The first question doesn't make any sense to me.

THERAPIST: Okay, then what?

PATIENT: I skip to the next question. I'm not sure of the answer.

THERAPIST: Then what?

PATIENT: I keep going until I find a question I know something about.

THERAPIST: Then what?

PATIENT: I guess I write the answer.

THERAPIST: Can you see yourself writing the answer?

PATIENT: Yes.

THERAPIST: Good. Then what?

PATIENT: I keep going until I find something else I can answer.

THERAPIST: Then what?

PATIENT: I go back to the first few questions, try to write something.

THERAPIST: Good. Then what?

PATIENT: Well, eventually I finish as much as I can.

THERAPIST: Then what?

PATIENT: I hand in the paper.

THERAPIST: And then?

PATIENT: I guess I go on to my next class.

THERAPIST: And then?

PATIENT: I sit down, get out the right notebook.

THERAPIST: And how are you feeling in the image now?

PATIENT: A little shaky still. I don't know how I did on the exam.

THERAPIST: Better than at the start when you were feeling blank and paralyzed?

PATIENT: Yes. Much better.

THERAPIST: Good. Let's review what you did. First, you recognized a distressing image, which you stopped at the absolute worst point. Then you kept imagining what would realistically happen next until you got to the point where you were feeling somewhat better. This is what we call "following the image to completion." (*pause*) Do you think it would help to practice this technique?

In the previous example, the patient is easily able to identify a reasonable outcome. In some cases, the therapist needs to suggest a modification of the scene:

THERAPIST: Can you picture what happens next? ... If you're looking around and seeing the other students, are you actually paralyzed?

PATIENT: I don't know. I *feel* paralyzed.

THERAPIST: What do you see happening next?

PATIENT: I don't know. I just keep sitting there, feeling paralyzed.

THERAPIST: Do you want to imagine yourself moving around a little in the chair, taking a breath, looking out the window?

PATIENT: Uh-huh.

THERAPIST: Do you want to rub the back of your neck and stretch, to make yourself less stiff?

PATIENT: Yeah.

THERAPIST: Okay, are you ready now in the image to read through the test until something seems familiar?

PATIENT: Yes.

THERAPIST: Are you picturing that? What do you want to imagine happens next?

PATIENT: I find an easier question.

THERAPIST: What do you want to imagine happens next?

Here I introduce a new element into the image to help Sally get "unstuck" and repeatedly ask her what she *wants* to imagine. I continue in this vein until she can continue on her own.

As mentioned above, sometimes the patient imagines a scene that worsens, often catastrophically. The therapist then asks questions to determine the meaning of the catastrophe and intervenes accordingly. This situation is exemplified by a different patient, Marie.

THERAPIST: Okay, Marie, so you see yourself in the car and it's starting to drift toward the guard rail of the bridge. Now, get as clear a picture in your mind as you can. Then what happens?

PATIENT: It's getting closer. It crashes through. (*Cries softly.*)

THERAPIST: (*gently*) Then what?

PATIENT: (*crying*) The car is totally wrecked.

THERAPIST: (*softly*) And you?

PATIENT: (*crying*) I'm dead.

THERAPIST: Then what happens?

PATIENT: I don't know. I can't see past that. (*still crying*)

THERAPIST: Marie, I think it'll help if we try to go a little further. What's the worst part about dying in this crash?

PATIENT: My kids. They won't have a mother anymore. They'll be just devastated. (*crying harder*)

THERAPIST: (*Waits a moment.*) Do you have an image of them?

In this example, following the image to completion leads to a catastrophe. I keep gently questioning so I can determine the special significance of the catastrophe. A later example in this chapter, inducing images to provide distance, illustrates one way to deal with this type of problem. In this case, a patient reveals that she has had a new image, of her children at her funeral, feeling utterly devastated. Once again, the patient has cut off an image at the worst point. (See pages 292–293 for an illustration of how the therapist will have the patient imagine her children [doing better] many years in the future.)

In summary, two outcomes are possible when following an image to completion. In one instance, the problem is eventually resolved, and the patient feels relief. In the second instance, the problem worsens to a catastrophe, at which point you ask for the meaning of or the worst part about the image, which helps you uncover a new problem. You can then help the patient induce a coping image, described later in this chapter.

Jumping Ahead in Time

At times, following an image to completion is ineffective because patients keep imagining more and more obstacles or distressing events with no end in sight. At this point, you might suggest that patients imagine themselves at some point in the near future.

THERAPIST: [summarizing] Okay, Sally, when you imagine getting started on this paper, you keep seeing how hard it is and how much effort it's taking and how many problems you're having with it. Realistically, do you think you'll eventually finish the paper?

PATIENT: Yeah, probably. I might have to work day and night for a long time, though.

THERAPIST: How about if you jump ahead in time and imagine finishing it. Can you picture that? What does that look like?

PATIENT: Well, I guess I see myself reading it over and making one last edit. Then I e-mail it to the professor.

THERAPIST: Wait a moment. Can you slow it down a little, really imagine the details?

PATIENT: Okay. I'm sitting at my desk in my dorm room. It's like 2 o'clock in the morning. It's hard to keep my eyes open, but I start at page 1 and proofread my work. I find a few mistakes and I fix them, then save it in a file. I open my e-mail and send it to my professor.

THERAPIST: How do you feel in the image now?

PATIENT: Relieved ... like a weight has been taken off my chest. Lighter.

THERAPIST: Okay, let's review what we did. You had an image of yourself starting to work on this paper and the more you imagined, the more problems you saw and the more anxious you were getting. Then you jumped ahead in time and saw yourself finishing it, which made you feel better. How about if we have you write something down about this technique—jumping ahead in time—so you'll be able to practice it at home, too.

Coping in the Image

Another technique is to guide patients so they can imagine they are coping with a difficult situation they have spontaneously envisioned.

THERAPIST: [summarizing] So you had an image of walking into the [elementary] school library with the student you've volunteered to tutor, and you're feeling at a complete loss? And then the kid acts up and starts making noise, and you feel as if he's out of control?

PATIENT: Yes.

THERAPIST: So once again, you've had an image and left yourself at the worst point?

PATIENT: I guess I did.

THERAPIST: Can we go through this image again, and this time, see if you can imagine coping with each problem as it arises?

PATIENT: Well, first the kid bangs open the library door. I guess I tell him, "Shh. There's another class in here."

THERAPIST: And then what?

PATIENT: He starts veering over to the books.

THERAPIST: So you ...

PATIENT: I guess I take his hand and guide him to a table.

The dialogue continues in this way until the patient has successfully coped in the image. If necessary, you can ask leading questions to help them devise solutions. ("Would you like to imagine that...?") You can also guide patients to imagine themselves using tools they have learned in therapy: for example, reading a coping card, using controlled breathing, and saying self-instructions aloud.

Changing the Image

Another technique involves teaching patients to reimagine a spontaneous image, changing the ending to alleviate their distress. The first example is a realistic change, the second, a "magical" change.

PATIENT: This morning I was thinking about spring vacation. I can't go home. I'll have to stay here. I was feeling really down about that.

THERAPIST: Did you have an image of what that would be like?

PATIENT: I was imagining myself just sitting at my desk, alone in my room, kind of slumped over, feeling really bad.

THERAPIST: Anything else?

PATIENT: No, just that it's so quiet. The dorm is deserted.

THERAPIST: And the image makes you feel ...

PATIENT: Sad. Real sad.

THERAPIST: Sally, you don't have to be at the mercy of this image. You can change it, if you want. It's as if you're a movie director: You can decide how you want it to be instead. You can change it in a magical way ... something that couldn't really happen. Or you can change it to a realistic image.

PATIENT: I'm not sure I understand how.

THERAPIST: Well, okay, you're sitting at your desk. What do you *wish* would happen next?

PATIENT: That my best friend calls me ... or it turns out there are more people in the dorm and someone comes knocking on my door, and we go to dinner together.

THERAPIST: Any other scenario?

PATIENT: Maybe that I remember there's some event on campus, like a softball game, and I go watch or play.

THERAPIST: Those *are* much better endings. How do you think you'd feel if you imagined those things happening?

PATIENT: Better. But how do I know they'll come true?

THERAPIST: Well, first of all, neither of us really knows if you'll actually end up sitting at your desk, crying. What we *do* know is *imagining* it makes you feel really sad now. Second, maybe we could talk about how to make it more likely that there really *is* a better ending. What could you do so your friend might call, or a dormmate might knock on your door, or you might go to a campus event?

Changing the image in this case leads to a productive discussion involving problem solving.

Some images lend themselves to change that is more "magical" in nature. Altering the image in this way also usually leads to a reduction in distress and allows the patient to act in a more productive way. An example follows:

THERAPIST: [summarizing, using Sally's own words] So you have an image of your professor standing very tall over you, scowling, speaking harshly, stomping his foot, being overbearing, and the image makes you very anxious?

PATIENT: Yes.

THERAPIST: Would you like to change the image? Imagine him in a different way?

PATIENT: How?

THERAPIST: I don't know ... He kind of reminds me of a 3-year-old having a tantrum. Can you imagine that he shrinks down in size but still is scowling, still stomping his foot?

PATIENT: (*Smiles.*) Yes.

THERAPIST: Describe him to me, in detail. (*Patient does so.*) And how do you feel now? As anxious?

PATIENT: No, less.

THERAPIST: Has it come down enough to let you go make an appointment with him?

PATIENT: Yes, I think so.

THERAPIST: Okay, let's review what we just did. We started with an image you had of your professor. It sounded as if this image was so distressing that it stopped you from doing what you need to do—make an appointment with him. Then you took control of the image by changing it and your anxiety came down, enough for you to go and meet with him. We call this technique "changing the image."

Reality Testing the Image

Here you teach patients to treat images like verbal automatic thoughts, using standard Socratic questioning.

THERAPIST: So you had an image of me frowning and looking disapproving when you told me you hadn't done part of your homework?

PATIENT: (*Nods.*)

THERAPIST: What's the evidence that I would frown and be disapproving? . . . Do you have any evidence on the other side?

In another situation, I teach Sally to compare a spontaneous image with what is really happening.

PATIENT: I was in the library late last night, and I had an image of the building being real deserted, and then I saw myself suddenly feeling really sick and passing out and having no one there to help me.

THERAPIST: Was it true that the library was completely deserted?

PATIENT: No. It was getting late, near closing time, but there were still a few people around.

THERAPIST: Okay. With this kind of image, when you're spontaneously imagining something happening right at the moment, you can do a reality check. You can ask yourself, "Is the library deserted? Am I actually feeling really sick right now?" If you had known to do that last night, what do you think would have happened to your mood?

PATIENT: I'd have felt less nervous.

In general, it is preferable to use techniques in imagery form when dealing with images, rather than the verbal techniques suggested in this section. However, patients who have many vivid, distressing images will benefit from a variety of techniques, and sometimes the verbal technique of a reality check is helpful.

Repeating the Image

The repetition technique can be useful when patients are clearly imagining exaggerated outcomes. You suggest that they keep imagining the original image over and over again, paying attention to whether the image and their level of distress change. Some patients seem to do an automatic reality check, and envision each succeeding image more realistically and with less dysphoria.

THERAPIST: Okay, Sally, so you had the image of asking your professor for an extension, and he clearly got quite upset, yelling at you, bending over close to you, waving his hands wildly, saying, "How dare you! You knew when it was due. Get out!"

PATIENT: Yes.

THERAPIST: I wonder, could you imagine this again? Start out the same way. See what happens.

PATIENT: (*Closes eyes.*)

THERAPIST: Finished? What happened?

PATIENT: He was pretty upset. He yelled at me, told me to get out.

THERAPIST: This time did he wave his hands, bend over too close to you?

PATIENT: No. He just stood up and stiffened his arms on his desk.

THERAPIST: Okay. Do the same thing again.

I ask Sally to repeat the scene three or four times. By the last repetition, her image has changed quite a bit: The professor leans back in his chair, gives Sally an annoyed look, and says no in an unkind but nonthreatening way. Sally's anxiety diminishes significantly.

Substituting Images

Substituting a more pleasant image has been extensively described elsewhere (e.g., Beck & Emery, 1985). It, too, must be regularly practiced in order for the patient to experience relief from distressing spontaneous images:

THERAPIST: Sally, another way of dealing with this kind of upsetting image is to substitute a different one. Some people like to imagine that the distressing image is a picture on a television set. Then they imagine changing the channel to a different scene, like lying on a beach, or walking through the woods, or recalling a pleasant memory. Would you like to try this technique? First, you'll picture the pleasant scene in as much detail as possible, using as many senses as possible; then I'll have you practice switching from a distressing image to the pleasant one. Now, what pleasant scene would you like to imagine?

INDUCING IMAGERY AS A THERAPEUTIC TOOL

At times, you will *induce* an image as opposed to help a patient respond to a spontaneous image. Covert rehearsal to uncover obstacles related to homework is one example (pages 303–305). Three other induced imaginal techniques are described next.

Rehearsal of Coping Techniques

You will use this technique to help patients practice using coping strategies in imagination. This technique differs from "coping in the image" because here you *induce* an image rather than having patients imagine how they would cope in a spontaneous image.

THERAPIST: Okay, you're predicting that you're going to have a rough time giving the oral report in class.

PATIENT: Yeah.

THERAPIST: When will you first notice your anxiety going up?

PATIENT: When I wake up.

THERAPIST: And what will be going through your mind?

PATIENT: I'm going to mess up. And I'll picture myself stammering and stuttering and being unable to talk.

THERAPIST: You mean in class?

PATIENT: Yeah.

THERAPIST: Okay, what could you do?

PATIENT: Tell myself to relax. Remind myself I've practiced this a lot.

THERAPIST: Okay, what then?

PATIENT: I could do some controlled breathing. That relaxes me some.

THERAPIST: Okay, can you see yourself doing that?

PATIENT: Yeah.

THERAPIST: Then what?

PATIENT: I feel a little better, but I'm still too nervous for breakfast. I just shower, get dressed, get ready to go.

THERAPIST: What's going through your mind?

PATIENT: What if I keep getting more and more nervous?

THERAPIST: How about imagining yourself reading the coping card [we made a few minutes ago] on the way to class? Can you imagine pulling it out and reading it?

PATIENT: Yeah ... I guess it helps some.

THERAPIST: As you get near class, how about if you imagine jumping ahead in time. You've finished the talk, and now you're sitting there listening to someone else ... How do you feel now?

PATIENT: Some relief. Still worried, but not as bad.

THERAPIST: Okay, now you're walking into class. What happens next, and what do you do?

The patient continues imagining herself realistically coping with the situation in detail. Then she writes down the specific techniques she predicts will help.

Distancing

Distancing is another induced imagery technique to reduce distress and help patients see problems in greater perspective. In the following example, I help Sally see that her difficulties are likely to be time limited.

THERAPIST: Sally, I know you're feeling kind of hopeless now, and you're predicting that these problems will go on and on. Do you think it would help if you could envision getting through this rough period?

PATIENT: I guess. But it's hard to imagine.

THERAPIST: Well, let's see. How about if you try to picture yourself a year from now?

PATIENT: Okay.

THERAPIST: Any idea what life is like?

PATIENT: I don't know. It's hard for me to think that far ahead.

THERAPIST: Well, let's be concrete. When do you wake up? Where are you?

PATIENT: Probably I wake up around 8:00 or 8:30. I guess I'm in an off-campus apartment.

THERAPIST: Living alone?

PATIENT: Maybe in a house with other students, some people from my floor this year. We've been talking about it.

THERAPIST: Okay, you wake up. What happens next?

PATIENT: I probably rush off to class. It'll take longer to get there if I'm not in a dorm.

THERAPIST: Do you see any of your housemates before you go? Do you go to class alone or with one of them?

PATIENT: I don't know.

THERAPIST: Well, it's your image. You decide.

PATIENT: Okay, I guess I'd walk over with one of them.

THERAPIST: What do you talk about on the way—or are you silent?

PATIENT: Oh no, we'd be talking about school or people we know. Something like that.

THERAPIST: Then what?

PATIENT: I'd go to class.

THERAPIST: A big lecture hall like most of your classes this year?

PATIENT: No, probably not, classes should be smaller next year.

THERAPIST: And what do you want to imagine happens in class? Do you interact or are you quiet?

PATIENT: Well, hopefully by then I'd know more people. I'd feel more comfortable. I'd probably still be quiet, but I might be participating more.

THERAPIST: How do you feel when you imagine this scene?

PATIENT: Good.

THERAPIST: How would you feel about finishing out this scene for homework? Then every time you have the thought, "I'll never get out of this," you could try switching to this scene to see if it has an effect on your mood.

PATIENT: I'll try.

THERAPIST: Now is this just the power of positive thinking, imagining this scene? Or could you really do some things to make it happen? In fact, aren't you already doing things to make it happen?

PATIENT: That's true.

Another distancing technique helps a patient deal with the imagined aftermath of a catastrophe. Marie, described previously, fears that her children would be devastated forever if she died. Her therapist has her imagine their realistic level of distress at different points in time, instead of just immediately after the accident. (This technique is similar to jumping ahead in time; it involves the passage of *years*, though, instead of minutes, hours, or days.)

THERAPIST: Marie, who do you imagine breaks the news of your death to the kids?

PATIENT: My husband.

THERAPIST: How does he do it?

PATIENT: (*sobbing*) He puts his arms around them. He says, "There's been an accident. Mommy's gone."

THERAPIST: And then?

PATIENT: They don't believe it, not really, at first. They start crying and saying, "No, it's not true. I want Mommy."

THERAPIST: They're feeling pretty bad?

PATIENT: Yeah. Real bad.

THERAPIST: (*Waits a moment.*) Can you jump ahead some? It's now 6 months later. What's going on now? Can you see them?

PATIENT: They're in school. Looking real sad. Bewildered. Kind of empty.

THERAPIST: How bad are they feeling?

PATIENT: Still pretty bad.

THERAPIST: Can we jump ahead 2 years? How old will they be?

PATIENT: Melissa will be 8. Linda will be 7.

THERAPIST: What do you see them doing?

PATIENT: Playing outside. It's our house. I don't think my husband would move.

THERAPIST: What are they playing?

PATIENT: They're jumping rope with the neighbor kids.

THERAPIST: How are they feeling now?

PATIENT: Okay, when they don't think about me.

THERAPIST: And when they do?

PATIENT: (*Tears up.*) They still cry sometimes. It's confusing.

THERAPIST: As bad as when they first found out?

PATIENT: No, not that bad.

The therapist gently leads Marie through a succession of images 5, 10, and 20 years after her imagined death. Through this exercise, Marie is able to see that the initial devastation her daughters feel eventually subsides to briefer periods of sadness and grief with which they are able to cope. Imagining in detail that her daughters grow up and create new families of their own significantly reduces Marie's fear of her own death in an automobile accident.

Reduction of Perceived Threat

A third type of induced image is designed to allow patients to view a situation with a more realistic assessment of actual threat. For example, I encouraged Sally to modify her image of her class presentation by imagining the encouraging faces of her friends in the room. Pam, a patient who feared undergoing a Caesarean section, envisioned all the life-saving equipment in the delivery room and the caring faces of the nurse and doctor behind their masks.

In summary, many if not most patients experience automatic thoughts in the form of spontaneous images. Persistent (though nonintrusive) questioning is often required to help patients recognize their images. Patients who do have frequent, distressing images benefit from regular practice of several imagery techniques. In addition, images may be induced for various therapeutic purposes.

Chapter 17

HOMEWORK

Homework is an integral, not optional, part of cognitive behavior therapy (Beck et al., 1979). A number of researchers have found that cognitive behavior therapy patients who carry out homework assignments progress better in therapy than those who do not (e.g., Kazantzis, Whittington, & Datillio, 2010; Neimeyer & Feixas, 1990; Persons, Burns & Perloff, 1988). You seek to extend the opportunities for cognitive and behavioral change *throughout the patient's week*. You prepare the patient for doing homework in the first session.

THERAPIST: Sally, I think it would be important for you to read this [statement about being depressed, not lazy] every day. Do you think you could do that?

PATIENT: Yes, I think so.

THERAPIST: In fact, reminding yourself of important things we talk about in session is one way you're going to get over your depression. Another way is by changing some of the things that you do. We've found that it's not enough for people to just come and talk. They need to make small changes in their thinking and behavior every day.

PATIENT: Okay.

THERAPIST: But we'll always make sure that you think the changes are a good idea and that you'll be able to do them. Now, what should we call these changes? Homework? Your action plan? Something else?

PATIENT: Homework, I guess.

THERAPIST: Okay, but I want you to remember that this isn't like school homework. This is homework that *you* think will help, that we'll design together, just for you.

Good homework assignments provide opportunities for patients to educate themselves further (e.g., through bibliotherapy), to collect data (e.g., through monitoring their thoughts, feelings, and behavior), to test their thoughts and beliefs, to modify their thinking, to practice cognitive and behavioral tools, and to experiment with new behaviors. Homework can maximize what was learned in a therapy session and lead to an increase in patients' sense of self-efficacy.

Many patients do homework quite willingly and easily; a few do not. It is important to note that even the most experienced therapists encounter difficulty with an occasional patient who, despite careful preparation, rarely does any *written* assignments. Nevertheless, you should initially assume that any patient (unless he or she is very low functioning) *will* do homework if you set it up properly. To enhance the probability that patients will comply, you need to take care, for example, to:

> * Tailor assignments to the individual,
> * Provide a sound rationale,
> * Uncover potential obstacles, and
> * Modify relevant beliefs.

This chapter is divided into four parts:

1. Setting homework assignments.
2. Increasing the likelihood of successful completion of homework.
3. Conceptualizing problems.
4. Reviewing completed homework.

SETTING HOMEWORK ASSIGNMENTS

There is no set formula for assigning homework. Rather, you tailor homework to the individual patient. How do you decide what to suggest? It depends on what you have discussed in session, which is influenced by your overall treatment plan and the patient's goals. You take into consideration individual characteristics of patients: their reading and writing abilities, their motivation and willingness to comply with homework, their current level of distress and functioning (cognitive, emotional, and behavioral), and practical constraints (e.g., of time), to name a few.

You may need to take the lead in suggesting homework assignments at the beginning of treatment but you begin, as soon as possible, to ask patients to devise their own assignments (e.g., "Now that we've finished talking about this problem with your roommate, what do you think would be helpful for you to remember this week? To do this week?"). Patients who routinely set their own homework by the end of therapy are more likely to continue doing so when treatment has ended.

In this first section, typical assignments are presented; then a sample of Sally's homework assignments are provided. The final portion of this chapter offers guidelines for increasing homework adherence.

Ongoing Homework Assignments

Typical ongoing homework assignments are discussed below.

1. *Behavioral activation.* Getting inactive, depressed patients out of bed or off the couch and helping them resume their normal activities (and engage in new activities) is essential. Activity scheduling benefits other patients as well.

2. *Monitoring automatic thoughts.* From the first session forward, you will encourage your patients to ask themselves, "What's going through my mind right now?" when they notice their mood changing, and remind themselves that their thinking may or may not be true. Initially they may jot down their thoughts (in their smartphone, on their computer, or simply on paper, in a notebook, or on an index card). Advise patients that monitoring their automatic thoughts can lead them to feel worse, if they accept them uncritically, and that you will do problem solving with them if their thoughts do turn out to be valid.

3. *Evaluating and responding to automatic thoughts.* At virtually every session, you will help patients modify their inaccurate and dysfunctional thoughts and write down their new way of thinking. An essential homework assignment is to have them read these therapy notes on a regular basis. Patients will also learn to evaluate their own thinking and practice doing so between sessions.

4. *Problem solving.* At virtually every session, you will help patients devise solutions to their problems, which they will implement between sessions.

5. *Behavioral skills.* To effectively solve their problems, patients may need to learn new skills, which they will practice for homework. For

example, you might teach relaxation skills to anxious patients, assertiveness skills to socially anxious patients, or organizational and time management skills to patients who would benefit from them.

6. *Behavioral experiments.* Patients may need to directly test the validity of automatic thoughts that seem distorted, such as "I'll feel better if I stay in bed"; "My roommate will get mad if I bring up the problem of noise"; "No one will talk to me at the meeting."

7. *Bibliotherapy.* Important concepts you are discussing in session can be greatly reinforced when patients read about them in black and white. It is usually valuable to have patients both read and note their reactions: what they agreed with, disagreed with, and had questions about.

8. *Preparing for the next therapy session.* The beginning part of each therapy session can be greatly speeded up if patients think about what is important to tell you before they enter your office. The Preparing for Therapy Worksheet (page 102) can help prepare them.

A Sampling of Homework Assignments for Sally

Some of the assignments below are helpful for almost any depressed patient; others were specifically designed for this particular patient.

Session 1

Read this list twice a day; set an alarm to remember.

1. If I start thinking I'm lazy and no good, remind myself that I have a real illness, called depression, that makes it harder for me to do things. As the treatment starts to work, my depression will lift, and things will get easier.
2. Read goal list and add others, if I think of any.
3. When I notice my mood getting worse, ask myself, "What's going through my mind right now?" and jot down the thoughts. Remind myself that just because I think something doesn't necessarily mean it's true.
4. Make plans with Allison and Joe. Remember, if they say no, it's likely that they'd like to hang out with me but they're too busy.
5. Read *Coping with Depression* booklet (optional).

Session 2

1. Daily: When I notice my mood changing, ask myself, "What's going through my mind right now?" and jot down my automatic thoughts (which may or may not be completely true).
2. If I can't figure out my automatic thoughts, jot down just the situa-

tion. Remember, learning to identify my thinking is a skill I'll get better at, like typing.

3. Ask Sean for help with Chapter 5 of Econ book.
4. Daily: Read therapy notes.
5. Continue running/swimming.
6. Plan two to three social activities.
7. Daily: Add to credit list (anything I do that is even a little difficult but I do it anyway).
8. (Tuesday morning): Review Preparing for Therapy Worksheet for 2 minutes.

Session 3

1. Daily: Read therapy notes.
2. Daily: When my mood changes, use Question List and answer mentally or in writing.
3. Daily: Add to credit list.
4. Daily: Follow activity chart.
5. Ask Lisa to study for Chem exam with me.
6. (Tuesday morning): Review Preparing for Therapy Worksheet.

Session 4

1. Daily: Read therapy notes.
2. Daily: When my mood changes, do first four columns of Thought Records in writing. Answer questions at bottom mentally.
3. Daily: Credit list.
4. Go for a walk or a run at least three days this week.
5. Make plans with friends.
6. Do activities we scheduled on activity chart.
7. Discuss late-night noise with Jane.
8. (Tuesday morning): Review Preparing for Therapy Worksheet.

Session 5

1. Daily: Read therapy notes.
2. Daily: Thought Records mentally or in writing.
3. Daily: Credit list.
4. Daily: Follow activity chart.
5. Ask Chem professor for help.

Session 6

1. Daily: Read therapy notes.
2. As needed: Thought Records.
3. Daily: Credit list.

4. Schedule activities.
5. Call Mom about summer plans.

Session 7

1. Daily: Read therapy notes.
2. As needed: Thought Records.
3. Daily: Credit list.
4. Schedule activities.
5. Make a comment or ask a question in class.

Session 9

1. Daily: Therapy notes.
2. As needed: Thought Records.
3. Daily: Credit list.
4. Schedule activities.
5. Fill in CBW.
6. Bring up clutter problem with Jane.
7. Go to Dr. Smith during office hours.

Session 12 (Penultimate Session)

1. Thought Record about termination.
2. Organize therapy notes from beginning.
3. Review notes on doing a self-therapy session.

INCREASING HOMEWORK ADHERENCE

Although some patients easily do the suggested assignments, homework is more problematic for others. Implementation of the following guidelines increases the likelihood that patients will be successful with homework and experience an elevation in mood:

1. Tailor the assignment to the individual. (Be 90–100% sure the patient can and will do the assignment.) Err on the side of devising assignments that are too easy rather than too hard.
2. Provide a rationale as to how and why the assignment might help.
3. Set homework collaboratively; seek the patient's input and agreement.
4. Make homework a no-lose proposition.
5. Begin the assignment (when possible) in session.
6. Help set up systems for remembering to do the assignment.

7. Anticipate possible problems; do covert rehearsal when indicated.
8. Prepare for a possible negative outcome (when applicable).

Tailoring Homework to the Individual

Successful completion of homework can speed up therapy and lead to an increased sense of mastery and improved mood. Rather than suggesting assignments according to a prescribed formula, you should consider the patient's characteristics (mentioned in the introduction to this chapter) and desires.

Matt, for example, was a patient who did not grasp the cognitive model in the first session and, indeed, became slightly irritated when his (novice) therapist kept pushing him to identify his automatic thoughts. He told his therapist, "You don't understand; I don't *know* what is going through my mind at the time; all I know is that I'm very upset." A homework assignment to jot down his automatic thoughts would have been inappropriate for this session. A second patient, Caitlin, on the other hand, had already read a popular book on cognitive behavior therapy and had an unusually good grasp of her automatic thoughts. Her initial homework assignment was to complete the first four columns of the Thought Record whenever she became upset.

While the type of assignment is important, so is the *amount* of homework. Sally was a motivated patient who was "in sync" with homework, as she was still a student. She was easily able to accomplish more between sessions than Matt, who was severely depressed and had been out of school for many years.

A third step in tailoring homework to the individual patient involves breaking down assignments into manageable steps. Examples include reading one chapter of a layman's cognitive behavior therapy book or school textbook, doing the first four columns of a Thought Record, spending 10–15 minutes paying bills, doing just one load of laundry, and spending just five minutes at a supermarket.

It is important to predict potential difficulties before assigning homework. Patients' diagnoses and personality styles can be a guide. Severely depressed patients, for example, initially will probably benefit more from behavioral (as opposed to cognitive) tasks. Avoidant patients shy away from behavioral assignments that they perceive as too challenging or likely to evoke a high level of dysphoria. Patients who are feeling anxious and overwhelmed might feel incapable of doing *any* assignment if you suggest too many tasks. It is much better to err on the side of providing homework assignments that are a little too easy. Failure to carry out an assignment, or to do it properly, often leads a patient to be self-critical or feel hopeless.

Providing a Rationale

Patients are more likely to comply with homework assignments if they understand the reason for doing them. I introduce a homework assignment to Sally in this way:

THERAPIST: Sally, research shows that exercise often helps people become less depressed. What do you think about taking a walk or a run a few times this week?

You will provide a brief rationale initially; later in treatment, you will encourage patients to think about the purpose of an assignment, for example, "Sally, what would be the point of checking with your roommate about her plans for this weekend?" or "Why might it be a good idea to continue keeping the credit list?" It is also important to emphasize that homework is an essential part of treatment:

THERAPIST: The way people get better is to make small changes in their thinking and behavior every day.

Setting Homework Collaboratively

Ideally, patients would set their own homework, but at the beginning of treatment they do not know which assignments would be beneficial. Instead, you will make suggestions and ensure they agree: "What do you think about asking your boss for time off?"; "Do you think it could help if you read this coping card before you leave the house?"; "Do you want to try [a particular technique] this week?"; "I think if you get in the shower as soon as you get up, you'll demonstrate to yourself that you can take control. What do you think? Is this something you want to try?" If patients are hesitant or skeptical, you will need to prepare them further. Either elicit and help them respond to their automatic thoughts and/or make the assignment much easier.

As therapy progresses, you will encourage patients to set their own assignments. "What would you like to do this week about [this problem]?"; "What could you do this week if you start getting uncomfortably anxious?"; "How will you handle [this problem] if it does arise?"

Making Homework a No-Lose Proposition

It is helpful when initially setting up assignments to stress that useful data can be obtained even if patients fail to complete their homework. Patients who do not do the homework are less likely to brand themselves as failures and thus feel more dysphoric:

THERAPIST: Sally, if you get this homework done, that's good. But if you have trouble doing it, that's okay—just see if you can figure out what thoughts are getting in your way, and we'll talk about those thoughts next time. Okay?

Sometimes patients fail to do a significant portion of their homework for two weeks in a row, or they do it immediately before the therapy session instead of daily. In these cases, you should uncover the psychological and/or practical obstacles that got in the way and stress how essential homework is, instead of continuing to make it a no-lose proposition.

Starting Homework in the Session

If you can, have patients begin assignments right in the therapy session itself; they will be far more likely to follow through at home. Continuing an assignment is much easier than initiating one. This is especially critical because patients often describe the hardest part of doing homework as the period *just before* they initiate it—that is, motivating themselves to get started. If you yourself find that you, too, occasionally have difficulty initiating a task (e.g., getting yourself to work on a paper, pay taxes, or start exercising), but find it much easier after a few minutes, you can self-disclose this to patients to normalize the experience and provide a role model for them to think about when they are procrastinating.

Remembering to Do Homework

It is vital to write down, or have patients write down, their assignments every week, starting with the first session. Ask them where they will keep the assignment list (or notebook) and how likely they think they might be to forget to look at the list on one or more days. If even slightly likely, you might suggest several strategies: You can ask patients to:

- Pair an assignment with another daily activity (e.g., "How about pulling out the activity chart at mealtimes and right before bed?").
- Post notes on their refrigerator, their bathroom mirror, or the dashboard of their car.
- Use their appointment book, smartphone, or computer to cue them.
- Ask another person to cue them.

You can also ask them how they remember to do other regularly scheduled activities, such as taking medication.

Anticipating Problems

To maximize the likelihood that you are suggesting reasonable assignments that patients are likely to do, consider the following:

> * Is the amount and degree of difficulty of homework reasonable for this patient, or will it feel overwhelming?
> * Is it related to the patient's goals?
> * How likely is the patient to do it?
> * What practical problems may get in the way (time, energy, opportunity)?
> * What thoughts may get in the way?

The single most important question to ask patients to assess the probability of adherence is:

> *How likely are you to do this, 0–100%?*

If patients are less than 90–100% confident, use one or more of the following strategies:

> 1. Covert rehearsal.
> 2. Change the assignment.
> 3. Do an intellectual/emotional role play.

These stategies are described below.

Covert Rehearsal

Covert rehearsal, illustrated below, uses induced imagery to uncover and solve potential homework-related problems.

THERAPIST: Sally, do you think anything will get in the way of your going to the teaching assistant for help?

PATIENT: I'm not sure.

THERAPIST: [getting her to specify and commit to a time] When would be a good time to go?

PATIENT: Friday morning, I guess. That's when his office hours are.

THERAPIST: Can you imagine it's Friday morning right now? Can you picture it? Can you imagine saying to yourself, "I really should go to the TA's office"?

PATIENT: Yeah.

THERAPIST: [asking for details so Sally will more easily be able to visualize the scene and accurately identify her thoughts and emotions] Where are you?

PATIENT: In my room.

THERAPIST: Doing what?

PATIENT: Well, I just finished getting dressed.

THERAPIST: And how are you feeling?

PATIENT: A little nervous, I guess.

THERAPIST: And what's going through your mind?

PATIENT: I don't want to go. Maybe I'll just read the chapter again myself.

THERAPIST: And how are you going to answer those thoughts?

PATIENT: I don't know.

THERAPIST: Do you want to remind yourself it's just an experiment, that we won't know what happens until you go? That if he's not helpful, we'll figure out Plan B together?

PATIENT: Yeah, I think so.

THERAPIST: Would it help to put that on a coping card you can read a few times between now and Friday?

PATIENT: Probably.

THERAPIST: Okay. Now can you imagine you're dressed and you're thinking, "I'll just read the chapter myself instead of going"? Now what happens?

PATIENT: I think, "Wait a minute. This is supposed to be an experiment. Now where's that coping card?"

THERAPIST: Oh, where is it?

PATIENT: Knowing me, I'd have to look for it.

THERAPIST: Is there someplace you could put it as soon as you get back today?

PATIENT: I don't exactly want my roommate to see it ... Maybe in the bottom drawer of my desk.

THERAPIST: Okay. And if you've already read it on Wednesday and Thursday, you'll probably remember where it is. Can you imagine pulling out the card and reading it?

PATIENT: Yeah.

THERAPIST: Now, what happens?

PATIENT: Probably I remember why I *should* go, but I still don't want to. So I decide to clean my room first.

THERAPIST: What could you remind yourself at this point?

PATIENT: That I may as well go and get it over with. That maybe it really will help. That if I stop and clean I may end up not going at all.

THERAPIST: Good. Then what happens?

PATIENT: I go.

THERAPIST: And then?

PATIENT: I get there. I ask him the question. I don't understand it all. I tell him what I'm confused about. He probably helps, at least some.

THERAPIST: And how do you feel at this point?

PATIENT: Better.

This kind of covert rehearsal helps you discover which practical obstacles and dysfunctional cognitions may hinder the completion of homework.

Changing the Assignment

Changing the assignment may be indicated if you judge that an assignment *is* inappropriate or if covert rehearsal has not been sufficiently effective. It is far better to substitute an easier homework assignment that patients are likely to do than to have them establish a habit of not doing what they had agreed to in session:

THERAPIST: Sally, I'm not sure you're ready to do this. [Or, "I'm not sure this assignment is appropriate."] What do you think? Do you want to go ahead and try or wait until another time?

You can also collaboratively decide to make certain assignments optional or to decrease the frequency or duration of a homework task. It is far better for patients to do less homework than no homework at all.

Intellectual–Emotional Role Play

An intellectual–emotional role play may help motivate reluctant patients when the therapist judges it is quite important for a patient to do a given assignment. This technique is not used early in therapy, as it can be perceived as somewhat challenging.

THERAPIST: I'm still not sure you'll actually pull out the coping card to get you going.

PATIENT: Probably not.

THERAPIST: Okay, how about if we do an intellectual–emotional role play about this? We've done this before. I'll be the intellectual part of you; you be the emotional part. You argue as hard as you can against me so I can see all the arguments you're using not to read your coping cards and start studying. You start.

PATIENT: Okay. I don't feel like doing this.

THERAPIST: It's true that I don't feel like doing it, but that's irrelevant. It doesn't matter if I feel like it or not. It's what I *need* to do.

PATIENT: But I can do it later.

THERAPIST: True, but my usual pattern is *not* to do it later. I don't want to reinforce a bad habit by putting it off. Here I have the opportunity to strengthen a new, better habit.

PATIENT: But it won't matter this one time.

THERAPIST: True. Any one individual time isn't all that crucial. On the other hand, I'll be better off in the long run if I strengthen this good habit as much as I can.

PATIENT: I don't know, I just don't want to.

THERAPIST: I don't have to pay attention to what I *want* to do now or *don't* want to do now. In the long run, I *want* to do things that I need to, so I can graduate, get a good job, and feel good about myself, and I *don't* want to constantly avoid things I don't feel like doing.

PATIENT: ... I've run out of arguments.

THERAPIST: Okay. Let's switch parts, then we'll get some of it down in writing.

Following role reversal, you have another choice point. You can collaboratively reassign the original homework task (e.g., "How do you feel *now* about trying [this assignment]?"). If patients do decide to keep the assignment, you and they can jointly write a coping card with some points mentioned in the role play above. If you believe it is unlikely that the patient will fulfill the assignment, however, you should suggest a change in homework or make the assignment optional.

Preparing for a Possible Negative Outcome

When devising a behavioral experiment or testing an assumption, it is important to set up a scenario that is likely to succeed. For example, Sally and I discussed which professor was most likely to be receptive to questions after class, what words she might use when negotiating late-night noise with her roommate, and how much help was reasonable to ask from her friend. It is a good idea, though, to have patients predict likely automatic thoughts or beliefs if the experiment does not turn out well.

THERAPIST: Now I suppose it *could* happen that Ross says he can't help you. If that happens, what will go through your mind?

PATIENT: That I shouldn't have asked. That he probably thinks I'm stupid for asking.

THERAPIST: [seeking an alternative explanation] What other reasons might he have for saying no?

PATIENT: That he was too busy.

THERAPIST: Or is it possible that he doesn't understand the material well enough to explain it to you? Or, that he simply doesn't like tutoring? Or, that he's preoccupied with something else?

PATIENT: I guess so.

THERAPIST: Do you have any evidence so far that he thinks you're stupid?

PATIENT: No, but we did disagree about politics.

THERAPIST: And did you get the idea that he thought your ideas were definitely stupid or that you simply had another point of view?

PATIENT: That we just felt differently about it.

THERAPIST: So as far as you know, he doesn't view you as stupid?

PATIENT: No, I don't think so.

THERAPIST: So even if he turns you down, it won't *necessarily* be that he's changed his view of you, based on your request for help?

PATIENT: No, I guess not.

THERAPIST: Okay, we've agreed that you'll approach him later today and ask for help. Either he'll help you, and that's good, or he'll say no, and then what will you remind yourself?

PATIENT: That it doesn't mean he thinks I'm stupid. He may just be busy or unsure of the stuff himself or not like to tutor people.

THERAPIST: Good, let's write that down, just in case.

Advance discussion of potential problems guards against dysphoria when an experiment does not turn out well.

CONCEPTUALIZING DIFFICULTIES

When patients have difficulty doing their homework, conceptualize why the problem arose. Was it related to:

- A practical problem?
- A psychological problem?
- A psychological problem masked as a practical problem?
- A problem related to the *therapist's* cognitions?

Practical Problems

Most practical problems can be avoided if you carefully set the assignment and prepare the patient to do it. Covert rehearsal (described earlier) can also ferret out potential difficulties. Four common practical problems and their remedies are described next.

Doing Therapy Homework at the Last Minute

Ideally, patients carry on the work of the therapy session *throughout the week.* For example, it is most useful for patients to catch and record their automatic thoughts at the moment they notice their mood changing and to respond to these thoughts either mentally or in writing. Some patients avoid thinking about therapy between sessions. Often, this avoidance is part of a larger problem, and you may first have to help patients identify and modify certain beliefs (e.g., "If I focus on a problem instead of distracting myself, I'll only feel worse" or "I can't change, so why even try?"). Other patients, however, need only a gentle reminder to look at their homework list daily.

Forgetting the Rationale for an Assignment

Occasionally, patients neglect an assignment because they do not remember *why* they were asked to do it. This problem can be avoided by having patients (who have demonstrated this difficulty) record the rationale next to an assignment.

PATIENT: I didn't do the relaxation exercises [or read the coping cards or practice controlled breathing or record my activities] because I was feeling fine this week.

THERAPIST: Do you remember what we said a few weeks ago—why it's helpful to practice this every day, regardless of how you're feeling?

PATIENT: I'm not sure.

THERAPIST: Well, let's say you don't practice your relaxation exercises for a couple of weeks. Then you have a very stressful week. How sharp will your skills be then?

PATIENT: Not very.

THERAPIST: Could we have you write down relaxation exercises for homework again this week with a reminder that you want to be really good at relaxation before you need to use it? (*pause*) Any other problems with practicing it?

Disorganization or Lack of Accountability

Many patients are more likely to do assignments when they have to mark off a daily checklist indicating whether they fulfilled an assignment. You or patients can draw a simple diagram (Figure 17.1) in session. Instruct patients to check off each assignment they complete each day. This technique both helps patients remember to do assignments and also makes them face what they are not doing.

Alternately, patients can write down assignments on a daily calendar or appointment book. (Do the first day together in the office and ask patients to write down the rest in the reception room after the session.) Later, after completing assignments, patients can check or cross them off.

A third technique, which you might use with patients whose adherence is likely to be low, is suggesting that they call your office to leave a message when they have completed an assignment. Knowing that you expect a message may motivate patients to do the homework.

	W	Th	F	Sat	Sun	M	T
1. Read therapy notes							
2. Do a credit list							
3. Do a Thought Record							
4. Ask a question in class							

FIGURE 17.1. Sample daily checklist for homework assignments.

As with any intervention, you should suggest these possibilities with a rationale and be sure that patients agree.

Difficulty with an Assignment

If you realize at a subsequent session that a homework assignment was too difficult or ill-defined (common problems with novice therapists), take responsibility. Otherwise patients may unfairly criticize themselves for not having successfully completed an assignment:

THERAPIST: Sally, now that we've talked about the problem you had with the homework, I can see that I didn't explain it well enough to you. [Or, "I can see that it was really too hard."] I'm sorry about that. What went through your mind when you couldn't [or didn't] do it?

Here you have an opportunity to (1) model that you can make and admit to mistakes, (2) build rapport, (3) demonstrate that you are concerned with tailoring therapy—and homework assignments—to the patient, and (4) help patients see an alternative explanation for their lack of success.

Psychological Problems

If patients don't do an assignment that was properly set up and which they had the opportunity to do, their difficulty may stem from one of the psychological factors described next.

Negative Predictions

When patients are in psychological distress, and particularly when they are depressed, they tend to assume negative outcomes. To identify dysfunctional cognitions that interfered with doing a homework assignment, ask patients to recall a *specific* time they thought about doing the assignment and then elicit related cognitions and feelings:

THERAPIST: Was there a time this week when you *did* think about reading the booklet on depression?

PATIENT: Yes. I thought about it on and off.

THERAPIST: Tell me about one of these times. Did you think about it last night, for example?

PATIENT: Yeah. I was going to do it after dinner.

THERAPIST: What happened?

PATIENT: I don't know. I just couldn't make myself do it.

THERAPIST: How were you feeling?

PATIENT: Down, sad, kind of tired.

THERAPIST: What was going through your mind as you thought about reading the booklet?

PATIENT: This is hard. I probably won't be able to concentrate. I won't understand it.

THERAPIST: Sounds like you were feeling pretty low. No wonder you were having trouble getting started. In fact, maybe we should have had you start reading it right in our session last week. (*pause*) I wonder how we could test this idea that you won't be able to concentrate and understand it.

PATIENT: I guess I could try it.

You might then ask patients to conduct an experiment right in session. Following a successful outcome, they might write down conclusions such as: "Sometimes my thoughts aren't true and I can do more than I think. Next time I feel hopeless, I can do an experiment, like I did with the booklet." (Note: If the experiment were unsuccessful, you would need to change the assignment to a more basic task.)

Patients can test other negative predictions (such as, "My roommate won't want to go to that meeting with me," or "I won't understand the material even if I ask for help," or "Doing homework will make me feel worse") through behavioral experiments. Again, it is important to prepare patients for their reaction to a possible negative outcome. You can help patients evaluate other thoughts, such as, "I can't do anything right," or "I might fail this course," with standard Socratic questioning.

When patients reveal ambivalence about the usefulness of doing an assignment, you should acknowledge that you do not know what the outcome will be: "I don't know for sure that doing this assignment *will* help. What will you lose if it doesn't work? What's the potential gain in the long run if it does work?" Alternatively, you and the patient could list advantages and disadvantages of doing the homework.

Finally, a patient may benefit from work at the belief level. Homework may activate beliefs such as:

> "I'm incompetent."
> "Having to do therapy homework means I'm defective."
> "I shouldn't have to put forth so much effort to feel better."
> "My therapist is trying to control me."

> "If I think about my problems, I'll feel worse and worse."
> "If I do homework and get better, my life will get worse."

These kinds of beliefs can be identified and modified through techniques described in Chapters 13 and 14.

Overestimating the Demands of an Assignment

Some patients overestimate how inconvenient or difficult it will be to do homework or do not realize that doing a therapy assignment will be time limited.

THERAPIST: What could get in the way of your doing a Thought Record a few times this week?

PATIENT: I'm not sure I'll find the time.

THERAPIST: How long do you think it will take each time?

PATIENT: Not that long. Maybe 10 minutes. But I'm pretty rushed these days, you know. I do have a million things to do.

You can then do straightforward problem solving to find possible time slots. Alternatively, you might propose an analogy, stressing that the inconvenience of doing assignments is time limited:

THERAPIST: It certainly is true; you *are* very busy these days. I wonder— this is an extreme example, I know—but what would you do if you had to take time every day to do something that would save your life [or your loved one's life]? What would happen, for example, if you needed a blood transfusion every day?

PATIENT: Well, of course I'd find the time.

THERAPIST: Now, it's obviously not life threatening if you don't do this assignment, but the principle is the same. In a minute, we can talk specifically about how you could cut back in another area, but first it's important to remember that this is *not* for the rest of your life. We just need you to rearrange some things for a little while until you're feeling better.

The patient who overestimates the *energy* an assignment benefits from similar questions. In the next example, the patient has a dysfunctional (and distorted) image of fulfilling an assignment.

THERAPIST: What could get in the way of your going to the mall every day this week?

PATIENT: (*Sighs.*) I don't know if I'll have the energy.

THERAPIST: What are you envisioning?

PATIENT: Well, I can see dragging myself into one store after another.

THERAPIST: You know, we talked about your going just for 10 minutes every day. How many stores would you actually get to in 10 minutes? I wonder if you could be imagining that this assignment will be more difficult than we had planned?

In a different situation, the patient has correctly recalled the assignment but again overestimates the energy it will require. I first help *specify the problem* by doing a modified, short version of covert rehearsal.

PATIENT: I'm not sure I'll have the energy to take Max to the park for 15 minutes.

THERAPIST: Will the problem be mostly getting out of the house, going to the park, or what you'll have to do *at* the park?

PATIENT: Getting out of the house. I have to get so much stuff together— his diaper bag, the stroller, a bottle, his coat and boots ...
[The therapist and patient then problem-solve; one solution is for her to gather all the necessities earlier in the day when she is feeling more energetic and less overwhelmed.]

In a third situation, I simply set up the assignment as an experiment.

PATIENT: I'm not sure I'll have the energy to make the phone calls.

THERAPIST: Since we've run short of time today, how about if we just set up this assignment as an experiment: Let's write down your prediction—"I won't have enough energy to make the calls"—and next session, you can tell me how accurate it was. Is that okay?

Perfectionism

Many patients benefit from a simple reminder that they should not strive for perfection when doing homework:

THERAPIST: Learning to identify your automatic thoughts is a skill, like learning the computer. You'll get better with practice. So, if you have any trouble this week, don't worry. We'll figure out how to do it better at our next session.

Other patients with a strong underlying assumption about the necessity of being perfect may benefit from assignments that *include* mistakes:

THERAPIST: It sounds as if your belief about perfectionism is showing up in difficulty doing therapy homework.

PATIENT: Yeah, it is.

THERAPIST: How about this week if we have you do a Thought Record that is *deliberately* imperfect? You could do it with messy handwriting or not do it thoroughly or make spelling mistakes. We should also put a 10-minute time limit on it.

Psychological Obstacles Masked as Practical Problems

Some patients propose that practical problems such as lack of time, energy, or opportunity may prevent them from carrying out an assignment. If you believe that a thought or belief is also interfering, you should investigate this possibility *before* discussing the practical problem:

THERAPIST: Okay, so you're not sure you'll be able to do this assignment [because of a practical problem]. Let's pretend for a moment that this problem magically disappears. *Now* how likely are you do to the homework? Would anything else interfere? Any thoughts that would get in the way?

Problems Related to the Therapist's Cognitions

Finally, you should assess whether any of *your* thoughts or beliefs hinder you from assertively and appropriately encouraging a patient to do homework. Typical dysfunctional assumptions of therapists include:

> "I'll hurt his feelings if I try to find out why he didn't do the homework."
> "She'll get angry if I [nicely] question her."
> "He'll be insulted if I suggest he try a homework monitor."
> "She doesn't really need to do homework to get better."
> "He is too overburdened now with other things."
> "She's too passive–aggressive to do homework."
> "He's too fragile to expose himself to an anxious situation."

Ask yourself what goes through *your* mind when you think about assigning homework or exploring why a patient has not done homework. If you are having dysfunctional thoughts, you might do Thought Records or behavioral experiments or consult a supervisor or peer. Remind yourself that you are not doing patients a favor if you allow them to skip homework (which research shows is important) and do not make extensive efforts to gain adherence.

REVIEWING HOMEWORK

Before each session, you should prepare by reviewing the notes of the previous session and noting the patient's homework. A discussion of homework is typically the first item on the agenda, unless it is clearly inappropriate (e.g., the patient is grieving a recent, serious loss). Even if a patient is in crisis, it is still useful to spend a few minutes discussing homework later in the session or, in a different case, to collaboratively agree that the homework assigned at the previous session does not apply at the moment.

Deciding how much time to spend reviewing homework and discussing whether patients want to continue any assignment is part of the art of therapy. You will spend more time on homework when:

- It covers an important, ongoing problem that requires further discussion.
- Patients have not completed a task.
- You judge that it is important to discuss what patients have learned or to help them reach a new understanding of their problems.

For example, if severely depressed patients do not follow through with activity scheduling, you will likely spend significant time in session conceptualizing what happened and planning with them how they can be more successful in the coming week. Spending too little time reviewing homework may deprive patients of reinforcing important learning and skills. Spending too much time may deprive patients of discussing new problems thoroughly.

The time you devote to a review of homework will vary. At the beginning of treatment, you will reinforce what was in the therapy notes (e.g., asking patients how much they believe the adaptive responses they wrote in the past session(s) and at home). You may need to review and allow patients to practice skills they did not quite grasp. You will also collaboratively decide which assignments a patient will continue or modify for the coming week.

In summary, both you and your patients should view homework as an essential part of treatment. Homework, properly assigned and completed, speeds progress and allows patients to practice the techniques of therapy which they will need when therapy is over. Kazantzis, Deane, Ronan, and Lampropoulos (2005) and Tompkins (2004) are helpful resources.

Chapter 18

TERMINATION AND RELAPSE PREVENTION

The goal in cognitive behavior therapy is to facilitate remission of patients' disorders and to teach them skills they can use throughout their lifetime. The goal is not for you to solve all their problems. In fact, if you view yourself as responsible for helping patients with *every* problem, you risk engendering or reinforcing dependence and you deprive patients of the opportunity to test and strengthen their skills.

Therapy sessions are usually scheduled once a week, unless there are practical constraints. Patients with severe symptoms may benefit from more frequent sessions. Once patients have experienced a reduction in symptoms and have learned basic skills, you may collaboratively agree to taper therapy gradually, on a trial basis, to once every 2 weeks and then to once every 3 to 4 weeks. In addition, patients are encouraged to schedule "booster" sessions approximately 3, 6, and 12 months after termination. This chapter outlines steps to prepare patients for termination and possible relapse from the start of therapy to the final booster session.

EARLY ACTIVITIES

You will begin to prepare patients for termination and relapse even in the initial session, as you tell them that your goal is to make treatment as time limited as possible, with the aim of helping them become their own therapist. As soon as they start to feel better, it is important to have a discussion about the course of recovery. Patients benefit from a visual depiction (Figure 18.1) of the course of progress, with periods of improvement that are typically interrupted (temporarily) by plateaus, fluctuations, or setbacks. (Later you will stress that life after therapy may be marked by occasional setbacks or difficulties but that patients will be better equipped to handle them on their own.)

THERAPIST: I'm glad you're feeling a little better. But I should tell you that you may still have ups and downs. Most people go along feeling a little better and a little better, then at some point, they reach a plateau or have a setback. Then they feel a little better and a little better, and then there may be another plateau or setback. So it's *normal* to have ups and downs ... Can you see why it's important to remember that in the future?

PATIENT: I guess so I won't worry so much about the down parts.

THERAPIST: Exactly. You can remember this discussion where we predicted some low points. In fact, you might want to refer to a graph [Figure 18.1]. This is a rough idea of what might happen. Do you see that the setbacks usually get fewer and shorter and generally less severe as time goes on?

PATIENT: Uh-huh.

THERAPIST: It's important for you to remember this graph, because otherwise, when you have a setback, you might think that therapy doesn't work, that you'll never get better.

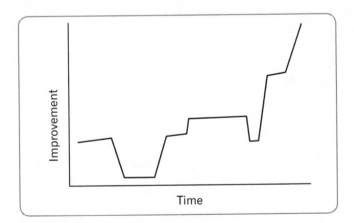

FIGURE 18.1. Progress in therapy. This graph, if skillfully drawn, can be made to resemble the southern border of the United States, with setbacks represented by "Texas" and "Florida." While striking some patients and therapists as humorous, this illustration may help patients recall that setbacks are normal.

PATIENT: Okay.

THERAPIST: You will probably have mild ups and downs even after therapy, because everyone does. Of course, by then, you'll have the tools you need to help yourself. Or you may want to come in again for a session or two. We'll discuss this toward the end of treatment.

ACTIVITIES THROUGHOUT THERAPY

Certain techniques should be used throughout treatment to facilitate relapse prevention.

Attributing Progress to the Patient

You should be alert at every session for opportunities to reinforce patients for their progress. When they experience an improvement in mood, find out why they think they are feeling better and reinforce the idea, whenever possible, that they have brought about changes in their mood by making changes in their thinking and behavior.

THERAPIST: It sounds as if your level of depression is lower this week. Why do you think that happened?

PATIENT: I'm not sure.

THERAPIST: Did you do anything differently this week? Did you go ahead and do the activities we scheduled? Or did you respond to your negative thoughts?

PATIENT: Yeah. I actually exercised every day, and I went out with friends twice. A few times I really criticized myself but I read my coping cards.

THERAPIST: Is it possible you're feeling better this week because you did a number of things that helped?

PATIENT: Yes, I think so.

THERAPIST: So what can you say about how you made progress?

PATIENT: I guess when I do things to help myself, I *do* feel better.

Some patients initially believe that all the credit for feeling better goes to their therapist. An alternative attribution—that the *patient* is responsible for positive changes—can fortify the patient's sense of self-efficacy.

THERAPIST: Why do you think you're feeling better this week?

PATIENT: You really helped me last session.

THERAPIST: Well, I may have taught you *some* things, but who was it who actually changed your thinking and your behavior this week?

PATIENT: I guess *I* did.

THERAPIST: How much do you believe, then, that it's really *you* who deserves the credit?

Alternatively, patients may attribute all the improvement to a change in circumstance (e.g., "I'm feeling better because my boyfriend called me") or to medication. While you should acknowledge such external factors, you should also ask about changes in their thinking or behavior that could have contributed to or helped maintain their improvement. When patients persist in believing that they do not deserve credit, you might decide to elicit their underlying belief ("What does it mean to you that I'm trying to give you credit?").

Teaching and Using Tools/Techniques Learned in Therapy

When teaching patients techniques and tools, you will stress that these are lifelong aids the patient can use in a number of situations now and in the future—that is, these techniques are not specific to just one disorder such as depression, but they can be used whenever patients realize they are reacting in an overly emotional or dysfunctional way. Common techniques and tools that can be used during and after therapy include the following:

1. Breaking down big problems into manageable components.
2. Brainstorming solutions to problems.
3. Identifying, testing, and responding to automatic thoughts and beliefs.
4. Using Thought Records.
5. Monitoring and scheduling activities.
6. Doing relaxation exercises.
7. Using distraction and refocusing techniques.
8. Creating hierarchies of avoided tasks or situations.
9. Writing credit lists.
10. Identifying advantages and disadvantages (of specific thoughts, beliefs, behaviors, or choices when making a decision).

You should help patients understand how they can use these tools in other situations during and after therapy:

THERAPIST: So identifying your depressing thoughts and then questioning and responding to them really reduced how sad you felt?

PATIENT: Yes, it did. I was surprised.

THERAPIST: Did you know you could use these same tools whenever you feel you're overreacting—when you think you feel more anger, anxiety, sadness, embarrassment, and so forth—than the situation calls for?

PATIENT: I hadn't really thought about it.

THERAPIST: Now, I'm not saying you should try to get rid of *all* negative emotion—only when you think you might be *over*reacting. Can you think of any other situations that came up in the last few weeks where it might have helped to use a Thought Record?

PATIENT: (*Pauses.*) Nothing really comes to mind.

THERAPIST: Any situations coming up in the next few weeks where it might be helpful to use a Thought Record?

PATIENT: (*Pauses.*) Well, I know I'm going to be really angry at my brother if he decides to stay at school for the summer instead of coming home.

THERAPIST: What do you think of doing a Thought Record on this situation, writing down and then responding to your thoughts?

PATIENT: Okay.

Preparing for Setbacks during Therapy

As soon as patients begin to feel better, you will prepare them for a potential setback by asking them to imagine what will go through their mind if they start to feel worse. Common responses include: "I shouldn't be feeling this way"; "This means I'm not getting better"; "I'm hopeless"; "I'll never get well"; "My therapist will be disappointed"; or "My therapist isn't doing a good job"; "Cognitive behavior therapy doesn't work for me"; "I'm doomed to be depressed forever"; "It was only a fluke that I felt better initially"; or patients may report an image of themselves in the future, for example, feeling frightened, alone, sad, huddled in the corner of their bed. Coping cards and the Progress in Therapy graph (Figure 18.1) can help avoid these negative cognitions.

THERAPIST: Well, you've really been making nice progress. Your depression seems to be lifting quite a bit.

PATIENT: I *am* feeling better.

THERAPIST: Do you remember that we talked about setbacks a couple of weeks ago?

PATIENT: A little.

THERAPIST: Since it's possible you *could* have a setback, I'd like to discuss in advance how you could handle it.

PATIENT: Okay.

THERAPIST: I'd like you to imagine for a moment that you've had a bad week. Nothing seems to have gone well. Everything looks black again. You're really down on yourself. It seems hopeless. Can you get a picture of that in your mind?

PATIENT: Yes. It's like it was before therapy.

THERAPIST: Okay. Tell me what's going through your mind now.

PATIENT: (*Pauses.*) It's not fair. I was doing so well. This isn't working.

THERAPIST: Good. Now, how can you answer these thoughts?

PATIENT: I'm not sure.

THERAPIST: Well, you have a choice. You can continue to think these depressing thoughts. If you do, what do you predict will happen to your mood?

PATIENT: I'll probably feel worse.

THERAPIST: *Or* you can remind yourself that this is only a setback, which is normal and temporary. Then how would you feel?

PATIENT: Better, probably, or at least not worse.

THERAPIST: Okay. Having reminded yourself that setbacks are normal, what kinds of things have you learned to do in the past few weeks that could help you?

PATIENT: I could read my therapy notes or get my mind off of it by concentrating on what I have to do.

THERAPIST: Or both.

PATIENT: Right, or both.

THERAPIST: Is there a reason to expect that the tools which helped you before won't help you again?

PATIENT: No.

THERAPIST: So you can respond to your negative thoughts and start concentrating on something else. Do you think it's worth writing down what we just talked about—so you'll have a plan in case you do have a setback at some point?

NEAR TERMINATION ACTIVITIES

Responding to Concerns about Tapering Sessions

Several weeks before termination, you should discuss tapering sessions, as an experiment, from once a week to once every other week. Although some patients readily agree to this arrangement, others may become anxious. It is useful for this latter group of patients to list verbally and perhaps record in writing the advantages of trying to reduce the frequency of visits. When patients fail to see advantages, you should first elicit disadvantages, use guided discovery to help patients identify advantages, and then help them reframe the disadvantages (see Figure 18.2).

Advantages of tapering therapy

1. I'll have more opportunity to use and sharpen my tools.

2. I'll be less dependent on [my therapist].

3. I can use the therapy fee for other things.

4. I can spend more time [doing other things].

Disadvantages	**Reframe**
1. I might relapse.	If I'm going to relapse, it's better for it to happen while I'm still in therapy so I can learn how to handle it.
2. I may not be able to solve problems myself.	Tapering therapy gives me the chance to test my idea that I need [my therapist]. In the long run, it's better for me to learn to solve problems myself, because I won't be in therapy forever.
3. I'll miss [my therapist].	This is probably true, but I'll be able to tolerate it and it will encourage me to build up a support network.

FIGURE 18.2. Advantages and disadvantages (to Sally) of tapering therapy.

The following transcript illustrates how such a discussion might proceed:

THERAPIST: In our last session, we briefly discussed the possibility of experimenting with spacing our therapy sessions. Did you think about going to an every-other-week schedule on a trial basis?

PATIENT: I did. It made me a little anxious.

THERAPIST: What went through your mind?

PATIENT: Oh, what if something happens that I can't deal with? What if I start getting more depressed—I couldn't stand that.

THERAPIST: Did you evaluate these thoughts?

PATIENT: Yeah. I realized I was catastrophizing, that it wasn't the absolute end of therapy. And you did say I could call you if I needed to.

THERAPIST: That's right. Did you imagine a specific situation that might come up that would be difficult?

PATIENT: No, not really.

THERAPIST: Maybe it would help if we had you imagine a specific problem now.

PATIENT: Okay. [Sally imagines getting a low grade on a test, identifies her automatic thoughts, responds to the thoughts, and makes a specific plan for what to do next.]

THERAPIST: Now, let's talk about the second automatic thought you had about spacing our sessions—that you'd get more depressed and that you wouldn't be able to stand it.

PATIENT: I guess that may not be quite true. You've made me realize that I could stand to feel bad again. But I wouldn't like it.

THERAPIST: Okay. Now let's say you *do* get more depressed and it's still a week and a half before our next session. What can you do?

PATIENT: Well, I can do what I did about a month ago. Reread my therapy notes, make sure I stay active, do more Thought Records. Somewhere in my notes I have a list of things to do.

THERAPIST: Would it be helpful to find that list now?

PATIENT: Yeah.

THERAPIST: Okay. How about for homework if you find the list and write a Thought Record for these two thoughts: "Something might happen that I couldn't deal with," and "I couldn't stand it if I got more depressed."

PATIENT: Okay.

THERAPIST: Any other thoughts about spacing our sessions?

PATIENT: Just that I'd miss not having you to talk to every week.

THERAPIST: I'll miss that, too. Is there anyone else you could talk to, even a little?

PATIENT: Well, I could call Rebecca. And I guess I could call my brother.

THERAPIST: That sounds like a good idea. Do you want to write that down to do, too?

PATIENT: Okay.

THERAPIST: And finally, do you remember that we said we could *experiment* with every-other-week sessions? If it's not working well, I do want you to call me so you can come in sooner.

Responding to Concerns about Termination

When patients are doing well with biweekly sessions, you might suggest scheduling the next appointment for 3 or 4 weeks in the future, in preparation for termination. Again, tapering can be viewed as an experiment. At each succeeding session, you and the patient agree either to continue spacing sessions or to return to more frequent sessions.

As termination approaches, it is important to elicit patients' automatic thoughts about termination. Some patients are excited and hopeful. At the other extreme, some patients are fearful or even angry. Most have some mixed feelings. They are pleased with their progress but concerned about relapse. Often they are sorry to end their relationship with you.

It is important both to acknowledge what patients are feeling and help them respond to any distortions. It is often desirable for you to express your own genuine feelings, if you can honestly say that you regret the (gradual) ending of the relationship but feel pride in what they have achieved in therapy and that you believe they are ready to make it on their own. Responding to other automatic thoughts and examining advantages and disadvantages of termination can be carried out in the same way as was previously described in responding to thoughts about tapering sessions. Additional strategies to help patients who are concerned about termination can be found in Ludgate (2009).

Reviewing What Was Learned in Therapy

You will encourage patients to read through and organize their notes so they can easily refer to them in the future. For example, a good homework assignment is to write a synopsis of the important points and skills they learned in treatment.

Self-Therapy Sessions

Although many patients do not follow through with formal self-therapy sessions, it is nevertheless useful to discuss a self-therapy plan (see Figure 18.3) and to encourage its use. When patients try self-therapy sessions while regular therapy sessions are still being tapered, they are much more likely to do self-therapy after termination. And they can discover potential problems: not having enough time, misunderstandings about what to do, and interfering thoughts (e.g., "This is too much work"; "I don't really need to do it"; "I can't do it on my own"). In addition to helping patients respond to these problems, you can remind patients of the advantages of self-therapy sessions: They are continuing therapy, but at their own convenience and without charge; they can keep their newly acquired tools fresh and ready to use; they can resolve difficulties before they become major problems; they reduce the possibility of relapse; and they can use their skills to enrich their life in a variety of contexts.

A generic self-therapy plan is presented in Figure 18.3. You can review it with patients and tailor it to meet their needs. Many patients benefit from a brief discussion of a reminder system: "Initially, you might want to try a self-therapy session once a week, then taper it to once or twice a month, then to once a season, and eventually, to once a year. How could you remind yourself to pull out this self-therapy plan periodically?"

Preparing for Setbacks after Termination

As mentioned previously, you begin preparing patients for setbacks early in treatment. As you near termination, you should encourage them to compose a coping card specifying what to do if a setback occurs after therapy has ended. (See Figure 18.4 for a typical card.)

It is desirable for patients to attempt to resolve their difficulties on their own before calling you. If they do need another appointment, you can help them discover what got in the way of their handling the setback or problem independently, and together you can plan what the patient can do differently in the future.

1. *Review of past week(s)*

   - What positive things have happened? What do I deserve credit for?

   - What problems came up? What did I do? If the problem recurs, what, if anything, should I do differently?

2. *Review of homework*

   - Did I do what I had planned? If not, what got in the way (practical problems; automatic thoughts), and what can I do about that next time?

   - What should I continue to do this week?

3. *Current problematic issues/situations*

   - Am I viewing this problem realistically, or have I been overreacting? Is there another way of viewing this?

   - What should I do?

4. *Prediction of future problems*

   - What problems may come up in the next few days or weeks, and what should I do about them?

5. *Set new homework*

   - What homework would be helpful? Should I consider:

     o Doing Thought Records?

     o Scheduling pleasure or mastery activities?

     o Reading therapy notes?

     o Practicing skills such as relaxation?

     o Doing a credit list?

6. *Schedule the next self-therapy appointment*

FIGURE 18.3. Guide to self-therapy sessions. From *Cognitive behavior therapy worksheet packet.* Copyright 2011 by Judith S. Beck. Bala Cynwyd, PA: Beck Institute for Cognitive Behavior Therapy.

Reprinted by permission in *Cognitive Behavior Therapy: Basics and Beyond, Second Edition*, by Judith S. Beck (Guilford Press, 2011). Permission to photocopy this material is granted to purchasers of this book for personal use only (see copyright page for details). Purchasers may download a larger version of this material from *www.guilford.com/p/beck4*.

What I can do in case of a setback:
1. I have a choice. I can catastrophize about the setback, get myself all upset, think things are hopeless, and probably feel worse. Or I can look back over my therapy notes, remember that setbacks are a normal part of recovery, and see what I can learn from this setback. Doing these things will probably make me feel better and make the setback less severe.
2. Next, I should have a self-therapy session and plan what to do to solve my problems.
3. I should call [a specific friend or family member] if I need more help.
4. I can call [my therapist] to briefly discuss what to do or to schedule another session.

FIGURE 18.4. Sally's coping card about setbacks.

BOOSTER SESSIONS

You should encourage patients to schedule booster sessions after termination for several reasons. If any difficulties have arisen, you can discuss how patients handled them and assess whether they could have handled them in a better way. Together you can look ahead to the next several weeks and months and predict future difficulties that could arise. Then you can jointly formulate a plan to deal with these situations. Knowing that you will ask them about their progress doing self-therapy may motivate patients to do their cognitive behavior therapy homework and practice their skills. In addition, you can help patients determine whether their previously modified dysfunctional beliefs have been reactivated. If so, they can do cognitive restructuring in session and plan for continued belief work at home.

Booster sessions also afford you the opportunity to check on the reemergence of dysfunctional strategies (such as avoidance). Patients can express any new or previously unaccomplished goals and develop a plan to work toward them. Together you can evaluate their self-therapy program and modify as needed. Finally, when patients know they are scheduled for booster sessions after termination, their anxiety about maintaining progress on their own is usually alleviated.

To prepare for booster sessions, you may provide patients with a list of questions (see Figure 18.5).

As the following transcript indicates, the overall goal for the booster session is to check on the patient's well-being and plan for continued maintenance or progress.

THERAPIST: I'm glad you were able to come in today. It looks like, from the Beck Depression Inventory, that you're a little more depressed than the last time we met. Is that right?

PATIENT: Yes, my girlfriend recently broke up with me.

THERAPIST: I'm sorry to hear that. Do you think that situation accounted for the rise in your score?

PATIENT: I think so. I was feeling pretty good until last week.

THERAPIST: Is the breakup something you'd like to put on the agenda to talk about today?

PATIENT: Yes, that and my progress, or rather lack of progress, in looking for a new job.

THERAPIST: Okay. And I'd like to find out how things have been going for you generally, aside from the breakup: whether you encountered any other rough spots, how you dealt with them, how much cognitive behavior therapy homework you were able to do, any difficulties you think may arise in the next 2 or 3 months. Does that sound okay?

PATIENT: Yes.

THERAPIST: Would you like to start with the breakup? Can you tell me how it came about? (*We briefly discuss the breakup. I am concerned with how the patient reacted to the breakup, whether his previous dysfunctional beliefs have become activated.*) [summarizing] So things had begun to deteriorate, and she told you she wanted to start seeing other guys? When she told you that, what went through your mind?

PATIENT: That she didn't really love me.

THERAPIST: And what did that mean to you, that she didn't love you?

PATIENT: That there must be something wrong with me.

THERAPIST: And what did you think was wrong with you?

PATIENT: That I'm not very lovable.

THERAPIST: How much did you believe that you weren't very lovable right when she told you she wanted to see other men?

PATIENT: Oh, about 90%

THERAPIST: And how much do you believe it now?

1. Schedule ahead—make definite appointments, if possible, and call to confirm.

2. Consider coming as a preventive measure, even if you have been maintaining your progress.

3. Prepare before you come. Decide what would be helpful to discuss, including:

   a. What has gone well for you?

   b. What problems arose? How did you handle them? Was there a better way of handling them?

   c. What problem(s) could arise between this booster session and your next booster session? Imagine the problem in detail. What automatic thoughts might you have? What beliefs might be activated? How will you deal with the automatic thoughts/beliefs? How will you problem-solve?

   d. What cognitive behavior therapy work did you do? What cognitive behavior therapy work would you like to do between now and the next booster session? What automatic thoughts might get in the way of doing the cognitive behavior therapy work? How will you answer these thoughts?

   e. What further goals do you have for yourself? How will you achieve them? How can the things you learned in cognitive behavior therapy help?

FIGURE 18.5. Guide to booster sessions. From *Cognitive behavior therapy worksheet packet.* Copyright 2011 by Judith S. Beck. Bala Cynwyd, PA: Beck Institute for Cognitive Behavior Therapy.

Reprinted by permission in *Cognitive Behavior Therapy: Basics and Beyond, Second Edition*, by Judith S. Beck (Guilford Press, 2011). Permission to photocopy this material is granted to purchasers of this book for personal use only (see copyright page for details). Purchasers may download a larger version of this material from *www.guilford.com/p/beck4*.

PATIENT: Less, maybe 50%, 60%.

THERAPIST: What made the difference?

PATIENT: Well, part of me knows that we probably just weren't right for each other.

THERAPIST: So you were able to modify this old idea of not being lovable?

PATIENT: Somewhat.

THERAPIST: Right. Now what did you learn from therapy that you can do to damp down this unlovable idea further and strengthen the idea that you are lovable?

PATIENT: A Thought Record might help. And I know my therapy notes have a lot on it. I should have gone back and reread them.

THERAPIST: That might have helped. Did you think of doing that?

PATIENT: Yeah. I guess I thought it really wouldn't help.

THERAPIST: What do you think now?

PATIENT: Well, it helped me before, it should help me again.

THERAPIST: What would get in the way of going home and doing some work on it in the next couple of days?

PATIENT: Nothing. I'll do it. I think it probably will help.

THERAPIST: Now might this thought, "It won't help," pop up again the next time you're going through a rough spot?

PATIENT: It might.

THERAPIST: What could you do now so it would be more likely that you'd test that thought?

PATIENT: What could I do *now*?

THERAPIST: Yes. What could you do to remind yourself that you had the thought *this* time and then realized it might not be true?

PATIENT: I should write it down, maybe on a paper I keep in my desk.

THERAPIST: Okay, how about if you write down some of the things we just talked about—doing a Thought Record on being unlovable, reading through your therapy notes, writing a response to the thought "It won't help."

In this portion of the booster session, I assess the patient's level of depression, set the agenda, discuss an issue, and help him set homework for himself. I ascertain that he has only mild depressive symptoms that seem primarily related to the breakup of the relationship. (Had the depression been more severe, I would have spent more time assessing triggers and identifying and modifying dysfunctional beliefs, thoughts, and behaviors. We would also have discussed the advisability of additional sessions.)

This patient is easily able to express his automatic thoughts and underlying belief. He and I spend little time developing a plan to help him modify his ideas; he had already learned the tools during therapy. He needed the booster session to remind and motivate himself to use the tools.

In summary, relapse prevention is carried out throughout therapy. Problems in tapering sessions and in termination are addressed as any other problems, with a combination of problem solving and responding to dysfunctional thoughts and beliefs.

Chapter 19

TREATMENT PLANNING

A t any given moment in therapy, how do you decide what to say or do next? Partial answers to this question have been provided throughout this book, but this chapter provides a more comprehensive framework for making decisions and planning treatment. To keep therapy focused and moving in the right direction, you continually ask yourself, "What is the specific problem here, and what am I trying to accomplish?" You are cognizant of your objectives in the current portion of the session, in the session as a whole, in the current stage of therapy, and in treatment as a whole. This chapter outlines a number of areas essential to effective treatment planning:

- Accomplishing broad therapeutic goals.
- Planning treatment across sessions.
- Devising treatment plans.
- Planning individual sessions.
- Deciding whether to focus on a problem.
- Modifying standard treatment for specific disorders.

ACCOMPLISHING BROAD THERAPEUTIC GOALS

At the broadest level, your objectives are not only to facilitate a remission of patients' disorders but also to prevent relapse. To do the latter, you tell patients early in treatment that one of your goals is to teach them to become their own therapist. To achieve your objectives, you will:

---

1. Build a sound therapeutic alliance with patients.
2. Make the structure and the process of therapy explicit.
3. Teach patients the cognitive model and share your conceptualization with them.
4. Help alleviate their distress through a variety of techniques and problem solving.
5. Teach them how to use these techniques themselves, help them generalize the use of the techniques, and motivate them to use the techniques in the future.

PLANNING TREATMENT ACROSS SESSIONS

You develop a general plan for treatment and a specific plan for each individual session. Therapy can be viewed in three phases. In the beginning phase of treatment, you build a strong therapeutic alliance; identify and specify patients' goals for therapy; solve problems; teach patients the cognitive model; get patients behaviorally activated (if they are depressed and withdrawn); educate patients about their disorder; teach them to identify, evaluate, and respond to their automatic thoughts; socialize them (to do homework, set an agenda in therapy, and provide feedback); and instruct patients in coping strategies. In this first phase of therapy, you often take the lead in suggesting homework assignments.

In the middle phase of therapy, you continue working toward these objectives but also emphasize identifying, evaluating, and modifying patients' beliefs. You share your conceptualization of patients with them and use both "intellectual" and "emotional" techniques to facilitate belief modification. You teach patients the skills they need to accomplish their goals.

In the final phase of therapy, the emphasis shifts to preparing for termination and preventing relapse. By this point, patients have become much more active in therapy, taking the lead in setting the agenda, suggesting solutions to problems, taking therapy notes, and devising homework assignments.

CREATING A TREATMENT PLAN

You develop a treatment plan based on your evaluation of patients, their Axis I and Axis II symptoms and disorder(s), and their specific presenting problems and goals. Sally, for example, set five goals in the first therapy session: to improve her schoolwork, decrease her anxiety about tests, spend more time with friends, join school activities, and have more fun. Based on her intake evaluation and these goals, I devised a general therapy plan (see Figure 19.1). In each session, we worked on several of the areas specified in the plan based on what we had covered in the previous session(s), what Sally had done for homework, and what problems or topics Sally put on the agenda that day. You also take each individual problem or goal and do a critical analysis, either mentally or on paper (Figure 19.2).

Having formulated a general treatment plan, you adhere to it to a greater or lesser degree, revising it as necessary. Analyzing specific problems compels you to conceptualize patients' difficulties in detail and to formulate a treatment plan tailored for them. Doing so also helps you focus each session, grasp the flow of therapy from one session to the next, and become more cognizant of progress.

---

1. Problem-solve how to improve her concentration, seek needed help in her courses, schedule time with friends, and join activities.

2. Help her identify, evaluate, and respond to automatic thoughts about herself, school, other people, and therapy, especially those that are particularly distressing and/or hinder her from solving problems.

3. Investigate dysfunctional beliefs about perfectionism and seeking help from others.

4. Discuss her self-criticism and increase giving herself credit.

5. Increase productive activity.

FIGURE 19.1. Sally's treatment plan.

Problem Analysis

A. Typical Problem Situations

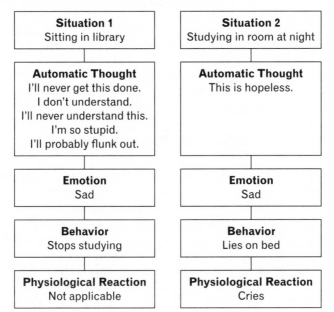

B. Dysfunctional Behaviors

Keeps going over and over same material when comprehension is poor or
  stops studying altogether.
Fails to respond to automatic thoughts.
Doesn't ask others for help.

C. Cognitive Distortions

Attributes problem to weakness in self rather than to depression.
Assumes future is hopeless.
Assumes she is helpless and can't do anything about the problem.
Possibly equates her worth with her achievement?

D. Therapeutic Strategies

1. Do problem-solving. Switch to another subject if comprehension is low
   after a second reading. Devise a plan to get formal or informal help from
   professors, teaching assistant, tutor, or classmate. Compose coping cards
   in session to be read before and during studying.
2. Monitor moods and behavior. Jot down automatic thoughts when mood
   gets worse or when she avoids.

(cont.)

FIGURE 19.2. Analysis of Problem 1: Difficulty studying.

3. Use Socratic questioning to evaluate automatic thoughts. Teach use of Thought Record.
4. Use guided discovery to uncover meaning of automatic thoughts; put in conditional (If ... then ...) format and test.
5. If applicable, use cognitive continuum to illustrate that achievement is on a continuum, rather than consisting of either perfection or failure.

FIGURE 19.2. *(cont.)*

PLANNING INDIVIDUAL SESSIONS

Before and during a session, you ask yourself a number of questions to formulate an overall plan for the session and to guide you as you conduct the therapy session. At the most general level, you ask yourself, "What am I trying to accomplish, and how can I do so most efficiently?" Experienced therapists automatically reflect on many specific issues. The following list of questions, while potentially daunting to the beginner, is a useful guide for more advanced therapists who wish to improve their ability to make better decisions about how to proceed within a therapy session. The list is designed to be read and considered before a therapy session as conscious contemplation of the questions during a session would undoubtedly interfere with the therapeutic process.

1. As you review your notes from the previous session *before the session*, you ask yourself:

   a. "What is the patient's disorder(s)? How, if at all, does standard cognitive behavior therapy need to be varied for treatment of this disorder and this patient in particular?"
   b. "How have I conceptualized the patient's difficulties? How, if at all, does standard cognitive behavior therapy need to be varied for this particular patient?"
   c. "At which stage of therapy are we (beginning, middle, final)? How many sessions do we have left (if there is a limit)?"
   d. "What progress have we made so far in the patient's mood, behavior, symptoms? Toward the patient's goals and major problems?"
   e. "How strong is our therapeutic alliance? What, if anything, do I need to do today to strengthen it?"
   f. "At which *cognitive* level have we primarily been working: automatic thoughts, intermediate beliefs, core beliefs, or a mixture? How much progress have we made at each level?"

g. "What behavioral changes have we been working toward? How much progress have we made?"

h. "What happened in the last few therapy sessions? What dysfunctional ideas or problems (if any) have hindered therapy? What skills have we been working on? Which one(s) do I want to reinforce? Which new skills do I want to teach?"

i. "What happened in the last session? What homework did the patient agree to do? What, if anything, did I agree to do (e.g., call patient's health care provider or find relevant bibliotherapy)?"

2. As you begin the therapy session and check on the patient's *mood*, you ask yourself:

a. "How has the patient been feeling since our last session compared to earlier in treatment? Which moods predominate (e.g., sadness, hopelessness, anxiety, anger, shame)?"

b. "Do objective scores match the patient's subjective description? If not, why not?"

c. "Is there anything about the patient's mood we should put on the agenda to discuss more fully?"

3. As the patient provides a *brief review of the week*, you ask yourself:

a. "How did this week go compared to previous weeks?"

b. "What signs of progress are there? What positive experiences did the patient have?"

c. "What problems came up this week?"

d. "Did anything happen this week (positive or negative) that we should put on the agenda to discuss more fully?"

4. As you check on the patient's *use of alcohol, drugs, and medication* (if applicable), you ask yourself:

a. "Is there a problem in any of these areas? If so, should we put it on the agenda to discuss more fully?"

5. As you and the patient *set the agenda*, you ask yourself:

a. "Which problem is most important to the patient? Which is the most solvable? Which one is likely to bring about symptom relief within today's session and in the coming week?"

6. As you and the patient *prioritize agenda items*, you ask yourself:

a. "How much time will each agenda item take? How many items can we discuss?"

b. "Are there any problems the patient could resolve alone, or with someone else, or bring up at another session? How much time should we allot to each chosen item/problem?"

7. As you and the patient *review the homework*, you ask yourself:

   a. "How is the patient's homework related to the agenda items? Should discussion of any of the homework tasks be postponed until we get to a specific agenda item?"
   b. "How much of the homework did the patient do? What, if anything, got in the way?"
   c. "How much does the patient agree with each statement in the therapy notes from last week? In therapy notes from previous weeks (if still relevant)? How relevant are the therapy notes to the problems on today's agenda?"
   d. "Was the homework useful? If not, why not? If so, what did the patient learn?"
   e. "Which homework tasks (if any) would be beneficial for the patient to continue in the coming week?"
   f. "How, if at all, should we modify homework assigned in this session to make it more effective?"

8. As you and the patient discuss the *first agenda item*, you ask yourself questions in four areas:

   Defining the Problem
   a. "What is the specific problem?"
   b. "In which specific situations did the problem arise? If it arose more than once, in which situation did the patient feel most upset or behave most dysfunctionally?"
   c. "Why does the patient believe he has this problem? Why do *I* think the patient has this problem?"
   d. "How does this problem fit into the overall cognitive conceptualization of the patient? How does it relate to his overall goals?"

   Devising a Strategy
   a. "What has the patient already done to try to solve the problem?"
   b. "What would *I* do if *I* were in the patient's position and had this problem?"
   c. "Can we do outright problem solving? What thoughts and beliefs might interfere with problem solving or carrying out a solution?"

   Choosing Techniques
   a. "What specifically am I trying to accomplish as we discuss this agenda item?"

b. "Which techniques have worked well for this patient (or for similar patients) in the past? Which techniques have *not* worked well?"

c. "Which technique should I try first?"

d. "How will I evaluate its effectiveness?"

e. "Will I employ the technique or employ it *and* teach it to the patient?"

Monitoring the Process

a. "Are we working together as a team?"

b. "Is the patient having interfering automatic thoughts about himself, this technique, our therapy, me, the future?"

c. "Is the patient's mood lifting? How well is this technique working? Should I try something else?"

d. "Will we finish discussion of this agenda item in time? If not, should we collaboratively decide to continue this item and curtail or eliminate discussion of another item?"

e. "What follow-up (i.e., homework assignment) might be beneficial?"

f. "What should we record for the patient to review at home?"

9. *Following discussion of the first agenda item*, you ask yourself:

a. "How is the patient feeling now?"

b. "Do I need to do anything to reestablish rapport?"

c. "How much time is left in the session? Do we have time for another agenda item? What should we do next?"

10. *Before closing the session*, you ask yourself:

a. "Did we make progress? Is the patient feeling better?"

b. "Is the patient committed to doing the homework we agreed on?"

c. "Do I need to probe for negative feedback? If there was negative feedback, how should I address it?"

11. *After the session*, you ask yourself:

a. "How should I refine my conceptualization?"

b. "What do I want to remember to address in the next session? Future sessions?"

c. "Do I need to attend to our relationship?"

d. "How would I score myself on each item of the Cognitive Therapy Rating Scale [Appendix C]? If I could do the session over again, what would I do differently?"

DECIDING WHETHER TO FOCUS ON A PROBLEM

A critical decision in every therapy session is which problem (or problems) to pursue. Although you collaborate in making this decision with patients, you nevertheless guide therapy toward discussion of problems that are distressing and ongoing (or recurrent) and toward which you judge you will be able to make some progress during the session. You tend to limit discussion of problems that:

- Patients can solve themselves,
- Are isolated incidents unlikely to recur, and/or
- Are not particularly distressing.

Having identified and specified a problem, you do several things to help you decide how much time and effort to spend on the problem. You:

1. Gather more data about the problem.
2. Review your options.
3. Reflect on practical considerations.
4. Use the stage of therapy as a guide.
5. Change the focus when necessary.

These five steps are described below.

Gathering More Data about a Problem

When patients first bring up a problem or when the existence of a problem becomes apparent in the midst of a session, you assess the nature of the problem to determine whether it seems worthwhile to intervene. For example, Sally has put a new problem on the agenda: Her father's business is failing, and Sally feels sad. I question her to assess how useful it will be to devote a significant portion of therapy time to this problem.

THERAPIST: Okay, you said you wanted to bring up something about your dad and his business?

PATIENT: Yeah. His business has been pretty rocky for a while, but now it looks as if it may go bankrupt.

THERAPIST: [gathering more information] If it does go bankrupt, how will that affect you?

PATIENT: Oh, nothing directly. I just feel so bad for him. I mean, he'll still have enough money but ... he's worked really hard for this.

THERAPIST: [trying to discover whether there is a distortion in Sally's thinking] What do you think will happen if it does go bankrupt?

PATIENT: Well, he's already started looking for a new business. He's not the type to just lie around or take time off.

THERAPIST: [still assessing whether Sally is thinking dysfunctionally] What's the worst part of this to you?

PATIENT: Just that he probably feels bad.

THERAPIST: How do *you* feel when you think about his feeling badly?

PATIENT: Bad ... sad.

THERAPIST: How sad?

PATIENT: A medium amount, I guess.

THERAPIST: [testing whether Sally can take a long view] Do you have a sense that though he may feel badly initially, he won't stay that way indefinitely? That he'll probably get involved in another business and feel better?

PATIENT: Yeah, I think that'll probably happen.

THERAPIST: Do you think you're feeling "normal" sadness over this? Or do you think this is affecting you *too* strongly?

PATIENT: I think I'm having a normal reaction.

THERAPIST: [having assessed no further work on this problem is warranted] Anything else on this?

PATIENT: No, I don't think so.

THERAPIST: Okay. I'm sorry this happened to your dad. Let me know what happens.

PATIENT: I will.

THERAPIST: Should we turn to the next item on our agenda?

In another situation, you determine that a problem *does* require intervention.

THERAPIST: You wanted to talk about living arrangements for next year?

PATIENT: Yes. I'm pretty upset. My roommate and I have decided to live together again. She wants to live off campus. So we have to look for an apartment in West Philly or Center City. But she's going home for spring vacation so it's mostly up to me to find a place.

THERAPIST: When were you feeling the most upset about this?

PATIENT: Yesterday, when I agreed to start looking while she was away . . . Actually, it was last night when I realized I didn't know what to do.

THERAPIST: How were you feeling?

PATIENT: Overwhelmed . . . anxious.

THERAPIST: As you were thinking about this last night, what was going through your mind?

PATIENT: What am I going to do? I don't even know where to start.

THERAPIST: [seeking a fuller picture; determining whether there were other important automatic thoughts] What else was going through your mind?

PATIENT: I was feeling overwhelmed. I didn't know what to do first, like should I go to a real estate agent? Should I look online?

THERAPIST: [probing for additional thoughts] Were you having any thoughts about your roommate?

PATIENT: No, not really. She said she'd help when she got back. She said I didn't have to start looking until then.

THERAPIST: Were you making any predictions?

PATIENT: I don't know.

THERAPIST: [giving an opposite example] Well, were you thinking you'd easily find a great place with a cheap rent?

PATIENT: No . . . no, I was thinking, "What if I find a place and it turns out to be infested with cockroaches, or unsafe, or too noisy, or in really bad shape?"

THERAPIST: Did you have an image like that in your mind?

PATIENT: Yeah. Dark, smelly, dirty. (*Shudders.*)

Reviewing the Options

Now that I have a fuller picture, I mentally review my options. I could do one or more of the following:

1. Engage Sally in straightforward problem solving, helping her decide which steps seem the most reasonable and feasible.
2. Teach Sally problem-solving skills, using this problem as an example.
3. Use this situation as an opportunity to reinforce the cognitive model.
4. Use this situation as an opportunity to help Sally conceptualize her larger difficulty of *assuming* she is incompetent in a new situation and feeling overwhelmed instead of testing this belief.

5. Have Sally identify the most distressing thought and help her evaluate it.
6. Teach Sally how to do a Thought Record using this situation.
7. Use the image she described as an opportunity to teach her imagery techniques.
8. Make a collaborative decision with Sally to move on to the next agenda item (perhaps to an even more pressing problem) and to return to this problem later in the session or in a future session.

Reflecting on Practical Considerations

How do you decide which course to pursue? I took into account a number of factors, including:

1. What is likely to bring Sally substantial relief?
2. What do we have time to do? What *else* do we need to do in the session?
3. What skills would be valuable to teach or review with Sally for which this problem provides an opportunity?
4. What, if anything, could Sally do herself (i.e., for homework) to relieve her distress? For example, if Sally could do a Thought Record on this at home, we can spend session time on other things that will speed her progress.

Using the Stage of Therapy as a Guide

You are often guided by a patient's stage of therapy. For example, you may avoid tackling a complex (but non-emergency) problem in the first few sessions with depressed patients if it is unlikely that you will make much headway toward solving it. Focusing on easier problem that are solvable, or partially solvable, engenders hope in patients and makes them more motivated to work in therapy.

Changing the Focus in a Session

Sometimes you can't easily assess how difficult a problem will be or how likely it is that a particular discussion will activate a painful core belief. In these cases, you may *initially* focus on a problem but switch to another topic when you realize your interventions are not successful and/or the patient is experiencing greater (unintended) distress. Following is a transcript from an early therapy session.

THERAPIST: Okay, next on the agenda. You said you'd like to meet more people. (*We discuss this goal more specifically.*) Now, how could you meet new people this week?

PATIENT: (*in a meek voice*) I could talk to people at work.

THERAPIST: (*noticing that the patient suddenly looks downcast*) What's going through your mind right now?

PATIENT: It's hopeless. I'll never be able to do it. I've tried this before. (*Appears angry.*) All my other therapists have tried this, too. But, I'm telling you, I just can't do it! It won't work!

I hypothesize from the patient's sudden negative affect shift that a core belief has been activated. I recognize that continuing in the same vein at this time will likely be counterproductive. Instead of refocusing on the problem, I decide to repair the therapeutic alliance by eliciting the patient's angry automatic thoughts ("When I asked you how you could meet more people this week, what went through your mind?") and then helping her evaluate these thoughts. Later I gave the patient a choice about whether to return to this agenda item:

THERAPIST: I'm glad you can see that I hadn't intended to make you do things you're not ready for. Now, would you like to return to the topic of meeting new people, or should we come back to it another time [at another session] and move on to the problem you had this week with your friend Elise?

In summary, early in treatment you tend to guide discussion *away* from problems you are unlikely to be successful in solving or partially solving (if patients are agreeable to postponing discussion about them). At any point, you avoid focusing on problems that patients can resolve on their own, that they do not want to work on, or that are not particularly distressing to them.

MODIFYING STANDARD TREATMENT
FOR SPECIFIC DISORDERS

It is essential that you have a solid understanding of patients' current symptoms and functioning, presenting problems, precipitating events, history, and diagnosis before starting therapy. You will need to consult specialized texts for patients whose primary disorder is not a simple, unipolar depression to educate yourself about key cognitions and behavioral strategies for the various psychiatric disorders.

In summary, effective treatment planning requires a sound diagnosis, a solid formulation of the case in cognitive terms, and consideration of the patient's characteristics and problems. Treatment is tailored to the individual; you develop an overall strategy as well as a specific plan for each session, considering the following:

1. Patients' diagnosis(es).
2. A conceptualization of their difficulties (which you check out with patients for accuracy).
3. Their goals for therapy.
4. Their most pressing concerns.
5. Your goals for therapy.
6. The stage of treatment.
7. Patients' learning characteristics, their stage of life, developmental and intellectual level, gender, and cultural background.
8. Patients' level of motivation.
9. The nature and strength of the therapeutic alliance.

You develop and continually modify a general plan for treatment across sessions and a more specific plan before each session and within each session.

Chapter 20

PROBLEMS IN THERAPY

Problems of one kind or another arise with nearly every patient in cognitive behavior therapy. Even experienced therapists encounter difficulties at times in establishing a therapeutic alliance, correctly conceptualizing a patient's difficulties, or consistently working toward joint objectives. A reasonable goal is not to avoid problems altogether but rather to learn to uncover and specify problems, to conceptualize how they arose, and to plan how to remediate them.

It is useful to view problems or stuck points in therapy as opportunities for you to refine your conceptualization of the patient. In addition, problems in therapy often provide insight into problems the patient experiences outside the office. Finally, difficulties with one patient provide an opportunity for you to refine your own skills, to promote your flexibility and creativity, and to gain new understandings and expertise in helping other patients, as problems can arise not just because of the patient's characteristics but also because of the therapist's relative weaknesses. This chapter describes how to uncover the existence of problems and how to conceptualize and remediate problems at stuck points in therapy.

UNCOVERING THE EXISTENCE OF A PROBLEM

You can uncover a problem in a number of ways:

---

1. By listening to patients' unsolicited feedback.
2. By directly soliciting patients' feedback, whether or not they have provided verbal or nonverbal signals of a problem.
3. By reviewing recordings of therapy sessions alone or with a colleague or supervisor and rating the tape on the Cognitive Therapy Rating Scale (Appendix C).
4. By tracking progress according to objective tests and the patient's subjective report of symptom relief.

A problem obviously exists when patients provide you with negative feedback (e.g., "I don't think you understand what I'm saying," or "I understand what you're saying *intellectually* but not in my gut"). Many patients, however, allude *indirectly* to a problem (e.g., "I see what you're saying, but I don't know if I could do it any other way," or, "I'll try" [implying that they believe they will be unsuccessful in carrying out a task]). In these cases, you should question the patient further to ascertain whether a problem does indeed exist and to determine the dimensions of the problem.

Many times, however, the patient fails to relate, either directly or indirectly, a problem with therapy. You can discover problems if you adhere to the standard structure of the session (which includes asking the patient for feedback at the end of the session), by periodically checking on the depth of the patient's understanding during the session, and by eliciting the patient's automatic thoughts when you notice an affect shift during the session.

For example, on one occasion I sensed through Sally's nonverbal cues (a faraway look in her eyes, restless shifting in her seat) that she was not fully processing what I was saying or that she did not agree. I asked her what was going through her mind. I took other steps throughout our session to make sure that Sally and I shared an understanding. I took care either to summarize often during the session or to ask Sally to summarize. I also asked her to rate how much she believed the summary (e.g., "Sally, we've just been talking about the idea that you're not completely responsible for your mother's unhappiness even though you moved away from home ... How much do you believe that now?").

I further checked on Sally's understanding at different points during the session (e.g., "Is it clear to you why else your roommate might be reacting in this way? ... Could you put it in your own words?"). I also made sure to elicit feedback at the end of the session (e.g., "Anything I said today that bothered you? ... Anything you thought I didn't understand?"). Because I guessed that Sally might hesitate to give me negative feedback, I also asked very specifically for feedback about a *portion* of the session during which I suspected she might have had a negative reaction: "How about when I suggested that you might be able to be more assertive with your mother? Did that bother you? ... Do you think you would be able to tell me if it *had* bothered you?"

In summary, you should seek to allay or to uncover problems within a therapy session by checking on patients' understanding, by asking for feedback, and by raising suspected problems directly during the session itself. You may also ask patients to complete a written evaluation of a session (page 77) that you can review with them at the next session.

If you are a novice therapist, you may be unaware of the existence of a problem and/or be less able to specify a problem. You should solicit permission to record therapy sessions to review on your own or (preferably) with an experienced cognitive behavior therapist. Obtaining patients' consent is usually not a problem if you present it in a positive light: "I have an unusual opportunity for you that I'm only offering a few patients [or that I'm only offering to you]. You should feel free to say yes or no. I occasionally record therapy sessions so I can listen to them later and figure out how I might be able to help patients more. [If relevant, "I may play them to a colleague [or supervisor] to get feedback. I always find that two heads are better than one."] I'll delete or erase the recording immediately afterward. (*pause*) Is it okay with you if we start out taping the session? If it bothers you after a few minutes, we can always turn it off or get rid of the recording at the end."

Another clear indication of a problem is a lack of progress or deterioration in a patient's functioning and/or mood (identified through self-report or objective tests such as the Beck Depression Inventory [see Appendix B]. You might suggest this lack of progress as an agenda item and collaborate with the patient in planning a more effective direction for treatment.

Finally, you should continually try to put yourself in patients' shoes, to see how they view their world and to reveal what obstacles might inhibit their ability to take a more functional perspective of their difficulties (e.g., "If I were Sally, how would I feel during therapy? What would I think when my therapist said _____ or _____?").

CONCEPTUALIZING PROBLEMS

Having identified the existence of a problem, be alert for automatic thoughts blaming the patient (e.g., "He's resistant/manipulative/unmotivated"). These labels tend to alleviate a therapist's sense of responsibility for resolving the difficulty and interfere with problem solving. Instead, ask yourself:

> **"What has the patient said (or not said) or done (or not done) in session (or between sessions) that is a problem?"**

Next, you ideally would consult with a supervisor who has reviewed a recording of the therapy session. You will undoubtedly need help in determining whether the problem is due to the patient's pathology, errors you have made, treatment factors (such as the level of care, format of therapy, session frequency), and/or factors external to treatment (e.g., an organic disease, a psychologically toxic home or work environment, ineffective medication or deleterious side effects, an absence of needed adjunctive treatments; see J. S. Beck, 2005).

Having identified a problem that calls for a change in what you are doing, you will conceptualize the level at which the problem occurred:

> 1. Is it merely a *technical problem*? For example, did you use an inappropriate technique or use a technique incorrectly?
> 2. Is it a more *complex problem with the session as a whole*? For example, did you correctly identify a dysfunctional cognition but then fail to intervene effectively?
> 3. Is there an *ongoing problem across several sessions*? For example, has there been a breakdown in collaboration?

Typically, problems occur in one or more of the following categories:

> 1. Diagnosis, conceptualization, and treatment planning.
> 2. Therapeutic alliance.
> 3. Structure and/or pace of the session.
> 4. Socialization of the patient.
> 5. Dealing with automatic thoughts.
> 6. Accomplishing therapeutic goals in and across sessions.
> 7. Patients' processing of the session content.

The following questions can help you and your supervisor specify the nature of a therapeutic problem. Then you can formulate, prioritize, and select one or more specific objectives on which to focus.

Diagnosis, Conceptualization, and Treatment Planning

DIAGNOSIS

1. "Have I made a correct diagnosis on the five axes according to the latest DSM?"
2. "Is a medication consult indicated for this patient?"

CONCEPTUALIZATION

1. "Do I use a Cognitive Conceptualization Diagram [page 200] to identify the patient's most central dysfunctional cognitions and behaviors?"
2. "Do I continually refine my conceptualization as I get new data and share my conceptualization with the patient at strategically appropriate times? Does the conceptualization make sense and 'ring true' to the patient?"

TREATMENT PLANNING

1. "Have I based treatment on the cognitive formulation of the patient's disorder(s) and my individual conceptualization of the patient? Do I continually modify treatment when needed, based on my conceptualization?"
2. "Have I varied standard cognitive behavior therapy, when needed, for this patient's Axis I (and/or Axis II) disorder(s)?"
3. "Have I addressed the need for a major life change if it became apparent that improvement via therapy alone is unlikely?"
4. "Have I incorporated skills training when needed?"
5. "Have I included family members in treatment as appropriate?"

Therapeutic Alliance

COLLABORATION

1. "Have the patient and I truly been *collaborating*? Are we functioning as a team? Are we both working hard? Do we both feel responsible for progress?"
2. "Have we been covering the problems that are of most concern to the patient?"
3. "Have I guided the patient to an appropriate level of compliance and control in the therapy session?"
4. "Have we agreed on the goals for treatment?"
5. "Have I provided the rationale for my interventions and homework assignments?"

PATIENT'S FEEDBACK

1. "Have I regularly encouraged the patient to provide honest feedback?"
2. "Have I monitored the patient's affect during the session and elicited automatic thoughts when I noticed a shift?"

PATIENT'S VIEW OF THERAPY AND THERAPIST

1. "Does the patient have a positive view of therapy and of me?"
2. "Does the patient believe, at least somewhat, that therapy can help?"
3. "Does the patient see me as competent, collaborative, and caring?"

THERAPIST'S REACTIONS

1. "Do I care about this patient? Does my caring come across?"
2. "Do I feel competent to help this patient? Does my sense of competence come across?"
3. "Do I have negative thoughts about this patient or about myself with respect to this patient? Have I evaluated and responded to these thoughts?"
4. "Do I see problems in the therapeutic alliance as an opportunity for growth versus assigning blame?"
5. "Do I project a realistically upbeat and optimistic view of how therapy can help?"

Structuring and Pacing the Therapy Session

AGENDA

1. "Do we quickly set a complete and specific agenda toward the beginning of the session?"
2. "Do we prioritize the agenda topics and roughly decide how to split our time?"
3. "Do we collaboratively determine which topic to discuss first?"

PACING

1. "Do we allot and spend an appropriate amount of time for the standard session elements: mood check, brief review of the week, setting the agenda, homework review, discussion of agenda topic(s), setting new homework, periodic summaries, feedback?"
2. "Do we collaboratively decide what to do if more time is needed for a problem than we had allotted or if important topics arose that were not part of the original agenda?"

3. "Do I appropriately and gently interrupt the patient when needed, or do we spend too much time on unproductive discourse?"
4. "Do we leave enough time at the end of the session to ensure that the patient will remember the most important points and has understood and agreed with the new homework assignments? To ensure that the patient's core beliefs were deactivated so the patient left the session feeling emotionally stable?"

Socializing the Patient to Cognitive Behavior Therapy

GOAL SETTING

1. "Has the patient set reasonable, concrete goals? Does the patient keep these goals in mind throughout the week? Is the patient committed to working toward these goals? Are these goals under the patient's control? Is the patient trying to change someone else?"
2. "Do I periodically review progress toward the patient's goals?"
3. "Do I help the patient firmly keep in mind why it is worth it to work in therapy (i.e., to reach his goals)?"

EXPECTATIONS

1. "What are the patient's expectations for himself and for me?"
2. "Does the patient believe all problems can be solved quickly and easily? Or that I alone should solve his problems? Does the patient understand the importance of taking an active, collaborative role?"
3. "Does the patient understand the necessity of learning certain tools and skills and using them regularly between sessions?"

PROBLEM-SOLVING ORIENTATION

1. "Does the patient specify problems to work on?"
2. "Does the patient collaborate with me to solve problems instead of just air them?"
3. "Does the patient fear solving current problems because then he will have to tackle other problems (such as a decision about a relationship or work)?"

COGNITIVE MODEL

1. "Does the patient understand that automatic thoughts influence his emotions and behavior (and sometimes physiology), that some of his thoughts are distorted, and that he can feel better and behave in a more adaptive way if he evaluates and responds to his thinking?"

HOMEWORK

1. "Have we designed homework around the patient's key issues?"
2. "Does the patient understand how homework relates to the work of the therapy session and to his overall goals?"
3. "Does the patient think about our therapy work throughout the week and does he do homework thoroughly?"

Dealing with Automatic Thoughts

IDENTIFYING AND SELECTING KEY AUTOMATIC THOUGHTS

1. "Do we identify the actual words and/or images that go through the patient's mind when he is distressed?"
2. "Do we identify the range of relevant automatic thoughts?"
3. "Do we select key thoughts to evaluate (i.e., the thoughts associated with the most distress or dysfunction)?"

RESPONDING TO AUTOMATIC THOUGHTS AND BELIEFS

1. "Do we not only identify key cognitions, but also evaluate and respond to them?"
2. "Do I avoid assuming *a priori* that the patient's cognitions are distorted? Do I use guided discovery and avoid persuasion and challenge?"
3. "If one line of questioning is ineffective, do I try other ways?"
4. "Having collaboratively formulated an alternative response, do I check to see how much the patient believed it? Does his emotional distress decrease?"
5. "If needed, do we try other techniques to reduce the patient's distress? If needed, do we mark relevant cognitions for future work?"

MAXIMIZING COGNITIVE CHANGE

1. "Do we write down the patient's new, more functional understandings?"

Accomplishing Therapeutic Goals in and across Sessions

IDENTIFYING OVERALL AND SESSION-BY-SESSION OBJECTIVES

1. "Have I appropriately expressed to the patient that the objective of treatment is not only to get him better but also to teach him lifelong skills so he can stay better?"

2. "Do I help the patient identify one or more important problems to discuss in each session?"
3. "Do we devote time to both problem solving *and* cognitive restructuring?"
4. "Do we work on both behavioral change *and* cognitive change for homework?"

MAINTAINING A CONSISTENT FOCUS

1. "Do I use guided discovery to help the patient identify relevant beliefs?"
2. "Can I state which beliefs of the patient are most central and which are narrower or more peripheral?"
3. "Do I consistently explore the relationship of new problems to the patient's central beliefs? Are we doing consistent, sustained work on the patient's central beliefs at each session instead of only crisis intervention?"
4. "If we have discussed childhood events, was there a clear rationale for why we needed to do so? Have I helped the patient see how his early beliefs relate to his current problems and how such insight can help him in the coming week?"

INTERVENTIONS

1. "Do I choose interventions based on both my goals for the session and the patients' agenda?"
2. "Can I clearly state to myself both the patient's dysfunctional belief and a more functional belief toward which I am guiding him?"
3. "Do I check how distressed the patient felt and/or how strongly he endorsed an automatic thought or belief both before and after an intervention so I could judge how successful the intervention was?"
4. "If an intervention is relatively unsuccessful, do I switch gears and try another approach?"

Patients' Processing of the Session Content

MONITORING PATIENTS' UNDERSTANDING

1. "Have I summarized (or asked the patient to summarize) frequently during the session?"
2. "Have I asked the patient to state his conclusions in his own words?"
3. "Have I been alert for nonverbal signs of confusion or disagreement?"

CONCEPTUALIZING PROBLEMS IN UNDERSTANDING

1. "Have I checked out my hypotheses with the patient?"
2. "If a patient has difficulty understanding what I am trying to express, is it due to a mistake I have made? To my lack of concreteness? To my vocabulary? To the amount of material I am presenting in one chunk or in one session?"
3. "Is a difficulty in understanding due to the patient's level of emotional distress in the therapy session? To distraction? To automatic thoughts the patient is having at the moment?"

MAXIMIZING CONSOLIDATION OF LEARNING

1. "What have I done to ensure that the patient will remember key parts of the therapy session during the week and even after therapy has ended?"
2. "Have I motivated the patient to read his therapy notes daily?"

STUCK POINTS

At times, patients may feel better during individual sessions but fail to make progress over the course of several sessions. The experienced therapist, in lieu of the preceding questions, may first wish to rule in or rule out five key problem areas. Having determined that you have a correct diagnosis, conceptualization, and treatment plan tailored for the patient's disorder (and have correctly employed techniques), you assess the following, alone or with a consultant:

---

1. Do the patient and I have a solid *therapeutic alliance*?
2. Do we both have a clear idea of the *patient's goals* for therapy? Is he committed to working toward his goals?
3. Does the patient truly believe the *cognitive model*—that his thinking influences his mood and behavior, that his thinking at times is dysfunctional, and that evaluating and responding to dysfunctional thinking positively affect how he feels emotionally and how he behaves?
4. Is the patient *socialized* to cognitive behavior therapy—does he contribute to the agenda, collaboratively work toward solving problems, do homework, provide feedback?
5. Is the patient's *biology* (e.g., illness, medication side effects, or inadequate level of medication) or his *external environment*

(e.g., an abusive partner, an extremely demanding job, or an intolerable level of poverty or crime in his environment) interfering with your work together?

REMEDIATING PROBLEMS IN THERAPY

Depending on the identified problem, you might consider the advisability of one or more of the following:

1. Doing a more in-depth diagnostic evaluation.
2. Referring the patient for a physical or neuropsychological examination.
3. Refining your conceptualization of the patient and checking it out with him.
4. Reading more about the treatment of the patient's Axis I (and Axis II) disorder(s).
5. Seeking specific feedback from the patient about his experience of therapy and of you.
6. Reestablishing the patient's goals for therapy (and possibly examining the advantages and disadvantages of working toward and accomplishing them).
7. Identifying and responding to your own automatic thoughts about the patient or about your skill as a therapist.
8. Reviewing the cognitive model with the patient and eliciting any doubts or misunderstandings he may have.
9. Reviewing the treatment plan with the patient (and eliciting his concerns or doubts about it).
10. Reviewing the patient's responsibilities (and eliciting his reactions).
11. Emphasizing setting and reviewing homework in session and accomplishment of homework throughout the week.
12. Working consistently on *key* automatic thoughts, beliefs, and behaviors across sessions.
13. Checking on the patient's understanding of session content and having him record the most important points.
14. Based on the patient's needs and preferences, changing (in one direction or the other) the pace or structure of the session, the amount or difficulty of material covered, the degree of empathy

you have been expressing, the degree to which you have been didactic or persuasive, and/or the relative focus on problem solving.

You should monitor your own thoughts and mood when seeking to conceptualize and remediate problems in therapy because your cognitions may at times interfere with problem solving. It is likely that all therapists, at least occasionally, have negative thoughts about patients, the therapy, and/or themselves as therapists. Typical therapist assumptions that interfere with making changes to the therapy format include:

"If I interrupt the patient, he'll think I'm controlling him."
"If I structure the session with an agenda, I'll miss something important."
"If I record a session, I'll be too self-conscious."
"If my patient gets annoyed with me, she'll drop out of therapy."

Finally, when you encounter a problem in treatment, you have a choice. You can catastrophize about the problem and/or blame yourself or the patient. Alternatively, you can turn the problem into an opportunity to refine your skills of conceptualization and treatment planning and to improve your technical expertise and your ability to vary therapy in accordance with the specific needs of each patient.

Chapter 21

PROGRESSING AS A COGNITIVE BEHAVIOR THERAPIST

This chapter briefly outlines steps to initiate the practice of standard cognitive behavior therapy. You should gain experience with the basic techniques of cognitive behavior therapy by practicing them yourself before doing so with patients. (See Appendix B for information on obtaining patient worksheets, tests, and booklets.) Trying the techniques yourself allows you to correct difficulties in application and putting yourself in the patient's role affords you the opportunity to identify obstacles (practical or psychological) that interfere with carrying out assignments. At a minimum, if you wish to become proficient in cognitive behavior therapy, you should do the following (if you have not already done so):

1. Monitor your moods and identify your automatic thoughts when you experience dysphoria or anxiety, when you engage in maladaptive behavior, and/or avoid engaging in adaptive behavior.

2. Write down your automatic thoughts. If you skip this step, you deprive yourself of the opportunity to discover potential obstacles that your patients may have in writing down *their* thoughts: lack of opportunity, motivation, time, energy, and hope. When employing a technique such as assigning homework in session, you can then make a rapid comparison between yourself and the patient. You think, "Would *I* have difficulty doing this assignment? What would I need to become motivated? What would get in the way of *my* doing it? Do I need to present

it in a more step-by-step fashion?" In other words, your progress as a cognitive behavior therapist is facilitated if you bring an understanding of yourself and human nature in general to treatment.

3. Identify your automatic thoughts that interfere with carrying out the step above. Thoughts such as "I don't have to write my automatic thoughts down," or "I know this stuff. I can get by with doing this in my head," are likely to impede your progress. A good adaptive response would acknowledge the partial truth of these thoughts but emphasize the advantages of behaving otherwise: "It's true that I can probably get by without using cognitive behavior therapy tools on myself. But it's also true that I will probably learn considerably *more* if I go ahead and write things down. I'll better understand why my patients have difficulty if I myself go through the same process first to see what it feels like and spot potential trouble spots. What's the big deal anyway? It'll only take a couple of minutes."

4. Once you have become proficient at identifying your automatic thoughts and emotions, start doing one Thought Record a day when you notice your mood changing. If your thoughts are not distorted, though, or if you tend automatically to respond adaptively to your thoughts in your head, doing a TR may not lead to a change in your affect. (Remember that cognitive behavior therapists do not try to *eliminate* negative emotion; they try to reduce *dysfunctional* degrees of emotion.) However, whether or not you personally benefit from doing TRs, doing them will sharpen your skill in teaching your patients to do them.

5. Fill out the bottom half of the Cognitive Conceptualization Diagram using three typical situations in which you felt dysphoric or behaved in a maladaptive way. If you have difficulty specifying the situation, identifying your thoughts or emotions, or uncovering the meaning of your thoughts, reread the relevant chapters in this book.

6. Continue to fill in the top half of the Cognitive Conceptualization Diagram. When you feel distressed, see whether there is a theme in the category of helplessness, unlovability, or worthlessness underneath. Once you have identified a core belief, fill in the other boxes.

7. Next, using a core belief identified in the prior exercises, fill out a Core Belief Worksheet (page 243). Examine your interpretation of situations to determine whether you are distorting evidence to support a negative core belief and/or if you are ignoring or discounting evidence contrary to this core belief. Note: This exercise may not affect your belief system if you have positive, counterbalancing beliefs that are continuously activated, but completing the worksheet will at least make you more familiar with it and more likely to use it effectively with patients.

8. Try other basic techniques: activity scheduling, credit lists, responding to spontaneous imagery, acting "as if," writing and reading

coping cards, making functional self-comparisons, and writing down advantages and disadvantages when making a decision.

9. Having used some of the fundamental conceptual and treatment tools yourself, choose a straightforward, uncomplicated patient for your first attempt at cognitive behavior therapy. If you select a difficult patient, the standard treatment as described in this book may be inappropriate. The ideal patient for a first cognitive behavior therapy experience is one who has a simple unipolar depression or adjustment disorder, with no diagnosis on Axis II. It is preferable to start with a new patient, rather than one whom you have been treating for a time using a different therapeutic orientation. It is also desirable to treat this patient according to the guidelines presented in this book, in as pure a fashion as possible. A note of caution: Therapists who are experienced in a different modality are often tempted to fall back on previously acquired skills that hinder cognitive behavior therapy treatment. If it is more practical, however, you can start using cognitive behavior therapy techniques with a patient already in treatment with you. Be sure to explain what you would like to do, provide a rationale, and elicit the patient's agreement.

10. Obtain written consent for recording therapy sessions. Review of therapy tapes with a colleague or supervisor is essential to progress. An indispensable tool for evaluating your tapes is the Cognitive Therapy Scale and Manual (see Appendix C). It is used extensively by cognitive behavior therapy supervisors to help trainees evaluate their work and plan for improvement and by researchers to rate therapist competency.

11. Continue throughout this process to read more about cognitive behavior therapy. Also be sure to read booklets, articles, or books that are intended for patients so you will be able to suggest appropriate bibliotherapy to them.

12. Refer to Wright, Basco, and Thase (2006) for additional guidelines in becoming a competent cognitive behavior therapist.

13. Watch actual cognitive behavior therapy sessions conducted by master clinicians (see Appendix B).

14. Seek opportunities for training and supervision, either locally or through the Beck Institute for Cognitive Behavior Therapy (see Appendix B).

15. Finally, consider joining and attending conferences of the Academy of Cognitive Therapy, the official "home" for cognitive behavior therapists; clinicians and students may join as regular members or apply to become certified cognitive therapists. Attend local, national, and international conferences put on by other associations of cognitive behavior therapy, as well (see Appendix B).

Appendix A

COGNITIVE CASE WRITE-UP

The format for the following case write-up is used with the permission of the Academy of Cognitive Therapy. Instructions for such a case write-up and scoring information are available at *www.academyofct.org*.

I. CASE HISTORY

A. Identifying Information: Sally is an 18-year-old Caucasian female college student, living in a freshman dorm with one roommate.

B. Chief Complaint: Sally sought treatment for depression and anxiety.

C. History of Present Illness: Several months after starting her freshman year of college, Sally developed symptoms of depression and anxiety. At intake, her symptoms included the following:

- *Emotional symptoms*: sadness, anxiety, guilt, loss of pleasure and interest, hopelessness, loneliness.
- *Cognitive symptoms*: pessimism, difficulty concentrating and making decisions, mild catastrophizing, self-criticism.
- *Behavioral symptoms*: social withdrawal, avoiding situations perceived as challenging (talking to professor, roommate, persisting in schoolwork).
- *Physiological symptoms*: loss of energy, fatigue, lowered libido, crying, restlessness, inability to relax, decreased appetite, disturbed sleep.

Sally faced the usual stressors of college freshmen: especially being away from home for the first time and encountering academic challenges. She fit in well socially but after she became symptomatic, she began to isolate herself somewhat.

361

D. Psychiatric History: Sally has no prior psychiatric history.

E. Personal and Social History: Sally is the younger of two children in an intact family. Her brother is 5 years older than she and achieves more highly academically. Her mother was always highly critical of Sally. Her father was more supportive of Sally, but was away from home a great deal due to a demanding job. Her parents argued a considerable amount, but Sally doesn't believe that unduly affected her. Growing up, Sally feared harsh teachers and was anxious about her grades. She has long been critical of herself for not measuring up to her brother, although her relationship with him has been fine. Sally has always had several close friends and dated throughout high school. She has maintained a good academic record.

F. Medical History: Sally did not have any medical problems that influenced her psychological functioning or the treatment process.

G. Mental Status Check: Sally was fully oriented, with depressed mood.

H. DSM-IV-TR Diagnoses:

- Axis I: Major Depressive Episode, Single Episode, Moderate 296.22
- Axis II: None
- Axis III: None
- Axis IV: Severity of psychosocial stressors: mild (leaving home for first time)
- Axis V: GAF Current—60. Best in Past Year—85.

II. CASE FORMULATION

A. Precipitants: Sally's depressive disorder was precipitated by leaving home for college and experiencing some initial difficulty in her courses. Anxiety probably interfered with efficient studying; Sally then became quite self-critical and dysphoric. As she withdrew from activities and friends, the lack of positive input contributed to her low mood, as did her failure to solve academic difficulties.

B. Cross-Sectional View of Current Cognitions and Behaviors: A typical current problematic situation is that Sally has difficulty studying. While attempting to study, Sally has the automatic thoughts: "I can't do this; I'm such a failure; I'll never make it here." She also has an image of herself, weighed down by a heavy backpack, trudging aimlessly, looking downtrodden. These thoughts and image lead to feelings of sadness. In another situation, as she's studying for a test, she has the automatic thoughts: "This is too hard. What if the teaching assistant won't help me? What if I flunk?" and she feels anxious and then has difficulty concentrating. She also has the automatic thought: "I should be doing more." She then feels guilty. In all of these situations, she stops studying, lies on her bed, and sometimes cries.

C. **Longitudinal View of Cognitions and Behaviors:** Sally always had a mild tendency to see herself as incompetent. While her school performance was above average, she was never among the brightest students in her classes. Academic success was very important to her and she developed certain assumptions: "If I work very hard then maybe I'll do okay but if I don't, I'll fail"; "If I hide my weaknesses, I'll be okay [for the moment] but if I ask for help, I'll expose my incompetence." Her compensatory behavioral strategies included working excessively hard to live up to her potential and a tendency to avoid asking for help so she would not expose her weaknesses. Once she became depressed, she often used avoidance (of schoolwork, of confronting challenges, of social opportunities). For the most part, Sally's beliefs about other people were positive and functional; she tended to see others as well intentioned, although she was sometimes cowed by authority figures. She also believed that her world was relatively safe, stable, and predictable.

D. **Strengths and Assets:** Sally had high psychological mindedness, objectivity, and adaptiveness. She was intelligent and before depression set in, very hard working. She was motivated for therapy. She had the ability to form good, stable relationships with others.

E. **Working Hypothesis (Summary of Conceptualization):** For much of her life, Sally saw herself as reasonably competent, worthwhile, and likeable. She was always vulnerable, however, to perceiving herself as incompetent, for at least three reasons: (1) her mother was highly critical of her growing up; (2) her supportive father was often not at home; and (3) she had a tendency to compare herself unfavorably to others. For example, Sally continually compared herself unfavorably to her brother, who (because he was 5 years older) could do almost everything better than she could. Instead of recognizing that she would likely be able to meet his accomplishments when she reached the same age, she interpreted the vast differences between what she was able to accomplish at a given time with what he accomplished during that same time as signs of her own incompetence. She also compared herself to the best students in the class and found herself lacking.

Sally historically was vigilant for signs of incompetence in herself and sometimes discounted or failed to recognize signs of competence. She developed certain rules to ensure that her incompetence would not be exposed (e.g., "I must work very hard"; "I must live up to my potential"; "I must always do my best"). As a result, she developed the following compensatory strategies: she holds high expectations for herself, works very hard, is vigilant for shortcomings, and avoids seeking help. Until she reached college, her life was guided by related assumptions: "If I achieve highly, it means I'm okay." "If I hide my weaknesses, others will view me as competent."

Throughout high school, Sally was able to achieve highly enough (in her estimation), but in her freshman year of college, she started to struggle with her studies. She became quite anxious. Her core belief of incompetence became activated. She started to have fearful automatic thoughts about failure. Her anxiety interfered with effective studying and problem solving. She also began to withdraw from others and avoid schoolwork and other challenges. Then the corollary to her underlying assumptions dominated her thinking: "If I don't achieve highly, it means I'm incompetent." "If I ask for help, I'll be seen as incompetent." As she began to perform more poorly, she became convinced of her incompetence. Failing to be productive and failing to gain social support from others probably contributed to the onset of her depression.

III. TREATMENT PLAN

A. Problem List

1. Studying and writing papers
2. Volunteering in class and taking tests
3. Social withdrawal
4. Lack of assertiveness with roommate, professors
5. Spending too much time in bed

B. Treatment Goals

1. Decrease self-criticism
2. Teach basic cognitive tools, Thought Record, etc.
3. Decrease time in bed
4. Find healthier ways to have fun.
5. Do problem solving around studying, papers, tests.
6. Build assertiveness skills

C. Plan for Treatment: The treatment plan was to reduce Sally's depression and anxiety through helping her respond to her automatic thoughts (especially those connected with inadequacy and incompetence), increase her activities through activity scheduling, problem-solve difficulties with studying and homework, and build assertiveness through role-playing and modifying interfering beliefs.

IV. COURSE OF TREATMENT

A. Therapeutic Relationship: Sally easily engaged in treatment. She saw her therapist as competent and caring.

B. Interventions/Procedures

1. Taught patient standard cognitive tools of examining and responding to her automatic thoughts (which allowed the patient

to see her dysfunctional, distorted logic and thus significantly reduced depressive and anxious symptoms).

2. Had Sally conduct behavioral experiments to test her assumptions. This resulted in reduced avoidance and increased assertiveness.

3. Helped Sally schedule and increase pleasurable activities.

4. Did straightforward problem solving.

5. Role-played to teach assertiveness.

C. Obstacles: None

D. Outcome: Sally's depression gradually reduced over a 3-month period after we started therapy, until she was in full remission.

Appendix B

COGNITIVE BEHAVIOR
THERAPY RESOURCES

TRAINING PROGRAMS

The Beck Institute for Cognitive Behavior Therapy (*www.beckinstitute.org*) in suburban Philadelphia offers a variety of onsite, off-site, distance, and online training programs.

THERAPIST AND PATIENT MATERIALS AND REFERRALS

Information about the following can be found at *www.beckinstitute.org*:

Patient booklets
Worksheet packet
Cognitive Therapy Rating Scale and Manual
Books, DVDs, and tapes by Aaron T. Beck, MD, and Judith S. Beck, PhD
Educational catalog
Referrals to mental health professionals certified by the Academy of Cognitive
    Therapy

ASSESSMENT MATERIALS

The following scales and manuals may be ordered from Pearson (*www.beckscales.com*):

Beck Depression Inventory–II
Beck Depression Inventory—Fast Screen for Medical Patients

Beck Anxiety Inventory
Beck Hopelessness Scale
Beck Scale for Suicidal Ideation
Clark–Beck Obsessive–Compulsive Inventory
Beck Youth Inventories—Second Edition

COGNITIVE BEHAVIOR THERAPY
PROFESSIONAL ORGANIZATIONS

Academy of Cognitive Therapy (*www.academyofct.org*)
Association for Behavioral and Cognitive Therapies (*www.abct.org*)
British Association for Behavioural and Cognitive Psychotherapies (*www.babcp.
com*)
European Association for Behavioural and Cognitive Therapies (*www.eabct.
com*)
International Association for Cognitive Psychotherapy (*www.the-iacp.com*)

Appendix C

COGNITIVE THERAPY RATING SCALE

The following rating scale, used in major research studies and by the Academy of Cognitive Therapy as a measure of competency, is used with permission. The scale and the accompanying manual can be found at *www.academyofct. org.*

Therapist: _____   Patient: _____   Date of Session: _____

Tape ID#: _____   Rater: _____   Date of Rating: _____

Session# _____   ( ) Videotape   ( ) Audiotape   ( ) Live Observation

Directions: For each item, assess the therapist on a scale from 0 to 6, and record the rating on the line next to the item number. Descriptions are provided for even-numbered scale points. *If you believe the therapist falls between two of the descriptors, select the intervening odd number (1, 3, 5).* For example, if the therapist set a very good agenda but did not establish priorities, assign a rating of a 5 rather than a 4 or 6.

If the descriptions for a given item occasionally do not seem to apply to the session you are rating, feel free to disregard them and use the more general scale below:

0	1	2	3	4	5	6
Poor	Barely Adequate	Mediocre	Satisfactory	Good	Very Good	Excellent

Please do not leave any item blank. For all items, focus on the skill of the therapist, taking into account how difficult the patient seems to be.

Reprinted by permission in *Cognitive Behavior Therapy: Basics and Beyond, Second Edition*, by Judith S. Beck (Guilford Press, 2011). Permission to photocopy this material is granted to purchasers of this book for personal use only (see copyright page for details). Purchasers may download a larger version of this material from *www.guilford.com/p/beck4*.

PART I. GENERAL THERAPEUTIC SKILLS

_____ 1. AGENDA

    0   Therapist did not set agenda.

    2   Therapist set agenda that was vague or incomplete.

    4   Therapist worked with patient to set a mutually satisfactory agenda that included specific target problems (e.g., anxiety at work, dissatisfaction with marriage).

    6   Therapist worked with patient to set an appropriate agenda with target problems, suitable for the available time. Established priorities and then followed agenda.

_____ 2. FEEDBACK

    0   Therapist did not ask for feedback to determine patient's understanding of, or response to, the session.

    2   Therapist elicited some feedback from the patient, but did not ask enough questions to be sure the patient understood the therapist's line of reasoning during the session *or* to ascertain whether the patient was satisfied with the session.

    4   Therapist asked enough questions to be sure that the patient understood the therapist's line of reasoning throughout the session and to determine the patient's reactions to the session. The therapist adjusted his/her behavior in response to the feedback when appropriate.

    6   Therapist was especially adept at eliciting and responding to verbal and nonverbal feedback throughout the session (e.g., elicited reactions to session, regularly checked for understanding, helped summarize main points at end of session).

_____ 3. UNDERSTANDING

    0   Therapist repeatedly failed to understand what the patient explicitly said and thus consistently missed the point. Poor empathic skills.

    2   Therapist was usually able to reflect or rephrase what the patient explicitly said, but repeatedly failed to respond to more subtle communication. Limited ability to listen and empathize.

    4   Therapist generally seemed to grasp the patient's "internal reality" as reflected by both what the patient explicitly said and what the patient communicated in more subtle ways. Good ability to listen and empathize.

    6   Therapist seemed to understand the patient's "internal reality"

thoroughly and was adept at communicating this understanding through appropriate verbal and nonverbal responses to the patient (e.g., the tone of the therapist's response conveyed a sympathetic understanding of the patient's "message"). Excellent listening and empathic skills.

_____ 4. INTERPERSONAL EFFECTIVENESS

0   Therapist had poor interpersonal skills. Seemed hostile, demeaning, or in some other way destructive to the patient.

2   Therapist did not seem destructive, but had significant interpersonal problems. At times, therapist appeared unnecessarily impatient, aloof, insincere *or* had difficulty conveying confidence and competence.

4   Therapist displayed a *satisfactory* degree of warmth, concern, confidence, genuineness, and professionalism. No significant interpersonal problems.

6   Therapist displayed *optimal* levels of warmth, concern, confidence, genuineness, and professionalism, appropriate for this particular patient in this session.

_____ 5. COLLABORATION

0   Therapist did not attempt to collaborate with patient.

2   Therapist attempted to collaborate with patient, but had difficulty *either* defining a problem that the patient considered important *or* establishing rapport.

4   Therapist was able to collaborate with patient, focus on a problem that both patient and therapist considered important, and establish rapport.

6   Collaboration seemed excellent; therapist encouraged patient as much as possible to take an active role during the session (e.g., by offering choices) so they could function as a "team."

_____ 6. PACING AND EFFICIENT USE OF TIME

0   Therapist made no attempt to structure therapy time. Session seemed aimless.

2   Session had some direction, but the therapist had significant problems with structuring or pacing (e.g., too little structure, inflexible about structure, too slowly paced, too rapidly paced).

4   Therapist was reasonably successful at using time efficiently. Therapist maintained appropriate control over flow of discussion and pacing.

6   Therapist used time efficiently by tactfully limiting peripheral

and unproductive discussion and by pacing the session as rapidly as was appropriate for the patient.

PART II. CONCEPTUALIZATION, STRATEGY, AND TECHNIQUE

_____ 7. GUIDED DISCOVERY

0   Therapist relied primarily on debate, persuasion, or "lecturing." Therapist seemed to be "cross-examining" patient, putting the patient on the defensive, or forcing his/her point of view on the patient.

2   Therapist relied too heavily on persuasion and debate, rather than guided discovery. However, therapist's style was supportive enough that patient did not seem to feel attacked or defensive.

4   Therapist, for the most part, helped patient see new perspectives through guided discovery (e.g., examining evidence, considering alternatives, weighing advantages and disadvantages) rather than through debate. Used questioning appropriately.

6   Therapist was especially adept at using guided discovery during the session to explore problems and help patient draw his/her own conclusions. Achieved an excellent balance between skillful questioning and other modes of intervention.

_____ 8. FOCUSING ON KEY COGNITIONS OR BEHAVIORS

0   Therapist did not attempt to elicit specific thoughts, assumptions, images, meanings, or behaviors.

2   Therapist used appropriate techniques to elicit cognitions or behaviors; however, therapist had difficulty finding a focus *or* focused on cognitions/behaviors that were irrelevant to the patient's key problems.

4   Therapist focused on specific cognitions or behaviors relevant to the target problem. However, therapist could have focused on more central cognitions or behaviors that offered greater promise for progress.

6   Therapist very skillfully focused on key thoughts, assumptions, behaviors, etc., that were most relevant to the problem area and offered considerable promise for progress.

_____ 9. STRATEGY FOR CHANGE (*Note*: For this item, focus on the quality of the therapist's strategy for change, not on how effectively the strategy was implemented or whether change actually occurred.)

0   Therapist did not select cognitive-behavioral techniques.

2   Therapist selected cognitive-behavioral techniques; however, either the overall strategy for bringing about change seemed vague *or* did not seem promising in helping the patient.

4   Therapist seemed to have a generally coherent strategy for change that showed reasonable promise and incorporated cognitive-behavioral techniques.

6   Therapist followed a consistent strategy for change that seemed very promising and incorporated the most appropriate cognitive-behavioral techniques.

_____10. APPLICATION OF COGNITIVE-BEHAVIORAL TECHNIQUES (*Note*: For this item, focus on how skillfully the techniques were applied, not on how appropriate they were for the target problem or whether change actually occurred.)

0   Therapist did not apply any cognitive-behavioral techniques.

2   Therapist used cognitive-behavioral techniques, but there were *significant flaws* in the way they were applied.

4   Therapist applied cognitive-behavioral techniques *with moderate skill*.

6   Therapist *very skillfully* and resourcefully employed cognitive-behavioral techniques.

_____11. HOMEWORK

0   Therapist did not attempt to incorporate homework relevant to cognitive therapy.

2   Therapist had significant difficulties incorporating homework (e.g., did not review previous homework, did not explain homework in sufficient detail, assigned inappropriate homework).

4   Therapist reviewed previous homework and assigned "standard" cognitive therapy homework generally relevant to issues dealt with in session. Homework was explained in sufficient detail.

6   Therapist reviewed previous homework and carefully assigned homework drawn from cognitive therapy for the coming week. Assignment seemed "custom-tailored" to help patient incorporate new perspectives, test hypotheses, experiment with new behaviors discussed during session, etc.

PART III. ADDITIONAL CONSIDERATIONS

12. _____a. Did any special problems arise during the session (e.g., nonadherence to homework, interpersonal issues between therapist and patient, hopelessness about continuing therapy, relapse)?

YES   NO

_____b. *If yes*:

0   Therapist could not deal adequately with special problems that arose.

2   Therapist dealt with special problems adequately, but used strategies or conceptualizations inconsistent with cognitive therapy.

4   Therapist attempted to deal with special problems using a cognitive framework and was *moderately skillful* in applying techniques.

6   Therapist was very skillful at handling special problems using cognitive therapy framework.

13. Were there any significant unusual factors in this session that you feel justified the therapist's departure from the standard approach measured by this scale?

YES (Please explain below)   NO

PART IV. OVERALL RATINGS AND COMMENTS

14. How would you rate the clinician overall in this session, as a cognitive therapist?

0	1	2	3	4	5	6
Poor	Barely Adequate	Mediocre	Satisfactory	Good	Very Good	Excellent

15. If you were conducting an outcome study in cognitive therapy, do you think you would select this therapist to participate at this time (assuming this session is typical)?

0	1	2	3	4
Definitely Not	Probably Not	Uncertain–Borderline	Probably Yes	Definitely Yes

16. How difficult did you feel this patient was to work with?

0	1	2	3	4	5	6
Not Difficult–Very Receptive			Moderately Difficult			Extremely Difficult

17. COMMENTS AND SUGGESTIONS FOR THERAPIST'S IMPROVEMENT:

18. OVERALL RATING:

Rating Scale:	0	1	2	3	4	5
	Inadequate	Mediocre	Satisfactory	Good	Very Good	Excellent

Using the scale above, please give an overall rating of this therapist's skills as demonstrated on this tape. Please circle the appropriate number.

REFERENCES

Alford, B. A., & Beck, A. T. (1997). *The integrative power of cognitive therapy*. New York: Guilford Press.

American Psychiatric Association. (2000). *Diagnostic and statistical manual of mental disorders* (4th ed., text rev.). Washington, DC: Author.

Antony, M. M., & Barlow, D. H. (Eds.). (2010). *Handbook of assessment and treatment planning for psychological disorders* (2nd ed.). New York: Guilford Press.

Arnkoff, D. B., & Glass, C. R. (1992). Cognitive therapy and psychotherapy integration. In D. K. Freedheim (Ed.), *History of psychotherapy: A century of change* (pp. 657–694). Washington, DC: American Psychological Association.

Barlow, D. H. (2002). *Anxiety and its disorders: The nature and treatment of anxiety and panic* (2nd ed.). New York: Guilford Press.

Beck, A. T. (1964). Thinking and depression: II. Theory and therapy. *Archives of General Psychiatry, 10*, 561–571.

Beck, A. T. (1967). *Depression: Causes and treatment*. Philadelphia: University of Pennsylvania Press.

Beck, A. T. (1976). *Cognitive therapy and the emotional disorders*. New York: International Universities Press.

Beck, A. T. (1987). Cognitive approaches to panic disorder: Theory and therapy. In S. Rachman & J. Maser (Eds.), *Panic: Psychological perspectives* (pp. 91–109). Hillsdale, NJ: Erlbaum.

Beck, A. T. (1999). Cognitive aspects of personality disorders and their relation to syndromal disorders: A psychoevolutionary approach. In C. R. Cloninger (Ed.), *Personality and psychopathology* (pp. 411–429). Washington, DC: American Psychiatric Press.

Beck, A. T. (2005). The current state of cognitive therapy: A 40-year retrospective. *Archives of General Psychiatry, 62*, 953–959.

Beck, A. T., & Beck, J. S. (1991). *The personality belief questionnaire*. Bala Cynwyd, PA: Beck Institute for Cognitive Behavior Therapy.

Beck, A. T., & Emery, G. (with Greenberg, R. L.). (1985). *Anxiety disorders and phobias: A cognitive perspective.* New York: Basic Books.

Beck, A. T., Freeman, A., Davis, D. D., & Associates. (2004). *Cognitive therapy of personality disorders* (2nd ed.). New York: Guilford Press.

Beck, A. T., Rush, A. J., Shaw, B. F., & Emery, G. (1979). *Cognitive therapy of depression.* New York: Guilford Press.

Beck, A. T., Wright, F. D., Newman, C. F., & Liese, B. S. (1993). *Cognitive therapy of substance abuse.* New York: Guilford Press.

Beck, J. S. (2001). A cognitive therapy approach to medication compliance. In J. Kay (Ed.), *Integrated treatment of psychiatric disorders* (pp. 113–141). Washington, DC: American Psychiatric Publishing.

Beck, J. S. (2005). *Cognitive therapy for challenging problems: What to do when the basics don't work.* New York: Guilford Press.

Beck, J. S. (2011). *Cognitive behavior therapy worksheet packet* (3rd ed.). Bala Cynwyd, PA: Beck Institute for Cognitive Behavior Therapy.

Bennett-Levy, J., Butler, G., Fennell, M., Hackman, A., Mueller, M., & Westbrook, D. (Eds.). (2004). *Oxford guide to behavioral experiments in cognitive therapy.* Oxford, UK: Oxford University.

Benson, H. (1975). *The relaxation response.* New York: Avon.

Burns, D. D. (1980). *Feeling good: The new mood therapy.* New York: Signet.

Butler, A. C., Chapman, J. E. Forman, E. M., & Beck, A. T. (2006). The empirical status of cognitive-behavioral therapy: A review of meta-analyses. *Clinical Psychology Review, 26,* 17–31.

Chambless, D., & Ollendick, T. H. (2001). Empirically supported psychological interventions. *Annual Review of Psychology, 52,* 685–716.

Chiesa A., & Serretti, A. (2010a). Mindfulness based cognitive therapy for psychiatric disorders: A systematic review and meta-analysis. *Psychiatry Research.*

Chiesa A., & Serretti, A. (2010b). A systematic review of neurobiological and clinical features of mindfulness mediation. *Psychological Medicine, 40,* 1239–1252.

Clark, D. A., & Beck, A. T. (2010). *Cognitive therapy of anxiety disorders: Science and practice.* New York: Guilford Press.

Clark, D. A., Beck, A. T., & Alford, B. A. (1999). *Scientific foundations of cognitive theory and therapy of depression.* Hoboken, NJ: Wiley.

Clark, D. M. (1989). Anxiety states: Panic and generalized anxiety. In K. Hawton, P. M. Salkovskis, J. Kirk, & D. M. Clark (Eds.), *Cognitive-behavior therapy for psychiatric problems: A practical guide* (pp. 52–96). New York: Oxford University Press.

D'Zurilla, T. J., & Nezu, A. M. (2006). *Problem-solving therapy: A positive approach to clinical intervention* (3rd ed.). New York: Springer.

Davis, M., Eshelman, E. R., & McKay, M. (2008). *The relaxation and stress reduction workbook* (6th ed.). Oakland, CA: New Harbinger.

DeRubeis, R. J., & Feeley, M. (1990). Determinants of change in cognitive therapy for depression. *Cognitive Therapy and Research, 14,* 469–482.

Dobson, D., & Dobson, K. S. (2009). *Evidence-based practice of cognitive-behavioral therapy.* New York: Guilford Press.

Dobson, K. S., & Dozois D. J. A. (2009). Historical and philosophical bases of the cognitive-behavioral therapies. In K. S. Dobson (Ed.), *Handbook of cognitive-behavioral therapies* (3rd ed., pp. 3–37). New York: Guilford Press.

Edwards, D. J. A. (1989). Cognitive restructuring through guided imagery: Lessons from Gestalt therapy. In A. Freeman, K. M. Simon, L. E. Beutler, & H. Arkowitz (Eds.), *Comprehensive handbook of cognitive therapy* (pp. 283–297). New York: Plenum Press.

Ellis, A. (1962). *Reason and emotion in psychotherapy.* New York: Lyle Stuart.

Evans, J. M. G., Hollon, S. D., DeRubeis, R. J., Piasecki, J. M., Grove, W. M., Garvey, M. J., et al. (1992). Differential relapse following cognitive therapy and pharmacology for depression. *Archives of General Psychiatry, 49,* 802–808.

Feeley, M., DeRubeis, R. J., & Gelfand, L. A. (1999). The temporal relation of adherence and alliance to symptom change in cognitive therapy for depression. *Journal of Consulting and Clinical Psychology, 67,* 578–582.

Foa, E. B., & Rothbaum, B. O. (1998). *Treating the trauma of rape: Cognitive-behavioral therapy for PTSD.* New York: Guilford Press.

Frisch, M. B. (2005). *Quality of life therapy.* New York: Wiley.

Garner, D. M., & Bemis, K. M. (1985). Cognitive therapy for anorexia nervosa. In D. M. Garner & P. E. Garfinkel (Eds.), *Handbook of psychotherapy for anorexia nervosa and bulimia* (pp. 107–146). New York: Guilford Press.

Goldapple, K., Segal, Z., Garson, C., Lau, M., Bieling, P., Kennedy, S., et al. (2004). Modulation of cortical–limbic pathways in major depression. *Archives of General Psychiatry, 61,* 34–41.

Goldstein, A., & Stainback, B. (1987). *Overcoming agoraphobia: Conquering fear of the outside world.* New York: Viking Penguin.

Greenberg L. S. (2002). *Emotion focused therapy: Coaching clients to work through their feelings.* Washington, DC: American Psychological Association.

Hayes, S. C., Follette, V. M., & Linehan, M. M. (Eds.). (2004). *Mindfulness and acceptance: Expanding the cognitive-behavioral tradition.* New York: Guilford Press.

Holland, S. (2003). Avoidance of emotion as an obstacle to progress. In R. L. Leahy (Ed.), *Roadblocks in cognitive-behavioral therapy: Transforming challenges into opportunities for change* (pp. 116–131). New York: Guilford Press.

Hollon, S. D., & Beck, A. T. (1993). Cognitive and cognitive-behavioral therapies. In A. E. Bergin & S.L. Garfield (Eds.), *Handbook of psychotherapy and behavior change: An empirical analysis* (4th ed., pp. 428–466). New York: Wiley.

Hollon, S. D., DeRubeis, R. J., & Seligman, M. E. P. (1992). Cognitive therapy and the prevention of depression. *Applied and Preventive Psychiatry, 1,* 89–95.

Jacobson, E. (1974). *Progressive relaxation.* Chicago: University of Chicago Press, Midway Reprint.

Kabat-Zinn, J. (1990). *Full catastrophe living.* New York: Delta.

Kazantzis, N., Deane, F. P., Ronan, K. R., & Lampropoulos, G. K. (2005). Empirical foundations. In N. Kazantzis, F. P. Deane, K. R. Ronan, & L. L'Abate (Eds.), *Using homework assignments in cognitive behavior therapy* (pp. 35–60). New York: Routledge.

Kazantzis, N., Whittington, C., & Dattilio, F. (2010). Meta-analysis of homework effects in cognitive and behavioral therapy: A replication and extension. *Clinical Psychology: Science and Practice, 17,* 144–156.

Khanna, M. S., & Kendall, P. C. (2010). Computer-assisted cognitive-behavioral therapy for child anxiety: Result of a randomized clinical trial. *Journal of Consulting and Clinical Psychology, 78,* 737–745.

Kuyken, W., Padesky, C. A., & Dudley, R. (2009). *Collaborative case conceptualization:*

Working effectively with clients in cognitive behavioral therapy. New York: Guilford Press.

Layden, M. A., Newman, C. F., Freeman, A., & Morse, S. B. (1993). *Cognitive therapy of borderline personality disorder*. Needham Heights, MA: Allyn & Bacon.

Lazarus, A. A., & Lazarus, C. N. (1991). *Multimodal life history inventory*. Champaign, IL: Research Press.

Leahy, R. L. (2003). Emotional schemas and resistance. In R. L. Leahy (Ed.), *Roadblocks in cognitive-behavioral therapy: Transforming challenges into opportunities for change* (pp.91–115). New York: Guilford Press.

Leahy, R. L. (2010). *Beat the blues before they beat you: How to overcome depression*. Carlsbad, CA: Hay House.

Ledley, D. R., Marx, B. P., & Heimberg R. G. (2005). *Making cognitive-behavioral therapy work: Clinical process for new practitioners*. New York: Guilford Press.

Lewinsohn, P. M., Sullivan, J. M., & Grosscup, S. J. (1980). Changing reinforcing events: An approach to the treatment of depression. *Psychotherapy: Theory, Research, Practice, and Training, 17*(3), 322–334.

Linehan, M. M. (1993). *Cognitive-behavioral treatment of borderline personality disorder*. New York: Guilford Press.

Ludgate, J. W. (2009). *Cognitive-behavioral therapy and relapse prevention for depression and anxiety*. Sarasota, FL: Professional Resource.

MacPhillamy, D. J., & Lewinsohn, P. M. (1982). The pleasant events schedule: Studies on reliability, validity, and scale intercorrelation. *Journal of Consulting and Clinical Psychology, 50*, 363–380.

Martell, C., Addis, M., & Jacobson, N. (2001). *Depression in context: Strategies for guided action*. New York: Norton.

McCown, D., Reibel, D., & Micozzi, M. S. (2010). *Teaching mindfulness: A practical guide for clinicians and educators*. New York: Springer.

McCullough, J. P., Jr. (1999). *Treatment for chronic depression: Cognitive behavioral analysis system of psychotherapy*. New York: Guilford Press.

McKay, M., Davis, M., & Fanning, P. (2009). *Messages: The communication skills book* (2nd ed.). Oakland, CA: New Harbinger.

McKay, M., & Fanning, P. (1991). *Prisoners of belief*. Oakland, CA: New Harbinger.

McMullin, R. E. (1986). *Handbook of cognitive therapy techniques*. New York: Norton.

Meichenbaum, D. (1977). *Cognitive-behavior modification: An integrative approach*. New York: Plenum Press.

Needleman, L. D. (1999). *Cognitive case conceptualization: A guidebook for practitioners*. Mahwah, NJ: Erlbaum.

Niemeyer, R. A., & Feixas, G. (1990). The role of homework and skill acquisition in the outcome of group cognitive therapy for depression. *Behavior Therapy, 21*(3), 281–292.

Persons, J. B. (2008). *The case formulation approach to cognitive-behavior therapy*. New York: Guilford Press.

Persons, J. B., Burns, D. D., & Perloff, J. M. (1988). Predictors of dropout and outcome in cognitive therapy for depression in a private practice setting. *Cognitive Therapy and Research, 12*, 557–575.

Raue, P. J., & Goldfried, M. R. (1994). The therapeutic alliance in cognitive-behavioral therapy. In A. O. Horvath & L. S. Greenberg (Eds.), *The working alliance: Theory, research, and practice* (pp. 131–152). New York: Wiley.

Resick, P. A., & Schnicke, M. K. (1993). *Cognitive processing therapy for rape victims: A treatment manual.* Newbury Park, CA: Sage.

Riso, L. P., du Toit, P. L., Stein, D. J., & Young, J. E. (2007). *Cognitive schemas and core beliefs in psychological problems.* Washington, DC: American Psychological Association.

Rosen, H. (1988). The constructivist–development paradigm. In R. A. Dorfman (Ed.), *Paradigms of clinical social work* (pp. 317–355). New York: Brunner/ Mazel.

Rush, A. J., Beck, A. T., Kovacs, M., & Hollon, S. D. (1977). Comparative efficacy of cognitive therapy and pharmacotherapy in the treatment of depressed outpatients. *Cognitive Therapy and Research, 1*(1), 17–37.

Safran, J. D., Vallis, T. M., Segal, Z. V., & Shaw, B. F. (1986). Assessment of core cognitive processes in cognitive therapy. *Cognitive Therapy and Research, 10,* 509–526.

Salkovskis, P. M. (1996). The cognitive approach to anxiety: Threat beliefs, safety-seeking behavior, and the special case of health anxiety obsessions. In P. M. Salkovskis (Ed.), *Frontiers of cognitive therapy: The state of the art and beyond* (pp. 48–74). New York: Guilford Press.

Shadish, W. R., Matt, G. E., Navarro, A. M., & Phillips, G. (2000). The effects of psychological therapies under clinically representative conditions: A meta-analysis. *Psychological Bulletin, 126,* 512–529.

Simons, A. D., Padesky, C. A., Montemarano, J., Lewis, C. C., Murakami, J., Lamb, K., et al. (2010). Training and dissemination of cognitive behavior therapy for depression in adults: A preliminary examination of therapist competence and client outcomes. *Journal of Consulting and Clinical Psychology, 78,* 751–756.

Smucker, M. R., & Dancu, C. V. (1999). *Cognitive behavioral treatment for adult survivors of childhood trauma: Imagery rescripting and reprocessing.* Northvale, NJ: Aronson.

Stirman, S. W., Buchhofer, R., McLaulin, B., Evans, A. C., & Beck, A. T. (2009). Public–academic partnerships: The Beck initiative: A partnership to implement cognitive therapy in a community behavioral health system. *Psychiatric Services, 60,* 1302–1304.

Tarrier, N. (Ed.). (2006). *Case formulation in cognitive behaviour therapy: The treatment of challenging and complex cases.* New York: Routledge.

Tompkins, M. A. (2004). *Using homework in psychotherapy: Strategies, guidelines, and forms.* New York: Guilford Press.

Weissman, A. N., & Beck, A. T. (1978). *Development and validation of the Dysfunctional Attitude Scale: A preliminary investigation.* Paper presented at the annual meeting of the American Educational Research Association, Toronto, Canada.

Wenzel, A. Brown, G. K., & Beck, A. T. (2008). *Cognitive therapy for suicidal patients: Scientific and clinical applications.* Washington, DC: American Psychological Association.

Williams, J. M. G., Teasdale, J. D., Segal, Z. V., & Kabat-Zinn, J. (2007). *The mindful way through depression: Freeing yourself from chronic unhappiness.* New York: Guilford Press.

Wright, J. H., Basco, M. R., Thase, M. E. (2006). *Learning cognitive-behavior therapy: An illustrative guide.* Arlington, VA: American Psychiatric Publishing.

Wright, J. H., Wright, A. S., Salmon, P., Beck, A. T., Kuykendall, J., & Goldsmith, J. (2002). Development and initial testing on a multimedia program for computer-assisted cognitive therapy. *American Journal of Psychotherapy, 56,* 76–86.

Young, J. E. (1999). *Cognitive therapy for personality disorders: A schema-focused approach* (3rd ed.). Sarasota, FL: Professional Resource.

Young, J. E., & Klosko, J. (1994). *Reinventing your life: How to break free of negative life patterns.* New York: Dutton Press.

Young, J. E., Klosko, J. S., & Weishaar, M. E. (2003). *Schema therapy: A practitioner's guide.* New York: Guilford Press.

INDEX

Page numbers followed by *f* indicate figure and *t* indicate table

Academy of Cognitive Therapy, 11,
    360, 367
Acceptance, 184
Acceptance and commitment therapy,
    2
Accomplishment scale, 96
Activity charts, 87–88*f*, 97–99, 263
    to assess accuracy of predictions,
        97–98
    case example, 86, 90–93, 97–99
    to measure moods and behaviors,
        267
Adjustment disorder, 360
Affect. *See* Emotional functioning
All-or-nothing thinking, 181*f*
Anorexia, 11
Anxiety disorders, 5, 6, 10, 53, 263,
    265–267
Assertiveness, 267–268
Assessment
    case write-up, 361–364
    identifying core and intermediate
        beliefs, 205–209, 233–234
    individual conceptualization of
        patient and patient's problems, 7,
        11, 38–39
    of intensity of emotions, 164–166

medication adherence and effects,
    105
mood check, 62–63
ongoing nature of, 46–47
of patient commitment to treatment,
    52
patient resistance to forms, 127–128
principles of cognitive behavior
    therapy, 7
symptoms checklist, 62, 63
therapist resources for, 366–367
therapist skills for, 13
types of core beliefs, 231–232
See also Cognitive conceptualization;
    Evaluation session
Association for Behavioral and
    Cognitive Therapies, 367
Assumptions, 35
    changing rules and attitudes into
        form of, 211
    in cognitive conceptualization
        diagram, 201–203
    See also Intermediate beliefs
Attentional bias, 272
Attitudes, 35. *See also* Intermediate
    beliefs
Audio-recorded therapy notes, 191

Audio recording of therapy session, 348, 360
Automatic thoughts
  additional thoughts as reaction to stimulus, 147–148, 154*f*, 155
  alternative explanation for, 173
  alternative strategies for evaluating, 178–180
  alternative strategies for responding to, 197
  assessing outcomes of evaluation process, 176
  associated emotions, 138–139
  between-session responses to, 187, 192–197
  case example, 43, 138, 140–153, 155–157, 160–166, 168–169, 171–176, 178–179, 183, 185–186, 188, 192–194
  causes of suboptimal responding, 197
  characteristics of, 137–140
  clinical significance, 137
  in cognitive conceptualization diagram, 199, 201
  in cognitive model, 3, 5, 30–31
  common distortions in, 179–180, 181–182*f*
  core beliefs and, 34–35, 177
  decatastrophizing, 173–174
  eliciting, 83–84, 142–147, 156*f*
  embedded in therapeutic discourse, 151–152
  emotions versus, 159–162
  evaluating therapy effectiveness, 353
  evidence for validity of, 172–173
  formation of, 31
  full and precise expression of, 152–153
  getting distance from, 175
  goals of cognitive behavior therapy, 10
  guided discovery to explore, 23–25
  hierarchy of, 201, 203*f*
  homework assignments, 296
  homework review, 109–110
  identification of, 36
  identification of important thoughts, 167–169
  identifying height of distress caused by incident, 148
  identifying hot cognitions, 142–143
  identifying problematic situations, 148–150
  identifying underlying beliefs, 207–209
  as images. *See* Imaginal automatic thoughts
  intermediate beliefs and, 35
  interpretations versus, 150–151
  leading to depression, 43–44
  linkage to behavior, 36–40
  as obstacle to activity, 80–81
  as obstacle to feeling pleasure or achievement, 81
  patient's recognition and understanding of, 140–142, 155–157, 184–186
  psychological distress and, 137–138
  questions for evaluation of, 168, 170–176, 172*f*, 184
  reasons for delaying therapeutic focus on, 169–170
  reasons for not challenging, 170
  recording responses to, 187
  refocusing attention from, 260–263
  responding to patient's dysfunctional cognitions, 22–23
  reviewing therapy notes, 188–191
  role play to elicit, 145–146
  source of, 32–35, 153–155
  therapist cognitions interfering with therapy structure, 123–124
  therapist self-assessment, 14–15, 358–359
  therapist self-disclosure, 180
  therapist's evaluation of, 32, 139–140
  true, 182–184
  unarticulated beliefs behind, 177–178
  unsuccessful attempts to restructure, 176–178
  utility of, 139
  validity of, 139
  visualization to elicit, 144–145
Avoidance behavior, 265–266
AWARE technique, 197, 263

Axis I disorders, 201–203, 230, 239, 248, 251
Axis II disorders, 11, 18, 360

B

Beck Depression Inventory, 62, 63
Beck Institute for Cognitive Behavior Therapy, 360, 366
Behavior
  linkage of automatic thoughts to, 36–40
  linkage of beliefs to, 226
Behavioral activation, 2
  activity review, 81–83, 85–86
  automatic thoughts as obstacles to, 80–81, 83–84
  case example, 82–97
  educating patient about benefits of, 89–90
  homework assignment, 296
  identifying pleasurable activities, 94–99
  lack of mastery or pleasure in, 81
  patient's recognition of benefits of, 104–105
  therapeutic significance, 99
  therapeutic strategies for, 81–82
Behavioral experiments, 10
  case example, 84–85
  homework assignments, 297
  preparing for negative outcomes, 307–308
  purpose, 26
  to test beliefs, 217–218
Belief modification, 35–36
  "as if" technique, 226
  case example, 215–226
  cognitive continuum technique for, 218–220
  considering other people's beliefs for, 222–225
  Core Belief Worksheet for, 242–246
  course of, for core beliefs, 230–231
  developing and strengthening new core beliefs, 239–241
  early intervention, 230

historical testing of core belief for, 247–248
  identifying important beliefs for, 209–210, 227
  obstacles to, 230
  questioning technique for, 215–217
  resistance of core beliefs to, 230
  restructuring early memories for, 248–255
  role play for, 220–222
  strategies for, 214, 227, 241–242, 242*f,* 255
  therapist self-disclosure for, 227
  use of extreme contrasts for, 246–247
  using fictional characters and metaphors for, 247
Beliefs. *See* Core beliefs; Intermediate beliefs
Better/worse list, 104–105, 104*f*
Bibliotherapy, 239, 297
Booster sessions, 316, 327–331
Brief therapy, 3

C

Case write-up, 361–365
Catastrophic thinking, 173–174, 181*f*
Change
  attributing progress to patient, 318–319
  cognitive model of, 2, 3
  goals of cognitive behavior therapy, 10, 316
  as modification of dysfunctional beliefs, 35–36
  patient commitment to, 125
  step model for monitoring progress toward goals, 164–165, 165*f*
  See also Belief modification
Cognitive behavioral analysis, 2
Cognitive behavior therapy
  applications, 3, 4*t*
  basic principles, 6–11
  conceptual basis, 2, 3. *See also* Cognitive model
  goals, 8, 158–159, 316

Cognitive behavior therapy *(cont.)*
  origins and conceptual
    development, 1, 2–3, 5–6
  outcomes research, 4–5
  patient selection for first application
    of, 360
  resources for therapists, 366–367
Cognitive conceptualization
  case example, 37*f*, 40–44, 57–58,
    201–204
  childhood data in, 201
  coping strategies in, 203–204
  development of, 29–30, 38–40,
    44–45, 57
  diagram, 199, 200*f*, 201–205, 202*f*,
    359
  evolving formulation of, 30, 40, 45,
    121, 204
  presenting to patient, 204–205
  purpose, 29, 39–40, 45, 198, 199
  as source of problems in therapy,
    350
Cognitive continuum, 218–220
Cognitive distortions, 179–180,
  181–182*f*
Cognitive model
  automatic thoughts and behavior
    in, 36
  complex sequences in, 38–40
  conceptual basis, 3, 30–31
  educating patient about, 70–73,
    140–142
  monitoring patient's understanding
    of, 352, 355
Cognitive processing therapy, 2
Cognitive therapy. *See* Cognitive
  behavior therapy
Cognitive Therapy Rating Scale,
  368–374
Cognitive Therapy Scale and Manual,
  360
Collaborative empiricism, 10
Compensatory strategies, 363
Computer-assisted cognitive behavior
  therapy, 4
Consultation with supervisor, 349
Contrasting technique, 245

Coping card, 15–16, 25
Coping strategies, 204*f*
  case example, 42–43
  in cognitive conceptualization
    diagram, 203–204
  development of, 42–43
  exposure, 265–267
  for imaginal automatic thoughts,
    284–285, 289–290
  overuse of, 204
Core beliefs
  activation of, 32
  automatic thoughts and, 34, 177
  case example, 40–42, 229, 234,
    235–240, 242–253
  categories of negative, 228, 231–232,
    233*f*
  in cognitive conceptualization
    diagram, 199, 201
  definition, 32, 198
  developing and strengthening new,
    239–241
  formation of, 35, 40–41, 201, 228,
    229, 247–248
  hierarchy of, 201, 203*f*
  identifying, 205–209, 233–234
  information processing in
    maintenance of, 32–33, 41
  intermediate beliefs and, 35
  negative beliefs about others, 229
  patient understanding of,
    235–239
  resistance to modification, 230
  therapeutic focus on, 35–36, 120
  therapeutic goals, 35
  therapist self-assessment, 359
  See also Belief modification
Core Belief Worksheet, 223, 242–246,
  243*f*, 359
Credit lists, 274–276

D

Daily Record of Dysfunctional
  Thoughts, 192–193
Decision-making skills, 258–260

Depression, 360
activity scheduling for, 80, 99
behavioral activation techniques for, 82–97
effects of inactivity in, 80–81
etiology, 43–44
first session discussion of diagnosis of, 65–68
homework assignments, 297–299
information resources for patients with, 68
origins of cognitive therapy in research on, 1, 5–6
positive focus in therapy for, 26–27
therapeutic relationship as treatment factor for, 18–19
Developmental issues in therapy
assessment, 7
formation of core beliefs, 32–34, 35, 201, 228
formation of intermediate beliefs, 35
present focus of therapy and, 8–9
reconstructing early memories to modify core beliefs, 248–255
Diagnosis, first session discussion of, 65–68
Dialectical behavior therapy, 2
Dichotomous thinking, 220
Disqualifying positive perceptions, 181*f*
Distancing, 290–293
Distraction from automatic thoughts, 261–263
Downward arrow technique, 206–208, 234
Dreams, 5
Dysfunctional Attitude Scale, 209

E

Education of patient
about automatic thoughts, 140–142, 155–157, 184–186
about beliefs, 210–212
about cognitive model, 70–73
about core beliefs, 235–239
about evaluation session objectives and procedures, 47, 48–49
about first session structure and goals, 59
about homework, 294–295, 301
about imaginal automatic thoughts, 277–280
about session structure, 101
on benefits of activity, 89–90
expectations for treatment, 56
first session discussion of diagnosis, 65–68
introduction of cognitive behavior therapy approach, 13–14
monitoring patient's processing of session content, 354–355
presentation of cognitive conceptualization, 204–205
principles of cognitive behavior therapy, 9
for responding to automatic thoughts, 187–197
Embedded automatic thoughts, 151–152
Emotional functioning
cognitive model, 30–31
distinguishing thoughts from emotions, 159–161
dysfunctional, 158
effects of automatic thoughts, 138–139
goals of cognitive behavior therapy, 158–159
heightening, to elicit automatic thoughts, 143–144
identifying hot cognitions, 142–143
intensity of emotion, 164–166
labeling emotions, 162–163
mismatch of emotions and thoughts, 161–162
Emotional reasoning, 181*f*
Emotion Chart, 162*f*
Epictetus, 2
Etiology
case example, 43–44
cognitive model, 3

European Association for Behavioural
and Cognitive Therapies, 367
Evaluation session
assessment phase, 49–53
communicating initial impressions
from, 53
family member participation in, 53
goals of, 46, 47, 48
patient's understanding of, 47,
48–49
preparation for, 47, 48
treatment planning after, 57–58
Exposure therapy, 2, 265–267

F

Family of patient in evaluation session,
53
Feedback
case example, 76–79
eliciting, 20, 22, 76
importance of, 79
negative, 120, 136
potential problems in, 135–136
purpose of, 20, 22, 76, 79
second and subsequent sessions,
119–120
therapist self-evaluation questions,
351
Therapy Report for, 76, 77*f*, 359
uncovering problems in therapy,
347–348
First session
development of cognitive
conceptualization after, 199
discussion of diagnosis in, 65–68
end of session summary, 74
goals, 60, 79
homework assignment, 67–68, 74–76
mood check during, 62–63
obtaining an update in, 63–65
patient feedback, 76–79
preparation for, 59–60
problem identification in, 68
setting agenda in, 60–62
setting goals in, 69–70
structure, 60

G

Gestalt therapy, 11, 251
Goals
of cognitive behavior therapy,
158–159, 316
for effective therapy, 333
of evaluation session, 46, 47, 48
for homework assignments, 27–28,
295
of initial session, 60
initial treatment planning, case
example of, 54–55
pie chart formulation, 268–270, 269*f*
principles of cognitive behavior
therapy, 8
second and subsequent sessions, 101,
112
setting, in first therapy session,
69–70
step model for monitoring progress
toward, 164–165, 165*f*
therapy review for progress toward,
352, 353–354
for therapy sessions, 21–22, 27
Guided discovery, 10, 23–25, 371

H

Helplessness, 228, 231–232, 233*f*
Homework assignments
amount of, 300
anticipating problems in, 303–306
behavioral skills training, 296–297
case example, 297–299
changing, 303–305
checklist for, 309, 309*f*
clinical significance of, 294
conceptualizing difficulties in, 308
covert rehearsal for, 303–305
evaluating therapy effectiveness,
353, 372
first session, 67–68, 74–76
flexibility in assigning, 78–79
goals, 27–28, 295
individualization of, 300
ongoing assignment, 22, 296–297

patient education about, 294–295, 301

patient role in setting, 296, 301

planning, 28, 295–296, 300

potential problems, 133, 134–135

practical problems preventing completion of, 308–310

preparing for negative outcomes, 307–308

problem solving, 296

psychological obstacles to completion of, 310–312

remembering, 27, 75, 302

reviewing, 28, 108–110, 315, 338

starting in therapy session, 302

strategies to enhance compliance, 295, 299–306

striving for perfection in, 313–314

therapist cognitions as source of problems in, 314–315

Hot cognitions, 142–143

I

Imagery, to restructure early memories, 251–255

Imaginal automatic thoughts, 139, 146

changing, 285–287

distancing technique to reduce stress of, 290–293

following to completion, 280–283

identifying, 277–279

imagining coping with, 284–285

imagining future outcomes of, 284

induced images in response to, 289–293

patient's understanding of, 279–280

reality testing, 287–288

reduction of perceived threat of, 293

repetition technique for, 288

strategies for responding to, 280

substituting for distressing images, 288–289

Imipramine, 5–6

Individual conceptualization of patient and patient's problems, 38–39

homework assignment and, 300

as principle of cognitive behavior therapy, 7

treatment planning considerations, 345

Information processing

in maintenance of core beliefs, 32–33

model, 34*f*

negative bias, 272

Intermediate beliefs

advantages and disadvantages of, 211–212

in assumption form for patient understanding, 211

behavioral experiments to test, 217–218

case example, 42, 205–212

in cognitive conceptualization diagram, 199, 201–203

constructing alternatives to, 212–213

definition, 198

educating patient about, 210–212

formation of, 35

hierarchy of, 201, 203*f*

identifying, 205–209, 227

important, 209–210, 227

influence of, 35

therapeutic goals, 214

therapy notes, 214

See also Belief modification

International Association for Cognitive Psychotherapy, 367

Interpretation

automatic thoughts versus, 150–151

enduring patterns of, 7

Interrupting patient, 22, 124–125

M

Magical change to imaginal automatic thought, 186

Magnification/minimization, 181*f*

Mental filter, 181*f*

Mindfulness, 264

Monitoring automatic thoughts, 296

Mood check, 62–63, 102–105, 127–128

N

Neurophysiological changes associated
    with cognitive behavior therapy, 4
Nonverbal cues
    of hot cognitions, 142, 143

O

Obsessive thoughts, 260
Outcomes studies, 4–5
Overgeneralization, 182*f*

P

Pace of therapy session, 351–352
Panic disorders, 11
Personality Belief Questionnaire, 209
Personality disorders, resistance of
    core beliefs to modification in,
    230
Personalization, as thinking error,
    182*f*
Pharmacotherapy, review of, 105
Pie technique, 268–272, 269*f*
Pleasure
    automatic thoughts as obstacle to, 81
    identifying pleasurable activities,
    94–99
Pleasure and Mastery Rating Scale,
    95–96, 95*f*
Point–counterpoint, 220
Precipitating factors, 7
Preparing for Therapy Worksheet, 101,
    102*f*
Principles of cognitive behavior
    therapy, 6–11
Problem identification
    case example, 340–342, 344
    changing therapeutic focus in
    session, 343–344
    data gathering for, 340–342
    in first session, 68
    identifying problematic situations,
    148–150
    prioritizing problems, 110–112, 340

in second session, 101, 106
    treatment planning process, 340,
    342–343
Problems in therapy
    cognitive conceptualization as
    source of, 350
    conceptualizing, 348–349, 350
    evaluating possible sources of,
    349–351, 355–356
    likelihood of, 346
    monitoring patient's processing of
    session content, 354–355
    opportunities for therapeutic
    progress in, 346
    questions for identifying, 349–355
    review of therapy goals, 352
    strategies for remediating, 356–357
    therapeutic alliance as source of,
    350
    therapist's cognitions as source of,
    357
    treatment planning as source of, 350
    uncovering, 346–348
    See also Problems with therapy
    structure
Problem-solving skills training,
    256–258
    homework assignments, 296
Problem-solving therapy, 2
Problems with therapy structure
    in assigning homework, 134–135
    difficulties in eliciting automatic
    thoughts, 143–147
    in discussion of agenda items,
    133–134
    failure to make intervention, 134
    in homework review, 133
    identifying, 136, 351–352
    in making summaries, 135
    pacing issues, 134
    patient engagement-related, 125
    patient resistance to mood check,
    127–128
    rambling or unfocused updates,
    129–130
    in setting agenda, 130–133
    socialization-related, 125
    sources of, 123

therapeutic alliance-related, 126
therapist cognitions as source of, 123–124, 357
unfocused discussion, 133–134
unresolved distress at end of session, 135–136
in use of interruption, 124–125
See also Problems in therapy
Psychoanalysis, 1
origins of cognitive therapy, 5
Psychodynamic psychotherapy, 11

R

Rational emotive therapy, 2
Reality testing of imaginal automatic thoughts, 287–288
Refocusing, 260–263
Relapse prevention
booster sessions for, 327–331
initiation in therapy, 101
preparing for setbacks after termination, 325
principles of cognitive behavior therapy, 9
self-therapy sessions for, 325, 326*f*
strategies for, 318–322
Relaxation techniques, 263–264
Role play
clinical applications, 267
to elicit automatic thoughts, 145–146
to enhance homework adherence, 305–306
to improve social skills, 267, 268
intellectual–emotional, 305–306
to modify beliefs, 220–222, 224–225
to practice assertiveness, 267–268
reconstruction of early experiences in, 248–251
Rules, 35. *See also* Intermediate beliefs

S

Safety behaviors, 266
Schema, 33, 228
Schema diagrams, 239

Second and subsequent sessions
agenda, 100–101
final summary and feedback at close of, 118–120, 135–136
goals, 101, 112, 120–121
homework review, 108–110, 133
introductory part, 101
middle part, 112–117
mood check, 102–105, 127–128
patient preparation for, 101, 102*f*
periodic summarizing in, 117–118
prioritizing problems in, 110–112
problem identification in, 106–107, 130–133
refinement of cognitive conceptualization in, 121
shift of therapeutic focus, 120
update of week in, 107–108, 129–130
Self-comparison, 272–274
Self-help books, 257
Self-therapy sessions, 325, 326*f*
Session structure
basic objectives, 11–12, 17, 21–22
first session, 60
guide, 336–339
identifying problems in, 123
length, 3
pacing, 351–352
patient feedback, 22
patient understanding of, 101
planning, 21
as source of problems, 351–352
See also Evaluation session; First session; Second and subsequent sessions
"Should" and "must" statements, 182*f*
Socializing patient, 125, 352–353, 355
Social skills, 267–268
Socratic questioning, 140–141
case example, 193–194, 215–217
in cognitive behavior therapy, 10–11
to construct or modify beliefs, 213, 215–217, 227
to evaluate automatic thoughts, 170–171
for testing of imaginal automatic thoughts, 287–288
See also Guided discovery

Strengths orientation, 26–27
  changing self-comparison to, 272–274
  credit list assignment, 274–276
Substance abuse, 11
Suicidal ideation or behavior, 50, 63, 68, 102, 105
Supervision, 349, 360

T

Temporal focus, 8–9
Termination of therapy
  booster sessions after, 327–331
  early preparation for, 316–318
  patient concerns about tapering sessions, 322–324
  planning for, 333–334
  preparing patient for setbacks after, 325
  review of therapy sessions prior to, 324–325
  self-therapy plan after, 325, 326f
Testing Your Thoughts Worksheet, 187, 196–197, 196f
Therapeutic alliance
  clinical significance, 17, 21
  first session goals, 79
  good counseling skills for, 18–19
  patient response to interruption, 124–125
  principles of cognitive behavior therapy, 7–8
  role of patient feedback in strengthening, 79
  sensitivity to patient feedback, 20
  as source of problems in therapy, 350
  strategies for building, 17–21, 126
  strategies for strengthening, 126
  therapist disclosure of automatic thoughts, 180
  therapist disclosure of beliefs, 227
  in treatment planning, 19–20
Therapeutic techniques and processes
  behavioral activation, 81–97
  case write-up, 361–365

changing self-comparison, 272–274
Cognitive Therapy Rating Scale to evaluate, 368–374
dealing with difficult problems, 116–117
decision-making skills training, 258–260
emphasis, 11
exposure therapy, 265–267
formulating new beliefs, 212–213
graph of therapeutic progress, 317–318, 317f
identification of automatic thoughts, 36
identifying core and intermediate beliefs, 205–209
interrupting patient, 22, 124–125
introduction of cognitive behavior therapy approach, 13–14
patient engagement with, 125
patient resistance to forms, 127–128
patient socialization and, 125
pie technique, 268–272
positive orientation, 26–27, 107–108, 159
preparing for setbacks in, 320–322
principles of cognitive behavior therapy, 7–11
problem-solving skills training, 256–258
range of, 10–11
refocusing attention, 260–263
relapse prevention strategies, 318–322
relaxation techniques, 263–264
responding to imaginal automatic thoughts, 280–289
scope of, 16, 256
therapist cognitions interfering with therapy structure, 123–124
therapist expertise in, 12–13, 14–16, 358, 360
therapist notes, 121–122
therapist self-evaluation after session, 339
therapist's first application of cognitive behavior therapy, 360
third session and beyond, 120–122

See also Belief modification;
  Homework assignments; Problems
  with therapy structure; Session
  structure; Termination of therapy;
  Therapeutic alliance
Therapist qualities
  Cognitive Therapy Rating Scale to
    evaluate, 368–374
  developing expertise in cognitive
    behavior therapy, 12–13, 14–16,
    358, 360
  self-assessment for problems, 351
  self-assessment of cognitions and
    affect, 14–15, 124, 358–359
  therapist cognitions interfering with
    therapy structure, 123–124, 357
Therapy notes, 188–191
  on old and new beliefs, 214
Therapy Report, 76, 77*f*, 359
Therapy structure
  booster sessions, 316
  duration, 56
  frequency, 56, 316
  number of sessions, 39
  patient expectations, 56
  phases, 333–334
  principles of cognitive behavior
    therapy, 9–10
  tapering near termination, 322–324
  See also Problems with therapy
    structure; Session structure
Thought Record, 160, 187, 192–194,
  195*f*
Treatment planning
  after evaluation session, 57–58
  agenda setting in first session, 60–62
  basic process, 21–22

building therapeutic alliance in,
  19–20
case example, 54–55, 58
case write-up, 364
essential elements of, 332
goals, 21
individualization, 345
patient role in, 8, 55–56
phases, 333–334
problem analysis for, 334, 335–336*f*
problem identification and focus,
  340–344
revising, 334
session plans, 336–339
as source of problems in therapy,
  350, 351
for specific disorders, 344–345
therapeutic goals, 333
therapist expertise in, 13
See also Cognitive conceptualization
Tunnel vision, 182*f*

U

Unlovability, 228, 231–232, 233*f*

V

Visualization, to elicit automatic
  thoughts, 144–145

W

Worthlessness, 228, 231–232, 233*f*

Maria Henderson Library
Gartnavel Royal Hospital
Glasgow G12 0XH Scotland